ACADEMIC SCIENTISTS AND
THE PHARMACEUTICAL INDUSTRY

Academic Scientists
and the
Pharmaceutical Industry

COOPERATIVE RESEARCH IN
TWENTIETH-CENTURY AMERICA

John P. Swann

The Johns Hopkins University Press

BALTIMORE AND LONDON

The Johns Hopkins University Press
701 West 40th Street
Baltimore, Maryland 21211
The Johns Hopkins Press Ltd., London

The paper used in this publication meets the minimum requirements of American National Standard for Information Sciences—Permanence of Paper for Printed Library Materials, ANSI Z39.48–1984.

Library of Congress Cataloging-in-Publication Data

Swann, John Patrick, 1956-
   Academic scientists and the pharmaceutical industry : cooperative research in twentieth-century America / by John P. Swann.
      p.   cm.
   Bibliography: p.
   Includes index.
   ISBN 0-8018-3558-5 (alk. paper)
   1. Drugs—Research—United States—History
—20th century.   2. Medical scientists—United States—History—20th century.
3. Medicine—Research—United States—History—20th century.   4. Drug trade—United States—History—20th century.   5. Science and industry—United States. I. Title.
   [DNLM: 1. Drug Industry—history—United States.   2. Research—history—United States.   3. Universities—history—United States.
QV 711 AA1-S9a]
RS122.S93 1988
615.1′072073—dc19
DNLM/DLC   87-29303
for Library of Congress   CIP

Contents

➤➤➤➤➤➤➤➤➤➤- ⫷⫷⫷⫷⫷⫷⫷⫷⫷⫷

Illustrations

-}}-}}-}}-}}-}}-(((-(((-(((-(((-(((-

Preface

➤➤➤-➤➤➤-➤➤➤-➤➤➤-➤➤➤- ⫷⫷⫷-⫷⫷⫷-⫷⫷⫷-⫷⫷⫷-⫷⫷⫷

This book attempts to explore and interpret the growth of research interactions in the biomedical sciences between two major estates of science in America, academe and industry. The different functions and interests inherent in these estates of science, including the different needs of scientists and managers in each estate, necessitated collaboration. Interactions in turn produced circumstances and concerns not encountered when the estates carried out the research within academe or within industry alone. For example, patents on medical products resulting from joint research often yielded concern and confusion. From the standpoint of the manufacturer, a patent was a necessary reward for a research investment. But many academic biomedical researchers in the early twentieth century scorned and derided patents; research, they felt, served as its own reward. How times have changed. A successful collaboration really depended on the willingness of the academic or corporate representatives to accommodate the interests of their collaborators. Public health had a vital stake in cooperative research too; many of the drugs discussed in this study would have been seriously delayed without collaboration. This was certainly true, for example, in the cases of insulin and its use in diabetes, the application of Mapharsen in syphilis therapy, pentothal and its value in surgical anesthesia, and streptomycin as a treatment for tuberculosis.

This investigation began as a doctoral dissertation at the University of Wisconsin and continued as part of a postdoctoral research project at the Museum of American History of the Smithsonian Institution, with the final revisions completed while I was a research associate at the University of Texas Medical Branch. In the course of these migrations, many have contributed to this project in a variety of ways. Unfortunately, space permits a mere mention of names for most of these people—far too brief an acknowledgment of their importance to the preparation of this book.

Tremendous assistance in identifying the widely scattered unpublished,

published, and oral matter pertinent to my research was provided by James Liebig of the University of Wisconsin Archives; Richard Wolfe of the Francis A. Countway Library, Harvard; Anita Martin and Gene McCormick of Eli Lilly and Company; Wilbur McDowell and the late John T. Sheehan of E. R. Squibb and Sons; Frances James Dallett and the staff of the University of Pennsylvania Archives; Harold Averill and Marion Wyse of the University of Toronto Archives; Katharine Martyn of the Thomas Fisher Rare Book Library at the University of Toronto; William Helfand, formerly of Merck Sharp and Dohme; David Cowen of Rutgers University; Robert J. Moore of the Medical Research Council, London; Maynard Brichford of the University of Illinois Archives; the staff at the Archives Division of the State Historical Society of Wisconsin; Michael Harris, John Fleckner, and Robert Harding of the National Museum of American History, Smithsonian Institution; Walter Southern and Ernest Volwiler of Abbott Laboratories; Sheldon Hochheiser of the University of Minnesota; D. Stanley Tarbell of Vanderbilt University; Jeffrey Sturchio of the Center for History of Chemistry, Philadelphia, and John Heitmann, formerly of the center; Karl Niederer of the New Jersey State Division of Archives and Records Management; James H. Hutson of the Library of Congress Manuscripts Division; Martin L. Black of the Warner-Lambert Company; the staff at the History of Medicine Division of the National Library of Medicine; Dorothy Whitcomb of the Middleton Medical Library of the University of Wisconsin; and Jonathan Liebenau, formerly of the Technical Change Centre, London.

Without financial assistance from several sources, this project would have been delayed considerably. Hence I recognize fellowships provided by the American Foundation for Pharmaceutical Education, including the George V. Doerr Memorial Fellowship; the considerable assistance of the University of Wisconsin Graduate School to supplement my fellowship support, including a travel grant for my research; a grant for this research through the offices of William Helfand, formerly senior vice-president of Merck Sharp and Dohme International; and a postdoctoral research fellowship through the National Museum of American History of the Smithsonian Institution.

A number of colleagues read all or parts of the manuscript. For their many comments, criticisms, and suggestions I am most thankful to John Lesch, Glenn Sonnedecker, Ramunas Kondratas, John Burnham, Nathan Reingold, Stanley Goldberg, Michael Bliss, Harry Marks, James Hull, and R. G. Macfarlane. Thanks are also due the 1985–86 Smithsonian fellows at the Museum of American History, who challenged me to rethink several parts of the manuscript. Special mention should be made of Chester Burns, who generously allowed me time to revise the manuscript, and Pamela Robers, for teaching a dinosaur the intricacies of word processing.

It was my great fortune to have the ample and highly professional assistance of George Thompson and Therese Boyd, of the Johns Hopkins University Press, in processing the manuscript through publication, as well as the skillful and thorough editing of Joanne Allen. I am indebted beyond recompense to John Parascandola, who suggested this topic as a possible dissertation project and who offered comments and advice whenever approached. Of course, any errors are fully my own responsibility. Finally, and most important, I could not possibly have completed this without the caring and support of my family.

ACADEMIC SCIENTISTS AND
THE PHARMACEUTICAL INDUSTRY

Introduction:
The Context for the
Study of Collaborative Research

>>>->>>->>>->>>->>>- <<<-<<<-<<<-<<<-<<<

Cooperative biomedical research between universities and industry in America emerged as a general movement between the two world wars. The 1920s and 1930s were decades of intellectual, social, and economic upheaval in the history of the biomedical sciences in America. Physiology, biochemistry, pharmacology, and other sciences were in various stages of establishing disciplinary roots in academic institutions, which helped nurture and propagate biomedical knowledge. However, even though medicine and public health continued to reign over other research areas in attracting financial support from private foundations, more and more this support was failing to keep pace with the needs of these sciences during the period between the two wars. On the eve of this period, many American pharamaceutical companies were fiscally sound, but those firms with a promising scientific future were the exceptions. Several companies had a scientific staff, but these were devoted primarily to quality control. The growth of biomedical research programs in the pharmaceutical industry was a phenomenon of the 1920s and 1930s.

The status of the therapeutic armamentarium was an important parallel issue. By World War I this offered much for treating disease and suffering, but it was far from sufficient. For example, Salvarsan and Neosalvarsan were a boon for syphilis therapy, but they were by no means safe remedies. Patients with neurological disorders—especially epilepsy—responded to some drugs, such as sedatives; but the undesirable side effects of these drugs compromised their value. Surgery, too, was in need of a safe, short-acting anesthetic. There were no really useful treatments for metabolic diseases such as diabetes and pernicious anemia. The same was true of many bacterial infections including tuberculosis—the dreaded white plague. Between the two world wars, the joint efforts of biomedical re-

1

searchers from academe and industry helped to eliminate these and many other ailments of the public health. At the same time, the formation of these research links filled many of the intellectual, technical, and economic needs of the two estates.

These joint efforts are noteworthy because the pharmaceutical companies were not amorphous entities that poured capital willy-nilly into university laboratories. To be sure financial support was an important part of the interactions between the two estates, but it was just one part. For example, some firms became important pools of scientific talent that academic workers could not ignore. In some cases, companies represented opportunities for university scientists to map their agendas for research programs onto novel institutional settings. Interactions involved much more than money transactions, which perhaps was a major difference between the links that developed between universities and industry and those between universities and most private foundations.

This study explores and interprets how and why cooperative biomedical research developed, and it assesses the significance of cooperative research from the standpoint of the university, the commercial organization, and therapeutics. *Research*, as defined in the Oxford English Dictionary and assumed throughout this study, is "a search or investigation directed to the discovery of some fact by careful consideration or study of a subject." The essence of this definition is that research is a deliberate endeavor to uncover new knowledge, or new interpretations of existing knowledge. A literature review of a subject, for example, is not research as defined above; its purpose is not to discover new knowledge but to summarize what is already known about a topic. The molecular modification of a drug, on the other hand, is research, because it is a search for a new fact, in this case a new drug. Research is by no means the exclusive pursuit of scientists, no more than knowledge itself is restricted to sciences. History, music, philosophy, sociology, art, economics, and other fields depend on research for their progress, too.

This book focuses on the history of scientific research. Since my emphasis is on research in the biomedical sciences, medical schools and the pharmaceutical industry receive primary consideration, although I mention other academic settings for biomedical sciences, such as departments of chemistry and (to a lesser extent) pharmacy schools. Given the scope and character of this book, as well as my preference for presenting an interpretive rather than a comprehensive study, this investigation required some restrictions.

In the first place, the bulk of this study addresses the 1920s and 1930s. That collaborative research existed prior to this era and that it proliferated from the 1940s onward is uncontestable. But collaborative biomedical research emerged as a systematic endeavor in America between the two world wars. We can trace only scattered instances of collaboration prior to World War I, and after World War II collaboration between the leading pharmaceutical firms and universities in general was a *fait accompli*. Second, the biomedical sciences encompass many fields, several of which are mentioned in this book (e.g., mycology, bacteriology, hematology, and neurology), but this study is concerned mainly with pharmacology and chemistry, particularly medicinal chemistry. Pharmacology and chemistry were crucial to drug development in the period between the wars. Chemistry was important for synthesizing new drugs and isolating natural products such as insulin, liver extracts, and vitamins. Pharmacology was useful for designing new drugs for possible synthesis on the basis of anticipated therapeutic action and for testing experimental drugs in the laboratory. Chemistry and pharmacology were the most frequent foci of reseach interactions during this period.

Finally, I employ a series of representative case studies to illustrate the growth of collaborative research. I discuss three ideal typologies of cooperation, citing several research-based pharmaceutical firms and scientists representing many of the major research universities across the country as examples. Among the pharmaceutical companies I emphasize Abbott Laboratories of North Chicago, Eli Lilly and Company of Indianapolis, Merck and Company of Rahway, New Jersey, Parke Davis and Company of Detroit, and E. R. Squibb and Sons of New York. Among universities scientists from Harvard, Illinois, Pennsylvania, Rochester, Toronto, Virginia, and Wisconsin receive much of my attention. With the exception of perhaps one or two of these universities, the firms and institutions above occupied the upper research echelons in the pharmaceutical industry and academe during the 1920s and 1930s.

This investigation is by necessity interfacial, since it deals with topics relevant to the history of science and technology, the history of medicine, and the history of pharmacy. From the standpoint of science and technology, this study pays some attention to (1) the interaction of science and technology from the viewpoint of institutions belonging to two estates of science with quite different missions, (2) the history of chemistry and its applications to the health sciences, (3) the history of sciences supporting medicine and pharmacy, and (4) the funding, planning, and execution of scientific research. For example, pharmacologist Alfred Newton Richards of the University of Pennsylvania, who later became vice-president in charge of medical affairs at Pennsylvania, chairman of the wartime Committee on Medical Research of the Office of Scientific Research and Development, and president of the National Academy of Sciences, was a long-time consultant to Merck and Company. Richards counseled the company on the establishment and broad development of its research programs, served as a liaison between the company and the academic community, and was a member of Merck's board of directors for a decade—the only outsider on the board. His background as a researcher, his familiarity with biomedical researchers in academe, and his experience in the organization of research on both the institutional and the national level were important qualities for Merck to draw upon. Richards played a major role in Merck's transformation from an organization with a fledgling research program at best to a highly respected institution where an academic scientist could go and expect to be stimulated and supported by the research environment.

From the standpoint of medicine, parts of this study examine the therapeutics of a wide range of diseases and the evolution of some of the preclinical sciences in a different institutional locale, industry. For example, Abbot laboratories assembled a gifted staff of organic and medicinal chemists, beginning with Ernest Volwiler, the first doctoral student of the renowned University of Illinois chemist Roger Adams. Volwiler and his coworkers, in collaboration with pharmacologists at the University of Wisconsin, developed a number of useful anesthetics and sedatives in the 1920s and 1930s, including pentobarbital and pentothal. Abbott's links with Wisconsin were crucial, because the firm did not have an experienced pharmacology staff to evaluate these anesthetics.

From the standpoint of pharmacy, this book must also occasionally look into the scientific and technical labor behind the discovery and development of certain drugs. A commitment to the marketing of new, science-based products formed the bedrock for the growth of the American pharmaceutical industry, which of course required a commitment to research. Only a few farsighted firms realized this prior to World War I. But during the 1920s and 1930s the managerial leadership of Merck, Abbott, Lilly, Squibb, and many other companies began to assemble their own research staffs with the assistance of academic scientists, to contract with universities for research services as needed, and to offer technical and economic support to academic researchers for the chance to capitalize on outsiders' therapeutic discoveries. For example, Lilly collaborated with the University of Toronto on the development of insulin. It was a collaboration that revolutionized Lilly's standing in the drug industry; in fact, Lilly has been the leader in the insulin market up to the present.

Certain functions and interests of universities and industry in general are implicit in my arguments. For example, companies ultimately depended for their survival on the accumulation of capital, a function that had to inform their interests in developing research links with academe. This is not to say that the executive officers of firms did not have philanthropic or purely scientific interests, because they did. But in the end, the pharmaceutical industry had to serve as its own endowment. Universities, ideally at least, were not-for-profit institutions dedicated to the pursuit of truth and the education of the citizenry. One certainly could argue that some activities, such as the pursuit of patents and patentable research, were hardly in line with these functions. Conversely, one could claim that such activities were necessary to support teaching and research programs if the state or private citizens were unwilling or unable to provide the perceived necessary funding for these programs. Nevertheless, one would be hard-pressed to argue that the primary mission of the university was the accumulation of capital.

Ironically, their fundamentally different priorities created opportunities for mutual benefit when academe and industry collaborated, but collaboration also created problematic situations for both estates of science. This was true, too, of the impact of cooperative research on the public. On the one hand, collaborative biomedical research was symbiotic. Companies with new in-house research programs had to maintain open channels of communication with universities in order to remain at the forefront of research. Even firms with established programs could not possibly cover every field of study, so they, too, depended on academic workers in some ways. University researchers in the interwar period needed to find support for their research programs at a time when the federal government had not yet initiated its mega-support of research in academe. As mentioned above, companies were increasingly a source of both financial and intellectual support for academic scientists. From the standpoint of public health, collaborative efforts produced numerous valuable therapeutic agents, such as hormones, vitamins, anticonvulsant drugs, anesthetics, sedatives, chemotherapeutic agents, and other drugs. Without collaboration, the introduction of many of these drugs would have been seriously delayed and perhaps never would have come about.

On the other hand, cooperative research had disadvantages as well. The attraction of a source of funding led more than a few academic scientists to focus on industrial problems in which they otherwise had little or no interest. Also, the proprietary nature of the collaborative research certainly created some concern about the possibility of inhibiting the exchange of research with colleagues through publications, student theses or dissertations, or informal dialogues at professional meetings or on other occasions. Essentially, this was a question of whether collaboration (or collusion, depending on one's viewpoint) was consistent with the traditional freedom in academe to pursue and disseminate research, a question of the viability of *Lehrfreiheit* and *Lernfreiheit*. Collaboration had disadvantages for companies as well. Sharing proprietary information with outsiders carried with it a risk of intelligence leaks. Also, a firm could possibly damage the development of an in-house research program by relying too heavily on contracted research. Finally, from the standpoint of the public, university workers and companies often entered into exclusive arrangements whereby the collaborating firm was entitled to a monopoly on any discoveries made by the academic researcher. Arguably, such exclusive agreements could inflate drug prices.

This work is divided into five chapters. Chapter 1 discusses the evolution of biomedical research in America and the growing interest of various industries in research in general. Basically, collaborative biomedical research awaited the emergence of biomedical sciences in America, and it awaited the recognition among industrial concerns that success was a function of their cultivation of research. Many biomedical sciences established a foothold in American universities by the late nineteenth century. By the early twentieth century an increasing number of chemical, pharmaceutical, electrical, communications, and petroleum firms established research laboratories. World War I fueled both an interest among companies in establishing in-house research programs and an interest among universities and firms in combining their resources. A few pharmaceutical companies, most notably Parke-Davis and the H. K. Mulford Company of Philadelphia, were among the first American firms to entertain an interest in research of both an in-house and a collaborative nature—as early as the 1890s. However, pharmaceutical firms, like companies in other industries, carried out joint work with academe on an ad hoc basis. Industries and academe did not pursue collaborative research systematically until after World War I.

Chapter 2 lays out the context for the following chapters by discussing general trends in the emergence of cooperative biomedical research. Cooperative research faced some formidable ideological barriers that delayed its growth as a general movement in the United States. On the one hand, by the late nineteenth century many biomedical scientists in universities had developed a mindset that convinced them to avoid contacts with drug companies. Their emphasis on fundamental research—which they understood to be research for its own sake, to contribute to the sum knowledge in a field—and their traditional deprecation of the patenting of medical discoveries imbued many academic biomedical scientists with a tainted image of the drug industry. Industry itself contributed to this image through questionable trade practices. During the 1920s and 1930s, however, some of the leading pharmaceutical firms eventually helped erode this image by developing in-house research programs, by hiring prominent scientists from academe as researchers and research directors, by establishing special institutes and laboratories devoted to research, and by fostering at least some fundamental work in industry. Consequently, companies and academic scientists developed increasingly frequent research contracts, and by the early 1940s some firms had devised elaborate networks to maintain connections with university workers.

Chapters 3, 4, and 5 address typologies of collaborative research, with several examples. I do not contend that these are the only typologies; rather, they are the most obvious typologies I have been able to cull from my investigation. Each chapter includes an introductory section that characterizes the typology and presents a few examples of the interaction in brief. Chapter 3 discusses the general consultantship as exemplified principally by the relations between Richards and Merck and between Adams and Abbott. In this typology, a single university scientist counseled a firm on a host of topics related to the broad development of its research programs. The general consultant advised the firm in the area of his personal specialty and several other areas, such as general company research policy, affairs requiring a liaison between the company and the academic community, and managerial aspects of the company's operations. Such consultants typically served their firm over many years and became so intimately involved in its internal affairs that they could eventually become members of its board of directors. Richards and Adams each acted as general consultant to a firm for thirty years or longer and served on that firm's board for several years.

Chapter 4 discusses a different breed of consultant, the specialist-consultant. The interactions of two pharmacologists at the University of Wisconsin—Arthur Loevenhart and Arthur Tatum—with a number of drug companies illustrate this typology, and I mention other examples in the introductory section to chapter 4. Unlike the general consultantship, the specialist-consultantship involved interactions of one or more university workers with several firms, on a considerably narrower basis. In his contact with companies the specialist-consultant rarely trespassed beyond his sphere of scientific expertise. Typically, the company engaged this consultant (often through a fellowship or a grant-in-aid) as an expert in a particular branch of chemistry, pharmacology, microbiology, or some other field.

Chapter 5 deals with another typology of cooperative research, the specific project collaboration, in which a university group and a single pharmaceutical firm cooperated for the express purpose of developing a specific therapeutic agent. Once they accomplished their task, the two sides terminated the collaboration. I discuss some of the problems that could arise in this typology, and how other project collaborations avoided these problems, in the cooperative ventures between Lilly and workers at the University of Toronto on insulin, between Harvard scientists and Lilly on a liver extract for pernicious anemia, and between Lilly and researchers at the University of Rochester on a liver extract for secondary anemia. Finally, in the epilogue I examine the changes in collaboration between these two estates of science after World War II, principally in the 1970s and 1980s. Today, many within and outside academe and industry look upon ties between universities and corporations as deliverance from a multitude of problems plaguing education, research, and American society in general. Consequently, a variety of plans linking the two estates are springing up throughout the country.

Considering this renewed interest in ties between business and academe in the past decade, it is a bit surprising that the historical literature lacks a synthetic treatment of cooperative biomedical research as an entity to itself. It is all the more surprising when we realize that such research clearly involved circumstances not encountered in research confined to academe alone or industry alone and that such research had a significant impact on therapeutics in the twentieth century. Some secondary works on the history of biomedical research and the history of the pharmaceutical industry have been useful for this project. However, the primary resources for this book were manuscript collections of pharmaceutical companies and the collected papers of scientists who worked with industry. The latter was a particularly important resource for information on firms, since few drug companies maintain archives (or admit that they do), and many of those do retain records do not necessarily permit outsiders to make use of them. Ample manuscript sources existed to relate in detail several case studies illustrating the emergence of cooperative research and to convey general trends in the growth of this type of research. Occasionally, when manuscripts and the published record did not shed sufficient light on an issue, several interviews with collaborating academic and industrial scientists helped fill in some details.

This project also relied, to a somewhat lesser extent, on patents and published scientific articles. Both were indispensable sources of information on the joint research per se. A history of biomedical research must utilize research publications. Published articles and books are the official transcripts of scientific research, and therefore the historian of biomedical research can ill afford to neglect these. Patents are a useful source as well. In the first place, they often related the highlights of the work in a way intelligible to the nonscientist. Also, patents themselves can be the source of disagreements and controversy within the academic and industrial communities, as well as between the two sides. Although it is impossible to avoid technical material in a work of this nature, I have tried to convey such material in a way understandable to a reader with little scientific background.

CHAPTER ONE

The Emergence of Biomedical and Industrial Research in America

->>>->>>->>>->>>->>>- (((- (((-((-(((-(((-

Development of the Biomedical Sciences

Cooperative biomedical research did not emerge on a broad scale in the United States until the twentieth century; indeed, the pharmacomedical sciences themselves did not emerge as distinct disciplines until the nineteenth century. The modernization of chemistry, for example, began under Lavoisier in the late eighteenth century, and alkaloidal chemistry arose in the early decades of the nineteenth century, principally through the efforts of Sertürner, Pelletier, and Caventou, as did organic and biological chemistry under Chevreul, Wöhler, Liebig, and other pioneers. Structural organic chemistry awaited the work of Kekulé, van't Hoff, and Le Bel in the middle decades of the nineteenth century. Other disciplines vital to pharmacomedical research can be traced to nineteenth-century Europe as well. Physiology flourished under many British (e.g., Sharpey and Foster) and Continental (Müller, Helmholtz, du Bois Reymond, Ludwig, Bernard) workers. Modern experimental pharmacology was a product of the nineteenth century too, principally through the efforts of Magendie, Bernard, Buchheim, and Schmiedeberg. Bacteriology emerged late in the century, following the discoveries of Pasteur, Koch and Behring.[1]

The major biomedical disciplines did not find a niche in American institutions until the last quarter of the nineteenth century. The social circumstances that facilitated the rise of these disciplines in Germany, such as a strong national system of secondary schools (the German Gymnasien), a widespread belief that higher learning was part of a nationalistic identity, and the active involvement, if not control, of the federal government in the policies and budgets of universities, were lacking in the United States.[2] Somewhat more direct influences also account for the delayed emergence of biomedical disciplines in America. For example, those within and outside the medical profession with antivivisectionist sentiments questioned the value of experimental biomedical research. The antivivisectionist movement was much stronger in Britain than in the United States; nonetheless, it led several states to pass laws hindering vivisection in the late nineteenth century, such as the New Jersey antivivisection act of 1880. Such opinion was a source of frequent concern for many biomedical scientists.[3] Also the longstanding conflict between laboratory workers and clinicians impeded a smooth and rapid transfer of German biomedical science to the United States and other countries.[4] However, American universities, medical schools, and agricultural colleges began fostering research in the biomedical sciences once biochemists such as Russell Chittenden, physiologists such as Henry Pickering Bowditch, and pharmacologists such as John Jacob Abel returned from periods of study in Germany. From the 1870s on, a growing group of the better universities, including Johns Hopkins, Harvard, Pennsylvania, Michigan, and Yale, established centers for biomedical research.

Harvard Medical School established the first laboratory for experimental physiology in America in 1871. Henry Pickering Bowditch, recently returned from a period of study in Europe under physiologists Claude Bernard and Carl Ludwig, headed the new laboratory. Five years later, in its inaugural year, Johns Hopkins appointed the Michael Foster–trained physiologist Henry Newell Martin to its biology chair. When William Henry Howell succeeded Martin in 1893, the biology chair became a physiology chair, reflecting physiology's increasing independence with respect to general biology. The University of Pennsylvania and the University of Michigan also opened laboratories of physiology in the 1870s.[5]

Modern biochemistry in America evolved from several sources. Russell Chittenden organized the first laboratory for experimental physiological chemistry in the Sheffield Scientific School at Yale in 1874. After a year of postgraduate work at Heidelberg, because he felt that "in 1878 any American student desirous of making progress in physiological chemistry had no recourse other than going to Germany for the knowledge and experience he needed to help him on his way,"[6] Chittenden moved into the first chair of physiological chemistry in the United States in 1882. His department at Yale was the dominant force in biochemistry for the next three decades. Although the Sheffield School had no formal clinical connections, modern biochemistry also had strong roots in medical schools; however, by the 1890s only the better medical schools, such as Hopkins, Pennsylvania, and Michigan, had a four-year course that permitted the establishment of preclinical disciplines such as biochemistry. In general, medical schools did not emerge as major centers for training and research in biochemistry until the first two decades of the twentieth century. At that time, more and more institutions were implementing the sweeping reforms in medical education that emphasized, among other things, the importance of a solid grounding in biochemistry and other sciences in the training of physicians. Finally, research in nutritional chemistry in agricultural experiment stations—particularly those stations in Wisconsin and Connecticut—was contributing significantly to the knowledge base of modern biochemistry by the late nineteenth and early twentieth centuries.[7]

Just as Chittenden was a leader in American biochemistry, John Jacob Abel was a leader in American pharmacology. Abel transformed the study of drugs in American medical schools from a didactic and descriptive exercise to a critical investigation of the action of drugs on tissues, on the basis of modern experimental chemistry and physiology. He had spent six years in Europe, including study under Oswald Schmiedeberg, before returning to the United States in 1891 to assume the first chair in modern experimental pharmacology at Michigan. Abel moved to Hopkins two years later, where he established a center for research and training in pharmacology. In addition, Abel played a prominent role in the formation of a national pharmacological society in 1908 and in the establishment of a journal devoted to pharmacology the following year.[8]

Insofar as the biomedical sciences emerged in America as functions of medical schools in the late nineteenth and early twentieth centuries,[9] their disciplinary status was closely tied to the reforms in American medical education in this period, as mentioned above. Institutions in the upper echelons of medical education initiated reforms by the 1880s, and many of the rank-and-file medical schools joined in the reforms in the first two decades of the twentieth century. The American Medical Association, the Association of American Medical Colleges, and a few private foundations, such as the Rockefeller and Carnegie foundations, spearheaded these changes. First, when higher entrance requirements caused medical school enrollments to plunge, schools had to align themselves with universities for economic support, since student fees were no longer sufficient to subsidize faculty salaries and expensive laboratory facilities. University administrations thus assumed many of the duties formerly performed by the medical faculties, such as guidance over budgets, hiring, and other policy matters. Second, the traditional position of faculty members as part-time teachers and part-time outside practitioners (fees were inadequate for the faculty to rely on the former alone for support) changed; they became professor-researchers. In part, this was a move to accommodate the new scientific medicine. Finally, after 1890 an increasing number of medical schools expanded their curriculum to four years and instituted minumum requirements for admission—at least two years of college work. This elevated the M.D., so that it resembled a graduate degree, and allowed specialized study of preclinical biomedical sciences apart from clinical work. Thus, medical reforms in the late nineteenth and early twentieth centuries institutionalized biomedical sciences, enabling them to avoid purely service functions and flourish on their own as independent disciplines.[10]

The Rise of Industrial Research

The development of industrial research in America depended, first, on progress in the natural sciences. The nineteenth century was a period of considerable growth for physics, chemistry, and biology. Synthetic organic chemistry, electricity and magnetism, and bacteriology, for example—the application of which established many industries on a solid scientific basis—made great strides during the nineteenth century. Of course, research in different industries did not progress at the same rate, simply because the sciences supporting these industries did not develop at a parallel pace. But the chemical, electrical, pharmaceutical, petroleum, and other industries had a vast scientific base to draw on by the late nineteenth century.

Second, an institutional network was necessary to facilitate the application of science. In the United States such a network had been growing since the second quarter of the nineteenth century, through the founding of several schools of applied science and technology. Beginning with the United States Military Academy at West Point, the American Literary, Scientific, and Military Academy in Norwich, Vermont, and the Rensselaer Polytechnic Institute in Troy, New York, in the first quarter of the nineteenth century, such institutions were established in the 1840s (the Sheffield Scientific School at Yale and the Lawrence Scientific School at Harvard), the 1860s (the Massachusetts Institute of Technology, the Columbia University School of Mines, and the Worcester Polytechnic Institute), and later in the century (the Case School of Applied Science and the Throop Polytechnic Institute, now the California Institute of Technology). In addition, many government-supported schools of applied agriculture and mechanical arts arose in the second half of the century through the Morrill Land Grant Act of 1862, the Hatch Act (1887), and the second Morrill Act of 1890.

Finally, the development of industrial research depended on (1) the ability of industrialists to recognize the importance of science and how this could relate to the success of their companies and (2) the willingness of scientists to work on a full- or part-time basis with firms. American industrialists, to be sure, could draw on many precedents in modern history that illustrated the value of organized scientific research in industry, such as the mobilization of French scientific resources in the late eighteenth century, which contributed significantly to military and communications technology; the application of science to improve optical technology, principally under Carl Zeiss in Germany; and most notably, the rapid growth of the German synthetic chemical industry in the final third of the nineteenth century, which gave birth to the modern industrial research laboratory. Because industries were able to offer academic scientists higher salaries and better equipment than universities, an increasing number of university scientists were drawn to industry, although some academic workers resisted these attractions.[11]

Until about the turn of the twentieth century, American industrial research was generally the province of the lone scientist and inventor; occasionally firms called on outside consultants for their expertise. Examples of the independent workers and consultants who developed innovations for various industries abound throughout the nineteenth century. The discoveries of several of these scientists revolutionized some industries. Benjamin Silliman, Jr., of the Sheffield Scientific School, examined petroleum samples from a Pennsylvania site for speculators in the 1850s and found that one of the distillates could serve as an excellent and comparatively inexpensive illuminating agent, thus giving rise to petroleum refining. Soon after the Civil War, John Wesley Hyatt, with formal background in chemistry, developed the versatile plastic celluloid. In the late 1880s Charles M. Hall discovered a commercially viable method to produce aluminum, which eventually benefited many industries. Other contributions by independent workers, such as those of Elias Howe to the textile industry and Alexander Graham Bell to communications, are too well known to recount here. The point is that industrial research, for the most part, was unorganized during the nineteenth century. Most industrialists believed that the manufacturer's job was to manufacture; new ideas to improve manufacturing could be purchased or otherwise appropriated. Typically, managers offered little support for research until they had evidence that a worker's results indicated likely commercial application. While some highly successful results derived from these solitary researchers, by and large their work was inefficient and duplicative and had little direction.[12]

There were some exceptional cases. For example, the Pennsylvania Railroad hired chemist Charles Benjamin Dudley as an analyst in 1875. On the basis of his analyses, Dudley developed specifications for many of the materials vital to Pennsylvania Railroad, including tallows used in locomotive cylinders, lard oil for signal lights, and the steel used to make the firm's rails. The value the company placed on Dudley's work was reflected in the growth of his laboratory at Pennsylvania Railroad, which expanded from a staff of about two untrained assistants when he accepted the position to nearly three dozen trained chemists when he retired.

In 1834 physician-chemist Samuel Luther Dana established what was probably the first industrial research laboratory in America for the Merrimack Manufacturing Company, a textile firm in Lowell, Massachusetts. Among his many contributions to Merrimack and the textile industry in general, Dana improved the processes of calico printing and the bleaching of cotton prior to printing. The most notable example of an organized industrial laboratory of the nineteenth century was Thomas Edison's facility at Menlo Park, New Jersey, established in 1876. The continuously high level of activity of his laboratory is partially explained by the dozens of workers Edison employed to design, build, and test apparatus.[13]

The modern industrial research laboratory emerged in America in the early twentieth century (see fig. 1). As the government enforced the Sherman Antitrust Act actively after the turn of the century, thereby throttling some established competitive mechanisms in industry, corporate research emerged as a new weapon to guarantee dominance over weaker firms. Those industries born in the laboratory and those firms big enough to afford research programs were the first to establish research facilities:

It is significant that most of the early laboratories appeared in industries such as electricity or chemicals. Not only were they relatively new industries, with no traditional inertia from the past, but in these industries there were large firms with sufficient financial resources and stability to support the laboratories; and a rapidly changing, competitive technology made successful research imperative for the sponsoring firm. Older industries, such as iron and steel, and those where no giants existed were relatively slow to bring science into their activities, and a great differential still exists.[14]

From the turn of the century up to World War I, firms from the chemical, pharmaceutical, electrical, and petroleum industries founded research laboratories: General Electric, Bell Telephone, Parke-Davis, Du Pont, Westinghouse, Standard Oil, and Eastman Kodak. World War I had a significant impact on the development of industrial research in the United States. New industrial research laboratories arose and extant laboratories expanded to replenish increasingly scarce imported commodities and to meet the technological needs of a wartime government.

Industrial research laboratories took part in many projects during the war. General Electric and Western Electric, for example, worked closely with university and government scientists in the development of an effective listening device for submarine detection. Industry also played an important part in the production of high-quality optical glass to replace the interrupted supply from German companies. American chemical companies, Du Pont in particular, managed to alleviate shortages of many goods for which America had depended on Germany in the past. Chemical firms developed means to process naturally occurring nitrates that were essential to explosives, and they produced synthetic materials used in smokeless

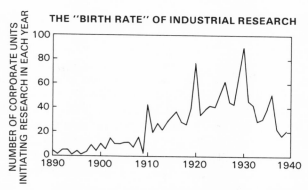

Figure 1. Graph of the "birth rate" of industrial research in the United States, showing the number of companies in all industries that established research as a recognized function in each year from 1890 through 1939 (adapted from Franklin S. Cooper, "Location and Extent of Industrial Research," 176).

powder. Pharmaceutical firms supplied many therapeutic agents that theretofore had been controlled by German firms, such as anesthetics, sedatives, and antimicrobial drugs.

The pressing wartime needs called for emergency measures, which industry actively carried out. The secretary of the navy established the Naval Consulting Board in 1915 to help organize vital research. The board included some members from academe and government, but most of its members were from industry. Although its major activity was the screening of inventions submitted by the public, the board facilitated the involvement of major firms in such problems as submarine detection. Industrial researchers also worked on many of the problems that the National Research Council (NRC) organized. Overall, research-based mass production came of age during the war, and a significant proportion of American industry thereafter increasingly manifested an interest in research.[15]

Industrial research grew significantly between the two world wars. As shown by the following figures, derived from fairly comprehensive surveys of all industries by the NRC, the interwar expansion of industrial research was set back only temporarily by the Depression. From the mid-1920s to World War II the total number of industrial laboratories more than doubled, and the total research staff tripled.[16]

Year	Laboratories	Research Staff
1927	1,000	19,000
1931	1,625	32,000
1933	1,575	27,000
1938	1,769	44,000
1940	2,264	58,000

For comparative purposes, the change in total research staff for 200 companies existing throughout the period of these surveys was as follows: 1927, 10,000; 1931, 14,000; 1933, 11,000; 1938, 16,000; 1940, 18,000. The NRC surveys clearly suggest an overall growth of interest in research within American industry.[17] The number of large industrial research laboratories increased during the period between the wars. In 1921 only 15 firms had research staffs of at least fifty, but by the late 1930s this group swelled to 120 companies. A handful of these firms, representing 1 percent of all companies listed in the 1938 NRC survey, employed one-third of all research personnel by that year.[18] There were also disparities in the level of research activity from industry to industry, as measured by the proportion of research personnel among an industry's total employees. The chemical industry (including the pharmaceutical industry) was by far the leader here throughout the interwar period. Moreover, the same four industries—petroleum, rubber products, electrical machinery, and instruments—were consistently the most research-intensive industries behind the chemical industry from 1920 to 1940.[19] Thus, by the end of this period, research had become a function of much of American industry, although a small number of firms in the chemical, electrical, and other industries cultivated research much more intensively than the rest.

Interactions between Academe and Industry

In-house laboratories satisfied many, but by no means all, of industry's requirements. For example, firms used independent research organizations such as Arthur D. Little, the Mellon Institute, and the Battelle Institute to complement their own research programs. Most of this contractual research concerned analytical work and improvement of extant products or processes.[20] For development of new products, among other functions, companies relied on their own facilities and academic laboratories.

At the turn of the twentieth century some university scientists were acting as consultants to industry; by and large, however, the main means by which universities and industries maintained contact was through graduates who had become industrial employees. As more and more firms developed an interest in research during the early decades of the twentieth century, different avenues opened to foster links. The industrial fellowship was the most frequent source of contact. Chemist Robert Kennedy Duncan pioneered the systematic use of industrial fellowships in academe at the University of Kansas in 1907. The seriously inefficient state of American industry, which Duncan attributed to the failure of industry to make use of research, and the manufacturer's lack of experience in scientific research convinced the chemist to institute the research fellowships. Typically the fellow, a graduate student working under the direction of Duncan, devoted nearly all of his time (with the exception of a few hours

one could determine the amount of that component in samples of crude ergot. By 1883 Parke-Davis had introduced twenty chemically assayed fluidextracts of botanical drugs. A few other firms, such as Lilly and G. D. Searle, followed suit in the 1880s. For example, J. K. Lilly went to work in the laboratory of his father's firm immediately after graduating from the Philadelphia College of Pharmacy in 1882; within a decade Lilly hired a chemist and a botanist to assist in control work.[33]

Science moved further into the pharmaceutical industry in the 1890s, when firms began manufacturing diphtheria antitoxin following Emil Roux's announcement in 1894 that he had developed a method to produce the antitoxin on a large scale. In the process, companies initiated early links with academic researchers. Mulford and Parke-Davis were the early leaders. Late in 1894 Mulford president Milton Campbell hired Joseph McFarland, a member of the Philadelphia Board of Health and the Medico-Chirurgical College, to produce diphtheria antitoxin and possibly other biologicals. This move was "the first direct effort on Campbell's part to enact a policy of active product development through laboratory science." McFarland soon acquired the assistance of faculty members of the University of Pennsylvania Veterinary School to produce the drug, and Mulford arranged for the Laboratory of Hygiene at Pennsylvania to test the antitoxin. By 1900 Mulford was producing nearly a dozen different biologicals through these arrangements, including tetanus antitoxin, antistreptococcus serum, and rabies vaccine.[34]

Parke-Davis also developed an interest in diphtheria antitoxin soon after Roux's announcement and, like Mulford, tapped a nearby academic institution for assistance. The Detroit firm had maintained some contact with the University of Michigan, particularly through Lyons, a Michigan graduate, so Parke-Davis turned to this university for assistance in producing diphtheria antitoxin. Michigan was also a logical place to seek advice because the dean and a faculty member of the medical school had attended the meeting at which Roux announced his discovery. Elijah M. Houghton, a research assistant in pharmacology at Michigan, joined Parke-Davis early in 1895, and Charles McClintock, a research assistant in bacteriology, followed Houghton the next year.

The firm immediately established a research laboratory in biology, in which McClintock served as director of research and Houghton as assistant director of Research. The two were able to produce diphtheria antitoxin within a few months. Thereafter, Houghton focused on biological standardizations of various botanical drugs—a field he pioneered—while McClintock turned his attention to the production of other biologicals. Biological research dominated Parke-Davis until the 1920s, when the firm established a separate department of chemical research. Parke-Davis's

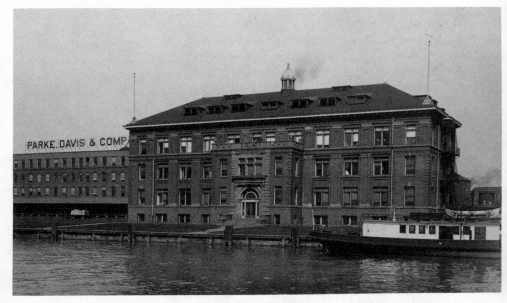

Figure 2. The Parke, Davis and Company Research Laboratory, established in Detroit in 1902. This was the first building in American industry to be erected as a research facility (from Parke, Davis and Company, *Parke-Davis at 100* [Detroit, n.d.], courtesy of Parke-Davis).

early commitment to research is indicated also by its construction of a separate building for research in 1902, one of the first among all industries in America (see fig. 2).[35]

Interest in biologicals also thrust Lederle Laboratories, of Pearl River, New York, into research activity. In 1906 chemist Ernst Joseph Lederle, a former president of the Board of Health of New York City, assembled a small but well-trained staff to enter his company into the field of biologicals. However, Lederle's interest came well after Parke-Davis's and Mulford's work in this area.[36]

A few other firms established scientific staffs and facilities in the late nineteenth and early twentieth centuries. Smith, Kline and French, of Philadelphia, set up an analytical laboratory headed by chemist Lyman Kebler in 1893. The firm soon built up the equipment and staff of the laboratory, but the company accomplished little in the way of original investigations before World War I. Kebler's group primarily provided a testing laboratory rather than a development laboratory. Upjohn, of Kalamazoo, Michigan, hired the Yale-trained chemist Frederick Heyl in 1913 to direct its new research division. Heyl and his colleagues carried out some studies on new products, but their chief responsibility was control work. Lilly's small scientific staff grew enough that the firm constructed a Scientific Building in 1911. By the following year the Indianapolis company had as many as a score of its personnel engaged in research on such topics as new synthetic drugs.[37]

By World War I, then, a few firms had assembled at least the rudiments of a research staff. Efforts at cooperative research in this period existed on a rudimentary level as well. Generally, companies dealt with only one or two academic institutions and typically contracted with university workers for control work. Thus H. A. Metz Laboratories, of New York, hired two Columbia biochemists as consultants to run occasional quality-control checks on its products. Mulford engaged the Laboratory of Hygiene at Pennsylvania as a biologicals testing laboratory, and pharmacologist Torald Sollmann, a consultant to the firm, worked out a process to increase the potency and shelf life of Mulford's products. Charles LaWall of the Philadelphia College of Pharmacy was a consultant to Smith, Kline and French periodically from 1895 to 1905. Parke-Davis occasionally worked with University of Michigan scientists. Mulford, Parke-Davis, and perhaps a few other companies arranged for regional hospitals to test their products, a measure that was voluntary in this period.[38]

Cooperative research was still a fledgling enterprise before the war, with little resemblance to the systems and networks of contacts that emerged in the 1920s. In part this was because research itself was relatively undeveloped and unorganized among firms with an interest in research.

CHAPTER TWO

The Rise of University-Industry
Interactions in Biomedical Research

→))-→))-→))-→))-→))- ((←-((←-((←-((←-((←

Cooperative biomedical research did not emerge on a systemic basis in America until the 1920s and 1930s. Certain mindsets and circumstances that collectively put the academic biomedical researchers in a unique position compared with other faculty in the university had impeded cooperation between academe and the pharmaceutical industry. In the first place, an increasing number of academic researchers in the last quarter of the nineteenth century repudiated applied work in favor of original and fundamental work. This was in part a continuation of a trend present in some corners of American science for decades and in part a result of a sort of indoctrination into what these researchers perceived to be a Germanic emphasis on fundamental research. Such a frame of mind was incompatible with an enterprise as utilitarian as the pharmaceutical industry. Second, medical researchers were not inclined to work with the pharmaceutical industry because of American medicine's traditional disapproval of the patenting of health-related processes and products. Questionable practices by some drug companies also helped create a tainted image of this industry.

The industry itself, however, helped erode this image. Beginning around the turn of the twentieth century, but primarily after World War I, company executives increasingly emphasized the value of research, both in word and in deed. Research staffs in many companies grew significantly during the 1920s and 1930s, as did research budgets. Some firms began to foster in-house fundamental research programs, although the weight of industrial research interests was practical in nature. Pharmaceutical firms also helped elevate their status among academic workers by employing prominent scientists, often as research directors. Companies reinforced this new image of a research-conscious industry in the 1930s by establishing special laboratories and institutes devoted to research and by supporting some fundamental work in universities through direct grants-in-aid and awards administered by scientific societies.

As a result, from 1920 to 1940 more and more university workers turned to drug companies, and vice versa, for intellectual, technical, and economic support. Academic scientists and firms developed a variety of relationships. Cooperative endeavors often benefited both sides. University researchers enjoyed a variety of direct and indirect benefits, including a source of support for their research programs in an era prior to large-scale government involvement in the support of research. Companies depended on universities for research personnel and know-how, which were necessities for remaining competitive in the modern pharmaceutical industry. Collaboration produced many drugs that contributed appreciably to companies' sales and profits. Public health shared in the benefits of cooperative research. Many important anesthetics, hormones, sedatives, anticonvulsants, antiinfectives, and other therapeutic agents derived from joint work by universities and drug firms.

Barriers to Cooperative Research

Impediments to interactions between academic scientists and pharmaceutical companies existed on both sides. These obstacles slowly dissolved after the turn of the twentieth century,[1] in part because university researchers during the Progressive era were more willing than in the past to address their work to the needs of society. Also, after World War I many company managers realized the importance of research for success. Consequently, firms fostered research through large-scale research programs within industry and through contacts with academic research programs.

The roots of one of the more significant barriers within American universities rested in the concept of fundamental research as it emerged in the United States in the late nineteenth century.[2] Prior to this, American universities were typically religious in character and emphasized the improvement of all mental faculties by training them on difficult and abstract material, such as Greek, Latin, and mathematics. However, the subjects per se were not as important to the nineteenth-century educator as was their use in developing the faculties to function efficiently in whatever field the student chose to enter. Thus educator Joseph Payne remarked that the aim of education was "quickening and strengthening the powers of observation and memory, and forming habits of careful and persevering attention; it should habituate the pupil to distinguish points of difference and recognize those of resemblance, to analyze and investigate, to arrange and classify. It should awaken and invigorate the understanding, mature the reason, chasten while it kindles the imagination, exercise the judgement and refine the taste."[3]

This is not to say that science was absent from antebellum higher education, because science developed an important place in the American college early on.[4] By the late 1820s, colleges commonly had four professorships devoted to science—in chemistry, physics, mathematics, and geology—representing as many as half of all positions on the faculty. Colleges turned to an elective system to rescue their curricula from increasingly superficial courses; it was a situation largely created by, rather than created for, the sciences. Interestingly, the first half of the nineteenth century witnessed a taste of the fundamental and original versus applied and practical rhetoric among American scientists that blossomed in the last quarter of the century. Scientists within and outside of colleges, such as Denison Olmsted, Charles Baker Adams, and Alexander Dallas Bache, made use of service roles (e.g., geological surveys) to augment their income, among other reasons, but their public stance did not necessarily mirror their feelings about such work as confided to colleagues, which could amount to apologies.[5]

Research, specifically fundamental research, did not become a recognized function of universities in America until the last quarter of the nineteenth century. The intimate relationship between fundamental research and higher education was an innovation of German universities in the nineteenth century. This relationship spread to American universities as scientists and scholars returned from abroad infected with the notion of *Wissenschaft* as a "dedicated, sanctified pursuit" of phenomena, "not the study of things for their immediate utilities, but the morally imperative study of things for themselves and for their ultimate meanings." This concept of *Wissenschaft* as a search for ultimate meanings sprang from German idealism of the eighteenth and early nineteenth centuries, which maintained close connections with universities through Kant (at Königsberg), Schelling (at Jena and Berlin), Hegel (at Berlin), and others. Unlike French and English universities of the same period, the German philosophical faculty achieved a status equal to the faculties of law, medicine, and theology.[6] Prior to the emergence of the basic biomedical sciences like physiology and biochemistry in the early nineteenth century, the German idealists' search for certainty helped shape a philosophical science of medicine, beginning around the turn of the nineteenth century.[7]

As the basic sciences began to make their way into German universities, the empirical methods of the natural and physical sciences clashed with the idealists' a priori approach to understanding.[8] Eventually, the empirical approach to science developed by Justus von Liebig early in his career in chemistry, Johannes Mueller and Carl Ludwig in physiology, Wilhelm Wundt in psychology, and many others established this methodology for the many disciplines that arose in German universities in the nineteenth century. However, "the idealistic mood lingered over the German universities long after it was severed from the circumstances of its origin," and "pure" learning, characterized in part by scrupulous investigation, became a recognized pursuit of German academic research later in the century.[9]

Pure research was not the only pursuit of German academic researchers. For example, the growing synthetic chemical industry in Germany developed close connections with several universities up to the 1880s, when firms developed in-house research facilities. Firms provided university workers, from the institute director to the privatdozent, with raw materials, consulting fees, patent royalties, and other means of support. In exchange, the academic chemists supplied industry with inventions, new production techniques, manpower in the form of graduates, and even expert testimony in the case of patent litigation. Eventually, the German chemical industry managed to help refashion the university chemical curriculum, in part to introduce the chemistry student to the needs of industry. Firms developed especially close ties with several of the better academic laboratories:

Cooperation with university chemists was so actively sought by the various German companies that a veritable competitive struggle arose between them over the "control" of the most important academic laboratories; and in time each company managed to establish strong ties with certain schools to the exclusion of all other rivals. The Bayer firm had particularly close ties with [Wilhelm] Wislicenus at Würtzburg and with the University of Göttingen. Through the efforts of Carl Martius, the Agfa of Berlin had a virtual "monopoly" on [August Wilhelm von] Hofmann's findings and a first choice in the hiring of his students. Höchst and the Badische Anilin- und Soda-Fabrik competed, or sometimes cooperated, for the favor of Adolph Baeyer, who taught successively in Berlin, Strasbourg, and Munich, and of Baeyer's many gifted students, such as [Carl] Graebe, [Carl Theodor] Liebermann, Emil and Otto Fischer, and Ludwig Knorr.[10]

Clearly, such a situation was far removed from any sort of disinterested search for ultimate meanings or from the Veblenian cult of idle curiosity.

Thus, higher education in Germany wore two distinctly different masks. On the one hand, the state governments kept the technical schools apart from the universities to use the former to promote industrialization. Also, throughout the last quarter of the nineteenth century about three-quarters of the university lectureships—in chemistry at least—were devoted to "pure" fields.[11] However, the links between academe and industry obviously were close. This was the confusing situation when the Americans arrived.

Americans migrated to German universities primarily in the 1870s, 1880s, and 1890s. Peak migration came in 1895–96, when over five hundred Americans enrolled in German institutions. That study in Germany was cheaper (even when including the cost of travel) than study at some of the better universities in the United States played some part in a student's decision to spend time at a German university, but the intellectual challenge alone was overwhelmingly attractive for most. In the 1890s Harvard philosopher Josiah Royce reflected on the lure of study in Germany: "German scholarship was our master and our guide. . . . The air was full of suggestion. . . . One went to Germany still a doubter as to the possibility of the theoretic life; one returned an idealist, devoted for the time to pure learning for learning's sake, determined to contribute his *Scherflein* to the massive store of human knowledge, burning for a chance to help build the American University."[12] Several American universities—some new, such as Clark, Stanford, and Chicago, and some refurbished, such as Harvard, Yale, and Cornell—followed the lead of Johns Hopkins in 1876 by establishing graduate research programs based on the German model (without the ties to industry). By 1900 some state universities as well—Wisconsin, California, and Michigan—established graduate research programs. The number of doctorates conferred by American universities increased from none in 1861 to 164 in 1890, and the postgraduate population in America rose from about 200 students in 1871 to nearly 3,000 in 1890.[13]

Qualitatively, Americans brought back with them the fundamental component of the German research experience, which accelerated the extant attitudes in American scientific education about the value of original and basic research. An early *Register* of Johns Hopkins proclaimed that the Baltimore university "provides advanced instruction, *not professional*, to properly qualified students, in various departments of literature and science."[14] Clark University was established in 1888 as a graduate school alone, which was indicative of the feeling of some that the pursuit of pure learning did not benefit from the popular precept that bigger (enrollment) was better. Few American educators were as ardently supportive of fundamental research as psychologist G. Stanley Hall, the first president of Clark University. He likened research-oriented professors to prophets, freed from the "routine and rules of common college life," in an atmosphere devoid of the practical components of Francis Bacon's House of Solomon: "In the new 'House of Solomon' they should have the best equipment, the largest pay, the freest air; for thus not merely the university, but the nation, receives with due honor its anointed prophets." Hall's image of the university clearly was free of utilitarian considerations: "The common sense of it all is, that the university should rest solely on the love of knowledge, and the true investigator refines, and over and over returns to, his method and thought till it is simple and direct, great but easily mastered because [it is] stated in a way to present the least possible resistance."[15]

But what of the other, "industrialized" side of German higher education in the late nineteenth century and how it affected the Americans? To assume that this even had an immediate effect presupposes that the visiting Americans had some involvement in the links with the firms, which is doubtful. Their purpose in leaving the United States was to learn chemistry, or physiology, or pharmacology, not to find support for these fields. Yet, even if they had some exposure to the connections with firms, there was nothing in America with which such connections could be compared. In relation to their analogues in Germany, nineteenth-century American companies were by and large primitives in research. In fact, interactions between American companies and universities did not begin to approach the same level of sophistication and intensity that German academic-industrial ties exhibited until the period between the two world wars. Preliminary indications for the biomedical sciences suggest that there may have been some rather marked similarities in such ties in Germany and America, but much more work on the former remains to be done.[16]

Incontestably, fundamental research played an important part in the development of the American university in the late nineteenth century, but the latter also had a well-established utilitarian component.[17] For example, the Morrill Land Grant Act of 1862, the Hatch Act of 1887 (which established agricultural experiment stations), and the second Morrill Act of 1890 (which helped subsidize the agricultural colleges established under the 1862 act) provided for practical instruction in many universities. By the turn of the twentieth century the American university emerged as an amalgam of fundamental and applied research functions:

In the one view, research was an activity to be initiated and directed from within the university. The searcher was to be independent, not only with respect to his conclusions, but to his choice of an area of work. To fill the gaps in knowledge that continuing inquiry revealed, to conduct investigations as the logic of a discipline directed—these were to be the functions of academic inquiry. Practical results might be forthcoming, but inquiry should be allowed to push against any of the frontiers of knowledge, and not merely along that border where material benefits were promised. . . . [But] the graduate school in the American university was only one of a heterogeneous group of divisions. In the other schools and departments [e.g., agriculture, commerce, engineering, and business administration], research was often geared to external and ulterior purposes.[18]

Notwithstanding the presence of practical interests, the strength of fundamental research in universities probably played some part in the reluctance of biomedical researchers to collaborate with pharmaceutical companies. Many physiologists, biochemists, pharmacologists, and other biomedical scientists spent time in Germany in the late nineteenth and early twentieth centuries, including some of the most prominent workers in their fields. Pharmacologist John J. Abel of Johns Hopkins spent seven years in Germany; and physiological chemist Russell Chittenden of Yale and physiologist Jacques Loeb, who spent nearly twenty years at Chicago and Berkeley before moving to the Rockefeller Institute, also brought German ideals of pure learning to America. These disciplines certainly faced practical obligations in settings such as medical and agricultural schools,[19] but such "service roles" did not lead to the abandonment of pure learning in the biomedical sciences. For example, Hopkins physiologist Henry Newall Martin felt that physiology "should be cultivated as a pure science absolutely independent of any so-called practical affiliation." Chittenden, the father of American biochemistry, developed a successful modus vivendi between purely theoretical work and practical instruction at the Sheffield Scientific School. Abel, Chittenden's counterpart in pharmacology, believed that once established, pharmacology would "yield valuable results for the practical man." He emphasized, however, that pharmacology "is not therefore an applied science, like therapeutics, but is one of the biological sciences, using that word in its widest sense."[20]

It was one thing for biomedical researchers to spend time training physicians and other professionals, but working with industry was an entirely different matter. Until the early twentieth century, drug companies by and large had no interest in research. There were a few exceptions, such as Mulford and Parke-Davis, but even the exceptional cases had little or no interest in fundamental work. Even after research (including some fundamental studies) had become a recognized function for many pharmaceutical companies, Abel refused to do any work for drug firms: "I personally would not think of working on a problem suggested to me by any firm anywhere. Usually, problems of this nature could be worked out very well in the laboratories of the firms since they almost always concern questions of what I might call applied pharmacology. A pharmacologist of any training or ability should have so many problems of his own awaiting solution that he should not spend his time on matters of little theoretical importance for his science."[21]

The high value placed on fundamental research in American universities, therefore, helped impede any movement for collaboration with pharmaceutical firms on strictly applied work. Traditional disapproval of medical patents by physicians and biomedical scientists also presented a barrier to cooperative work from within academe. The code of ethics adopted by the American Medical Association in 1847 explicitly decried medical patents: "Equally derogatory to professional character is it, for a physician to hold a patent for any surgical instrument, or medicine."[22] Patenting of discoveries could also generate repugnance among some physical scientists, such as Joseph Henry, although most did not clamor against patents to the same extent as their biomedical colleagues did.[23]

Harvard bacteriologist Hans Zinsser proclaimed why physicians and medical researchers had such an aversion to medical patents:

The invention of an improvement in the mechanism of automobiles, or of a shoe-buckle, concerns matters of convenience or luxury, and can be dispensed with easily by those who are forced to do without them. The relief of the sick and the prevention of unnecessary sorrow by the maintenance of individual and public health are matters in a different category. As soon as we are in possession of the knowledge of principles or methods which can contribute to these purposes their free utilization becomes a public necessity; and any procedure which inhibits their most rapid and effective application to the needs of the community would seem to us as unjustified as the cornering of the wheat market or the patenting of the process of making bread.[24]

Abel, too, questioned the ethics of patenting medical discoveries: "I have always considered it unethical for a medical man, and especially for a research worker who is supported by a university and foundations, to take out patents."[25]

The American pharmaceutical industry did not make significant use of the patent system until after World War I. For example, Edward R. Squibb, founder of E. R. Squibb and Sons, proclaimed, "I do not myself think that anything should be patented by either physician or pharmacist; I am sure that the patient would not be benefited thereby." Indeed, the Squibb company held only one patent by 1920.[26] The German pharmaceutical industry held the vast majority of American patents on therapeutic agents prior to World War I. Several American firms received licenses to produce these patented drugs after the U.S. government abrogated German-owned patents under the Trading with the Enemy Act of 1917. Before the war, drug companies protected their processes through secrecy; the American Medical Association had long censured this means of protection as well as patenting.[27]

It may seem incongruous to conceive of an unwillingness within academe to cooperate with the pharmaceutical industry on the basis of anti-patent bias, given the actual paucity of patent activity by American firms. However, there was no reason for university scientists to doubt that American firms would turn to patents to protect their research investments—much as German industry did—once they established research programs.[28] To effect the latter, of course, required the cooperation of academic researchers. In a sense, with respect to collaboration with universities, drug companies in the late nineteenth and early twentieth centuries were damned if they did and damned if they did not. On the one hand, it was difficult for academic scientists to take firms seriously as potential collaborators until the companies developed an interest in research. On the other hand, once firms established research programs of their own, they would in all likelihood (based on the experience of German firms) become more aggressively patent-minded. As the relationship between university scientists and drug firms evolved in the early decades of this century, interest in research was a more important precondition to cooperation. Also, academic biomedical scientists themselves began seeking patents in the 1920s and 1930s.

The pharmaceutical industry itself was perhaps the biggest barrier to collaborative research. In the first place, the distant, embarrassing relatives of such respectable firms as Parke-Davis, Squibb, and Lilly—the manufacturers of Wendell's Ambition Pills, Old Sachem Bitters, William Radam's Microbe Killer, and other questionable nostrums—certainly did not help the image of respectable pharmaceutical companies. The companies discussed in this study were far removed (and they attempted to remove themselves) from the so-called patent medicine makers. However, when the latter began to mimic methods by which respectable firms advertised their products to physicians and in medical journals by the late nineteenth century, the situation for the comparatively small group of ethical firms worsened. In addition, even respectable firms marketed a fair share of dubious home health care items, which probably confused distinctions between nostrum makers and ethical firms. The efforts of muckraking journalists, the American Medical Association, the American Pharmaceutical Association, and others to expose the fraud of the "patent" medicine makers helped to differentiate respectable companies from the others.[29]

In the second place, while the ethical industry per se was not to blame for the inundation of "patent" medicines, it had its share of practices that seemed questionable to physicians and medical researchers. For example, as mentioned above, firms relied on secrecy to protect their products. Also, company researchers that published scientific papers rarely published anything negative about house products in this period before the war.[30] Even in the late 1930s, Merck pharmacologist Hans Molitor said that usually only positive results from industrial laboratories were published, although "non-publication of results, particularly of negative ones, is not necessarily due to a desire to keep them secret, but more often is caused by the impossibility of finding a periodical willing to allot sufficient space to the publication of data which interest only a small minority of its readers."[31] The type of experience Abel had with a firm could damage the reputation of an otherwise respectable drug company. According to the Hopkins pharmacologist:

Even reputable houses will do things that tend to damage men. About ten years ago [c. 1900] one of our large and reputable houses put on their labels and stated in pamphlets that their preparation of the suprarenal principle was made by a method of Professor John J. Abel, of the Johns Hopkins University, Medical School, etc. etc. My friends immediately called my attention to these labels and asked me if I had "supplied this firm with a method." I wrote to the firm at once stating that I should publish a card in every medical journal in the country calling attention to the injury that was being done to me in these statements which implied that I had given them a "method." [I] furthermore stated that while I could not and did not wish to keep manufacturers from making use of my work, I must insist that they should state in their literature that this method was obtained from my [published] papers.[32]

The firm soon acquiesced. It is not clear how extensively respectable firms made free use of the names of researchers in advertisements, but the publicity generated from just a few such affairs could damage a company's reputation among potential collaborators.

Given all of the above, it should not be surprising that by the beginning of the period between the two world wars academic scientists had a tainted image of industrial pharmaceutical work. As one indication of this image, consider the reaction of scientists when Max Gottlieb—the creation of Sinclair Lewis and bacteriologist Paul De Kruif, whom De Kruif based on Jacques Loeb—abandoned academic life to work for the fictional pharmaceutical firm Dawson T. Hunziker and Company, Inc. Scientists lamented, "How could old Max have gone over to that damned pill-peddler?" and "Of all the people in the world! I wouldn't have believed it! Max Gottlieb falling for those crooks. . . . I wish he hadn't gone wrong!"[33] *Arrowsmith* was a novel, but the depiction of the alarm and dismay of his academic colleagues when a respected scientist joined a drug company reflected the opinion of many biomedical scientists and physicians.

For example, around 1910 Cornell pharmacologist Robert A. Hatcher agreed to abstract all available literature on the physiological action of caffeine for the Coca-Cola Company; this involved neither personal comments nor original research by Hatcher. When Torald Sollmann, a pharmacologist at Western Reserve University, heard about the agreement between Hatcher and Coca-Cola, he informed Hatcher that his reputation would suffer a very severe shock if it became known that he had done the work for them and if the firm chose to misuse the abstracts.[34] Hatcher's friend Abel tried to assure the former that there was nothing improper in abstracting literature for a firm, but Hatcher nonetheless felt "certainly sicker of this thing than I have even been of anything I can recall. I never make resolutions, but I do hope I may not get into such a fix again."[35]

Like Hatcher, other pharmacologists sought Abel's advice from time to time about the propriety of collaborating with companies. For example, in the early 1930s Alfred Newton Richards, of Pennsylvania, approached the Hopkins pharmacologist for an enlightened opinion about an offer Merck had made to Richards to serve as a consultant to the firm. North Carolina pharmacologist William MacNider likewise sought Abel's counsel when a pharmaceutical company wanted MacNider to evaluate the therapeutic value of one of its new plant extracts. MacNider was seriously considering the offer, even though he normally was reluctant to cooperate with industry: "I must say that I have almost a phobia concerning becoming mixed up with commercial enterprises, and also receiving money for such work. My innate reaction is against it."[36] We have already seen that Abel personally opposed cooperative work on the basis that applied pharmacological research was more the province of industrial laboratories than universities. He also believed that if academic workers were less cooperative with industry, firms by necessity would have to establish their own research programs, which would be all the better for industry (and academic pharmacologists):

My own opinion in regard to professors of pharmacology doing work for firms is that they had better not. I mean to say that a man will be better satisfied with himself in the long run if he can keep out of it. The firms can get good men from abroad (for that matter, in this country), if they will treat them as scientifically trained men should be treated. If no reputable pharmacologist who holds a chair will do hack work or expert work for them, I think that they will get men of their own as the foreign firms do and as one of the large firms in this country has done.[37]

The circumstances surrounding medicinal chemist Edward Calvin Kendall's departure from, ironically, Parke-Davis bore out Abel's theme of industry's need to treat its researchers as scientifically trained people. Kendall joined the firm in 1910 and left soon thereafter, angered at being treated more like a factory worker than a scientist and depressed by the lack of any sort of scholarly atmosphere.[38]

Biomedical scientists and physicians collectively as well as individually took a stand against commercial work. For example, the American Medical Association censured the patenting of medicines. At its forty-eighth (1896) annual meeting in Atlanta the association refused a delegate permission to register because he had applied for a patent; he had not even obtained a patent. Prior to the period between the wars, members of the Society for Experimental Biology and Medicine introduced a stipulation into the society's constitution expelling anyone who published deliberately favorable analyses of foods and drugs for manufacturers. The society used this stipulation to remove one of its members.[39]

No scientific society in the United States took as strong a stance against industrial work as the American Society for Pharmacology and Experimental Therapeutics (ASPET), whose vast majority of members were M.D.'s. According to the original ASPET constitution, framed when Abel and a small group of pharmacologists established the society in 1908, "no one shall be admitted to membership who is in the permanent employ of a drug firm," and "entrance into the permanent employ of a drug firm shall constitute forfeiture of membership."[40] A decade later, however, a movement involving a handful of members (including Abel) was underfoot to eliminate the ASPET ban. This small group did not succeed, but sentiment to remove the clauses grew over the 1920s and 1930s, as the tainted image of the pharmaceutical industry slowly dissipated.

Erosion of the Tainted Image

Several developments within the pharmaceutical industry between World War I and World War II helped erase the academic biomedical community's disparaging view of this industry and thereby opened the way for widespread cooperation between industry and academe. The most significant developments were (1) a major change in attitude among many firms, emphasizing the value of research and an active application of this philosophy (including the support of some fundamental research); (2) employment of prominent scientists, often as directors of company research; and (3) establishment of special research laboratories and research institutes.

Some firms had developed an interest in research in the late nineteenth century. These companies—most notably Parke-Davis and Mulford—developed rudimentary research interactions with a few university scientists. However, research in the pharmaceutical industry did not emerge on a wide scale until after World War I.[41] Research in this period grew, not out of quality-control work,[42] but out of product development. While government regulation—through the Biologics Control Act of 1902 and the Pure Food and Drug Act of 1906—led to the introduction of science-based control work in a number of firms, such work was geared to the improvement of existing products and processes.[43] While necessary, control work simply could not add as much to a firm's capital as could new product research and development. The industry grew rapidly after World War I, when firms actively began turning out new therapeutic products. Research programs were essential to this new primary function of industry.

The neglect of product development by U.S. manufacturers became quite obvious once wartime conditions forced German firms to interrupt drug supplies to the United States. German pharmaceutical firms had introduced some of the leading analgesic, anesthetic, hypnotic, antimicrobial, and other agents, and they employed a variety of trade practices to maintain control of the markets for these drugs in the United States. As the war dragged on, a dearth of these drugs set in, and prices skyrocketed. After the government abrogated German patents near the end of the war, U.S. pharmaceutical firms soon filled the demand for these drugs, partly because many firms already had trained staff on hand for control work and partly because outside scientists assisted some firms, such as Roger Adams's cooperation with Abbott (see chap. 3). Essentially, this enabled many firms to get their collective foot in the product-development door.[44]

If U.S. firms learned anything from their German counterparts after the war, it was that research was fundamentally important if they were to remain at the cutting edge of practical therapeutics. Thus Alfred S. Burdick, president of Abbott Laboratories, proclaimed, "Research is fundamental and vital. Without it real progress is impossible, in spite of occasional evanescent success." According to Carleton Palmer, president of Squibb, his firm could not neglect in-house research: "We cannot afford to discontinue all research work even though we connect with the Mellon Institute and use their data to solve our bigger problems. Just whether we need any additional men or whether we do not possess men on our present staff sufficiently qualified to take charge of our research work I leave to you to decide. But I do feel that we should have a regular research department."[45]

Lilly president Josiah K. Lilly recognized the need for a solid foundation of chemists, pharmacologists, biologists, pharmacists, and clinicians "to insure a steady stream of useful and profitable specialties to Eli Lilly and Company."[46] From the time he became the chief executive of Merck and Company in 1925, George Merck planned a research laboratory of the highest order, on a level equal to the best academic laboratories: "To do research worthy of the name, to do research which will bring to industry true recognition of its contribution to the advance of knowledge, industry must have at its disposal genuinely creative minds so placed and so protected that their mental powers of thought, study, and imagination can concentrate on problems of great difficulty."[47]

These and other pharmaceutical company executives put their strong convictions about research into action. Abbott, for example, was appropriating about $100,000 annually for research by the late 1920s and had a research and control staff of twenty-nine by 1933. Upjohn's research staff had grown to a similar size by this time. Merck's research program grew slowly in the 1920s, but this changed in the next decade: from 1931 to 1940, Merck annual research expenditures ballooned from $146,000 to $906,000 (the latter sum was 4 percent of the company's total sales for 1940). Squibb had only a handful of researchers at the end of World War I, but by 1928 the firm's research staff totaled at least fifteen (not including scientific personnel at its biologicals laboratory), with a research budget of about $200,000 per year. Lilly had one of the largest research and control staffs in the industry by the mid-1930s. Its personnel in analytical, organic, and biochemistry; pharmacology; bacteriology and immunology; and other divisions amounted to over seventy, forty of whom held graduate or professional degrees.[48] Parke-Davis had built up such a research program

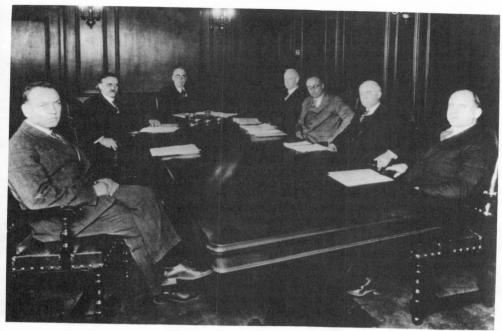

Figure 3. The Parke, Davis and Company Research Committee, sometime in the late 1920s. Members are, *clockwise from left foreground*: Oliver Kamm, director of chemical research; Frank O. Taylor, chief chemist; Elijah Mark Houghton, director of Biological and Research Laboratories; Wilbur L. Scoville, head of the Analytical Department; A. W. Lescohier, general manager; Walter E. King, assistant director of Biological and Research Laboratories; and Lawrence T. Clark, junior director of Biological and Research Laboratories (courtesy of the American Institute of the History of Pharmacy).

that in 1924 president Oscar W. Smith appointed a research committee, which included a physician, a Ph.D. in pharmacology, and a Ph.D. in organic chemistry (see fig. 3). Smith charged the committee to

decide what problems should be investigated; [devise] methods of keeping records; determine what practical results may be utilized from the investigators; . . . stimulate the best efforts of the individual research worker without in any way detracting from the initiative and originality of the worker. . . . I trust that this Committee will be able to push forward the selection of whatever problems may be decided upon as rapidly and conclusively as possible and in such a manner as to enhance the scientific standing and material welfare of Parke, Davis and Company. In carrying out its duties, I believe the Committee should meet regularly at a set time and place, perhaps as frequently as once a week or once in every two weeks.[49]

Not all of the leading pharmaceutical firms displayed a firm commitment to research during the period between the world wars. Smith, Kline and French, for example, had sales of $8–9 million by the mid-1930s (slightly higher than Abbott's sales in the same period), but the company employed only eight researchers, who received only $70,000 in support annually at this time. Most of the leading pharmaceutical companies, however, were becoming more and more aware of the value of research, and they were willing to invest in personnel, equipment, and facilities. When chemist Max Tishler moved from Harvard to Merck in 1937, he was most impressed by the industrial laboratory—its personnel, facilities, and the first-rate scientific work coming out of Merck at the time.[50]

Generally, industry had to rely on itself for present and future support of industrial research, as J. K. Lilly argued: "It should be recognized, also, that it must be a prosperous and reasonably profitable concern that essays to support, financially, extensive research. In short, [industry] must supply its own endowment." Thus, research had to pay its own way to have a future in industry; that is, it had to be translated into profit margins. Company executives, after all, were not going to invest hundreds of thousands of dollars in an enterprise without a return. Oscar Smith established a research committee at Parke-Davis, in part to "enhance the material welfare of Parke, Davis and Company"; and the general superintendent of Squibb emphasized that "I do not believe we are in [a] position at this time to spend money on research work concerning products we manufacture or might manufacture that would not be likely to yield profitable results in a business way."[51]

The director of research at Lilly, G. H. A. Clowes, suggested to president J. K. Lilly and vice-president Eli Lilly in 1929 that in the selection of in-house research projects and in the support of research proposals from outside the company, "our scientific reputation is now so firmly established that we can afford to be somewhat more exacting and discriminating than heretofore." Clowes outlined three categories of drug use, categories that he felt should be kept in mind when allotting research funds: (1) occasional use (e.g., antitoxins), (2) temporary use (e.g., ephedrine, a decongestant, and antisyphilitic arsenicals), and (3) regular use (e.g., insulin and liver extracts for pernicious anemia). Clowes felt that in terms of comparative consumption, regularly used drugs would turn more profit for the company than temporarily used medications, and the latter would be more profitable than occasionally used items. However, he went on to propose several other factors to be taken into account when considering a research proposal, such as the patentability of the drug or process, the prevalence of the disease for which a drug is to be used, and the projected cost to the patient.[52]

Research in the pharmaceutical industry was not entirely geared to immediate practical benefit. By 1921 Lilly supported fundamental research by Clowes in Indianapolis, and the company funded a unit at the Marine Biological Laboratory in Woods Hole, Massachusetts, where Clowes and other Lilly scientists took regular retreats in the summer. Some of the basic research in Indianapolis included studies of the physico-chemical nature of drug adsorption and the mechanisms of anesthesia. Clowes summarized his Lilly-sponsored research at Woods Hole as studies of "1) the mechanism underlying growth . . . and pathological growth as it occurs in cancer; 2) the mechanism underlying the penetration of drugs, anesthetics, germicides, etc., into living cells and the mode of action in the protoplasm of the cells; and 3) the mechanism underlying specificity, immunity, etc."[53] He recognized in this type of fundamental work an importance beyond the value of basic research in and of itself:

There is one point upon which considerable stress should be laid and that is the necessity of securing the recognition, respect and confidence of scientific and medical organizations and individuals all over the world. The greater the authority with which we can speak when we do speak, the greater will be our prestige and the more certain we shall be of establishing the scientific standing of the laboratory and improving the status of Eli Lilly and Company in the eyes of the medical profession. For this reason it may pay to spend a great deal of time on the scientific intricacies of problems from the solution of which there may be no immediate commercial return.[54]

Fundamental research became a battle cry for companies later in the period between the wars, when the pharmaceutical industry opened several research institutes and laboratories. It was not a case where firms were merely paying lip service to basic research in the presence of prominent academic scientists. Firms actually were engaging in more and more of this type of research by the end of the 1930s. The experience during the 1920s and 1930s established a fundamental research consciousness in the pharmaceutical industry that eventually thrust it ahead of other industries in terms of published output of this type of research.[55]

That company executives wanted to establish research programs is clear. That they really understood how to establish a research program was another matter. Carleton Palmer of Squibb was sure that he wanted his firm to have a research department, but he was not quite sure how or whether to add to his research staff. George Merck was solidly behind research at his firm. When he would walk around the laboratories, talking to the bench scientists, "he would get all excited about what people were telling him. He didn't understand it, but you could see he was getting all excited about it."[56] This is not surprising, since Palmer, Merck, and many other executives in the drug industry between 1920 and 1940 were businessmen, not scientists. Thus they, and even executives with some scientific background like the Lillys and Alfred Burdick of Abbott, turned to scientists to help them create research departments.

Several firms hired major scientists to head their research departments. John F. Anderson joined Squibb in 1915 as director of the Research and Biological Laboratories. Twelve years earlier, Anderson had been the first to identify Rocky Mountain spotted fever and had suggested the wood tick (*Dermacentor andersoni*) as the probable vector. He had served in the United States Public Health Service since 1901 and was the director of its Hygienic Laboratory from 1909 until the time he joined Squibb. Ernest Volwiler, Roger Adams's first Ph.D. student, joined Abbott as a research chemist the same year he graduated from Illinois, in 1918. Volwiler was named chief chemist in 1920, and he quickly assembled a string of impressive therapeutic discoveries, most notably in hypnotics and sedatives. He became director of research at Abbott in 1930. George Henry Alexander Clowes studied chemistry in his native England and took a Ph.D. in that field at Göttingen before emigrating to the United States in 1901. His first position in the United States was as a research chemist at the New York State Institute for the Study of Malignant Disease in Buffalo. Clowes soon developed an interest in cancer research and became part of a small circle of pioneering researchers in that field. He worked in the Chemical Warfare Service and at the Marine Biological Laboratory at Woods Hole from 1917 to 1919, when he accepted the Lillys' offer to organize a research program in Indianapolis as director of research.[57]

Other firms soon followed suit. Parke-Davis hired Oliver Kamm, an organic chemist on the faculty of the University of Illinois, as director of chemical research in 1920. Hoffman-La Roche was in the process of establishing a research program at its New Jersey plant, independent of its parent firm in Switzerland, when it appointed physiologist Friedrich Gudernatsch, who had received his Ph.D. from German University in Prague in 1910, as director of research laboratories in 1929. Gudernatsch had spent several years prior to this appointment on the faculty of the Cornell Medical College; throughout his directorship he was a visiting professor at New York University. George Merck, on the recommendation of Princeton physical chemist Hugh Taylor, invited a rising organic chemist at Princeton, Randolph Major, to head research at his firm.[58] Major joined Merck as director of pure research in 1930. Sharp and Dohme engaged pharmacologist John Krantz, of the University of Maryland School of Pharmacy, briefly (1927–30) as director of pharmaceutical research. A long-time faculty member at Johns Hopkins Medical School, George Harrop, became director of the Squibb Institute for Medical Research in 1937.

In addition to these well-respected research directors, many bright young scientists went to work for pharmaceutical companies in the 1920s and 1930s. Among those hired were pharmacologist David Macht (beginning in 1925) at Hynson, Westcott, and Dunning; biochemist George Cartland (1927) at Upjohn; pharmacologist K. K. Chen (1929) and biochemist M. E. Krahl (1933) at Lilly; pharmacologist Harry van Dyke (1938) at Squibb; and chemists William Ruigh (1930), Karl Folkers (1934), and Max Tishler (1937) and pharmacologist Hans Molitor (1932) at Merck.

The proliferation of research (including some basic research) and a growing migration of respected scientists to industry were the most significant factors in the erosion of the tainted image of industrial work between 1920 and 1940. On the other side of the collaboration, we cannot neglect the impact of the Progressive era. Those scientists not already inclined to consider the practical application of their work became increasingly mindful of the social relevance of their research in the early twentieth century. Even as stalwart a defender of research for its own sake as G. Stanley Hall accepted utilitarian research: "Fifteen years ago [1893] it was quite commonly assumed that pure science ranked not only far above, but must pedagogically precede applied science. . . . But I think that now, scientific values being equal or even approximately so, the problem that promises most useful results would always be preferred, even for pedagogic reasons."[59] Science, journalism, education, and other segments of American society increasingly addressed the needs of cities, factories, consumers, the infirm, and so on. Pharmacomedical scientists, no matter how staunchly devoted to fundamental research, were in a strategic position to contribute significantly to these causes through the eradication of disease. Cooperation between universities and industry for the good of society was entirely in line with Progressive thought.[60]

The Rise of Research Laboratories and Institutes

Several leading, research-conscious firms in the pharmaceutical industry established special research units in the 1930s, such as the Merck Research Laboratory, which included the Merck Institute for Therapeutic Research (founded in 1933), the Lilly Research Laboratories (1934), the Squibb Institute for Medical Research (1938), and the Abbott Research Laboratories (1938). Some companies, such as Parke-Davis and Lilly, had established research laboratories as early as the first decade of this century. The difference between these and the above-mentioned institutions founded in the 1930s was that the earlier laboratories only went so far as to establish a comparatively rudimentary level of science in the pharmaceutical industry, whereas laboratories established in the 1930s contributed to the general stream of pharmacomedical sciences.

The research laboratories and institutes typically opened with much fanfare. Major scientists and others from universities, the federal government, and private research foundations addressed assemblies of prominent scientists and physicians at the dedication ceremonies (see fig. 4).

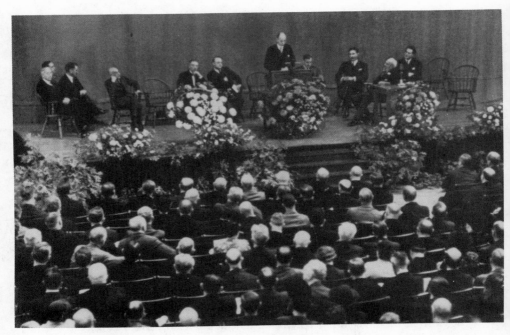

Figure 4. Dedication ceremonies for the Squibb Institute for Medical Research, held on the campus of Rutgers University, 11 October 1938. The speakers are, *left to right:* Robert Clarkson Clothier, president of Rutgers University; William H. Cole, professor of physiology at Rutgers; John F. Anderson, vice-president and director of the Squibb Biological Laboratories; Abraham Flexner, director of the Institute for Advanced Study at Princeton; August Krogh, professor of physiology at the University of Copenhagen; George A. Harrop, director of the Squibb Institute; George R. Minot, professor of medicine at Harvard Medical School *(at podium);* Russell M. Wilder, head of the Section on Internal Medicine at the Mayo Clinic; Carleton H. Palmer, president of Squibb; Theodore Weicker, chairman of the board at Squibb; and Lowell Weicker, also of Squibb (from *Field and the Work of the Squibb Institute for Medical Research* 1, no. 1 [1938], courtesy of Squibb).

The speakers at the Merck Research Laboratory dedication, for example, included Surgeon General Hugh S. Cumming, industrialist Lammot Du-Pont, and British pharmacologist Henry Dale. Dale, Irving Langmuir of the General Electric Research Laboratory, pharmacologist Carl Voegtlin of the United States Public Health Service, Frederick Banting of insulin fame, and the discoverers of the value of liver in anemias, George Minot and George Whipple, were among the speakers at the dedication of the Lilly Research Laboratories.[61]

In their addresses to these distinguished audiences, the executives and research directors of these firms emphasized the high level of scientific work, even fundamental work, to be expected from these research units, the need for closer cooperation between universities and the drug industry, and the separate status of these research units with respect to the business interests of the firms. George Merck informed his audience in Rahway, New Jersey, that the Merck Research Laboratory was made up of an applied research department, the Merck Institute of Therapeutic Research, and a "Pure Research division" devoted "to the study and preparation of new chemicals of scientific interest." G. H. A. Clowes reminded the Lilly audience of his company's support of basic research: "[J. K. Lilly] and Mr. Eli Lilly fully appreciated the value of fundamental research and were not only willing but eager and anxious that we should conduct investigations in certain fields in which there could be no possible hope of any commercial return. . . . What question could there possibly be regarding association with an organization directed by men holding such an enlightened point of view?"[62]

Abbott research director Ernest Volwiler touched on the need for closer cooperation between industry and universities: "Your presence here today to join in the dedication of this new research building shows your belief that new steps forward in hygiene must come about through the mutual efforts of the medical arts and all the accessory sciences; of the university and industry; of the individual worker in science and the highly organized group." J. K. Lilly, chairman of the board of the Indianapolis firm, recalled that many therapeutic agents—"adrenalin, tryparsamide, thyroxin, viosterol, insulin, liver extract, parathyroid extract, ephedrine"—all derived from collaborative work. George Merck proclaimed that the Merck Institute operated as a foundation independent of Merck and Company, a proclamation that president Carleton Palmer echoed five years later in his address at the dedication of the Squibb Institute: "In fact, this Institute for Medical Research stands separate and distinct from the business activities of Squibb. It replaces none of our manufacturing research. That goes on as before. The new Institute is an addition; it will be conducted in the interests of science only."[63]

The separate nature of the institutes of these two New Jersey firms warrants special attention, because interests outside of science proper forced Merck—and presumably Squibb—to detach these institutes legally from the firms. Merck had planned to establish a pharmacological research laboratory to test Merck products and conduct other research since 1931. The firm equipped the laboratory (see fig. 5) and engaged a Viennese pharmacologist, Hans Molitor, to head the program. However, when Molitor arrived in the United States to begin his work in September 1932, he discovered a most surprising turn of events: "Mr. [George] Perkins [vice-president of Merck] asked me today what really a "vivisection"

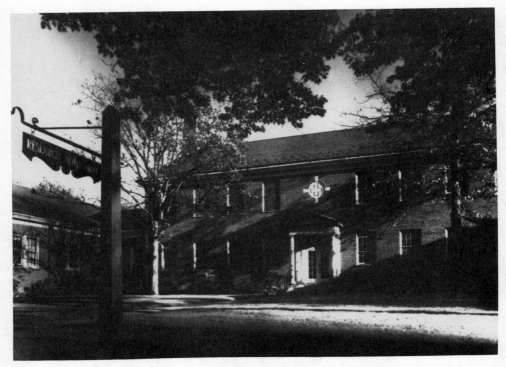

Figure 5. The Merck Research Laboratory, established in Rahway, New Jersey, in 1933. The laboratory housed the Division of Pure Research, the Division of Applied Research, and the Merck Institute for Therapeutic Research (from *Merck Sharp and Dohme International Review* 21, no. 2 [1983], courtesy of Merck and Company).

experiment means, and told me that the permit for performing such experiments, for which Dr. Major had applied, had been refused by the State of New Jersey. . . . It seems to me—speaking confidentially—a little bit of "Schildbürgerstreich" [i.e., a foolish act] to equip a new laboratory and engage a pharmacologist, without being sure that both of them will be permitted to work."[64]

The New Jersey legislature had passed an act for the prevention of cruelty to animals in 1880; it imposed a fine of up to $250 and a jail sentence of up to six months for violations.[65] According to an amendment to this act in 1915,

nothing in this act contained shall be construed to prohibit or interfere with any properly conducted scientific experiments or investigations, which experiments or investigations shall be performed only under the authority of the Board of

Health of the State of New Jersey, the said Board of Health being hereby granted power to authorize the conduct of such experiments or investigations by agricultural stations and schools maintained by the State or Federal government, medical societies, universities, colleges and philanthropic institutions having among their corporate purposes investigation into the causes, nature and mode of prevention and cure of diseases in men or animals.[66]

Thus, Merck and anyone else wishing to conduct experiments with animals in New Jersey had to seek a permit for such investigations. In other states, by comparison, some firms were not only working with animals but operating their own clinical research units.[67]

Merck applied for a permit in the late summer of 1932. Before granting the permit, the New Jersey Department of Health asked that Merck (1) inform the department as to how it proposed to use animals and (2) incorporate the pharmacology laboratory separately from the company. In the meantime, the consultant who originally suggested that Merck organize a laboratory for pharmacological research, pharmacologist A. N. Richards of the University of Pennsylvania, assured the president of the Department of Health that he was fully confident that Merck's pharmacology department would contribute significantly to therapeutics.[68] The Rahway firm incorporated its pharmacology laboratory separately from the firm, in line with the laws of the state of New Jersey and the wishes of the Department of Health.[69] On 10 January 1933, the day after Merck filed a certificate of incorporation with the New Jersey secretary of state, the Department of Health authorized the Merck Institute of Therapeutic Research to conduct experiments on animals. Molitor soon developed a policy in the Merck Institute of using dogs and cats as little as possible and reducing the number of experiments requiring animals to be sacrificed at the end of an investigation. He even designed a bloodless method for measuring peripheral circulation in animals.[70]

That these institutes were legally separated from the firms is certain. Economic separation was an entirely different matter. Neither the Merck Institute nor the Squibb Institute was self-sustaining. To be sure, the American Society for Pharmacology and Experimental Therapeutics felt that these institutes still were beholden to their parent companies. When ASPET member Harry van Dyke left academe to head the Division of Pharmacology of the Squibb Institute, the society expelled him from membership, in accordance with its constitution. The Squibb pharmacologist argued that he merely acted as a consultant to Squibb and that he had as much freedom to pursue his research as a university scientist. (ASPET had, by this time, formally permitted members to consult with industry through a constitutional amendment.) To support his contention, van Dyke cited Carleton Palmer's address at the Squibb Institute dedication, and he sent ASPET a letter from director Harrop reiterating that van Dyke's status "is quite analogous to that of a university professor and that as Director of the Squibb Institute I could assure him that both he and his staff would have the same freedom and support as the members of any university department." These arguments did not convince ASPET treasurer Charles Gruber. He felt that van Dyke was an employee of Squibb rather than a consultant, since he derived his full salary from the company. The executive council of ASPET must have concurred, because they unanimously rejected van Dyke's appeal for reinstatement in the society.[71]

For the present purposes, detailed examination of each of the research institutes and laboratories would be out of place. However, a brief discussion of the organization, evolution, and type of work at one of these research units, the Merck Institute, should convey some idea of how these units operated toward the end of the period under study and to what extent they contributed to the breakdown of barriers to collaborative work. While the Merck Institute had a board of trustees (consisting of Merck and Company executives), scientific directors (Molitor and other Merck scientists), and scientific advisers (outside scientists),[72] Molitor was given much freedom in setting up the institute. His goal was to build up the Merck Institute in such a way as to improve relations between universities and industry in biology and medicine: "At present the Merck Institute is probably still regarded by the outside world as a commercial laboratory; it will be my greatest success if this opinion can gradually be changed, and I shall do everything in my power to accomplish this task. I think that it can be done if the present management of Merck and Co. Inc. is not changed and its research policy remains unaltered."[73]

The Merck Institute struggled for space and personnel during the 1930s. Until it moved into its own three-story building in 1940, the institute was confined to three rooms (excluding animal quarters) in the Merck Research Laboratory, totaling about one thousand square feet. In addition to director Molitor, the institute had only one other employee with a degree, a chemical engineer. But Molitor was imaginative. First, he employed medical students during the summers. Second, most of his technicians were high-school youths. Molitor trained them himself and later on encouraged them to take classes on a part-time basis at area universities. He eventually arranged for a few of these technicians to do graduate work at New York University, which agreed to allow them to work on thesis topics relevant to their work at the Merck Institute. Finally, Molitor arranged for a consulting pathologist from an area hospital to work about one afternoon a week at the institute. By 1937 the institute employed another pharmacologist (Klaus Unna), and two years later Merck transferred a biochemist to the institute.[74]

The Merck Institute generally addressed three types of research problems: research having no immediate application to therapeutics, fundamental work; evaluation of experimental compounds submitted by Merck chemists and others, developmental research; and biological assays of established drugs, quality-control work. The institute typically conducted bioassays on such Merck products as tryparsamide, arsphenamines, B complex vitamins, vitamin K, and vinyl ether. Most of the institute's developmental research concerned experimental drugs from Merck chemists, but Molitor believed that this should be expected of a commercially supported laboratory. Still, Molitor's group spent a significant portion of their time testing experimental drugs for outsiders.[75] Molitor blamed himself for the steady decline of fundamental work in the early years at the Institute:

I would like to emphasize at this point again, that the Board of Trustees of the Merck Institute has not only never opposed research work of the abstract, fundamental type, but on the contrary has encouraged it. What I mentioned before in connection with pressure of urgent work [on the pharmacology, toxicology, and pathology of new drugs], represents entirely my own personal feeling. If anyone is to blame for the gradual sliding of the Merck Institute into developmental research it is I, and perhaps the circumstances; but certainly not our Board of Trustees.[76]

Some of the fundamental problems the Institute investigated were the influence of anesthetics on nerve currents, the mode of action of curare, the effect of pain on the circulatory system, and the influence of oxygen deficiency in arterial blood on the liver.[77]

As part of his goal to use the Merck Institute to improve relations between universities and industry, Molitor formed contacts with academic workers and publicized the work of the institute in a number of ways. He and other institute staff regularly presented papers at scientific and professional meetings, the cost of which Merck at least partially subsidized. For example, in 1937 alone institute personnel attended six major meetings, including meetings of the American Medical Association, the Federation of Biological Societies, and the American Chemical Society.[78] The institute actively published its results as well. Molitor's group produced over thirty papers in the first five years and about fifty papers from 1939 through 1941.[79] Molitor and another member of the staff presented lectures at the Rutgers College of Pharmacy on a regular basis, and Molitor made frequent visits to academic workers in a number of eastern and midwestern universities, particularly A. N. Richards's group at Pennsylvania.[80]

The most notable way the Merck Institute interacted with the academic community was by testing experimental drugs for university scientists. Molitor believed that such work was the province of the industrial pharmacology laboratory, not the university pharmacology department:

The determination of the toxicity of a new compound has become to a large extent a standardized procedure, offering little opportunity for startling discoveries, but requiring a great deal of time, expense and, particularly in chronic toxicity experiments, space for the housing of animals. . . . Such a procedure probably requires greater facilities than those existing in the majority of university laboratories and more time than many academic investigators are willing to spend on a problem of a semi-routine character. . . . The task of providing the required data remains therefore, rightly or wrongly, in most instances that of the manufacturer, and it is probably this type of work for which a non-academic research laboratory should primarily be prepared.[81]

A large portion of the institute's developmental research could be devoted to testing new drugs for university workers. In 1935, for example, Molitor and his coworkers tested thirty new drugs, sixteen of which came from outsiders. Apparently, the group did not test any one class of drugs preponderantly for university scientists, just a variety—chemotherapeutic agents, anticonvulsants, hypnotics, and so on.[82]

The growing interest in and support of research in the pharmaceutical industry, the slow migration of prominent academic scientists to industry to organize and direct company research programs, the movement of promising young scientists into industrial positions, the academic scientist's growing concern for the social relevance of his work in the Progressive era, and the sudden emergence of a cluster of industrial research institutes and laboratories, all helped erode the barriers to collaborative biomedical research between the two world wars. Successful collaborations early in this period, such as the work between Roger Adams and Abbott on barbital and procaine and the introduction of insulin through the joint efforts of the University of Toronto and Lilly, fueled the movement for cooperative work. Abbott President Alfred S. Burdick's address to the American Pharmaceutical Manufacturers' Association in the early 1930s testified to this change of venue in cooperative biomedical work:

There never was a time . . . when the university men were so eager to collaborate with commercial houses as they are now. I remember when we first started in, the average college professor working in the field was a haughty creature. He would not be tainted with commercialism in any form. His research was academic, for purposes of science. I may say that is all changed. They are just as eager to have friendly relations with commercial houses as any other type of men. In fact, they come to me almost every day or every few weeks—men connected with universities that are following certain lines of research, whose funds have run out

search staff annually visited scores of academic research centers across the United States and in Canada. This system of contacts helped keep Lilly apprised of research in universities, even if the contact were unable to spend more than one or two days at each institution. Every division within the company took part in this program: the Medical Department sent six representatives to visit seventy-five universities and independent medical colleges; seven representatives of the Biological Division contacted nineteen universities; two representatives from the Pharmacology Department visited eighteen medical schools; the Organic Chemistry Department put six representatives in contact with thirty-one academic institutions; and the Biochemistry Department sent four representatives to twelve universities.[104] It is not clear how cooperative the academic workers were with the Lilly representatives, but the firm built up many valuable research contacts with this program.

Fifth, Lilly established quotas of delegates to attend scientific and medical meetings. This gave the firm an opportunity to learn of the progress of its fellows, to keep abreast of the latest developments in various fields, to publicize the firm's own research achievements, and to encourage quality research among its staff. The Lilly Research Committee determined the quotas, and the department heads selected the delegates. The firm sent about one hundred delegates to thirty-eight different meetings and symposia from July 1942 to January 1944, including eighteen delegates for the joint meetings of the Federation of American Societies for Experimental Biology, nine delegates for the American Chemical Society meetings, and six to seven delegates for annual meetings of the American Medical Association and the American Pharmaceutical Association.

Sixth, Lilly initiated a series of monthly lectures at the firm, often by distinguished scientists, such as Cornell biochemist Vincent du Vigneaud. This gave at least some Lilly researchers the opportunity to interact with stars in biochemistry, pharmacology, organic chemistry, and other fields, and it allowed the firm to put its research programs on display—and perhaps to plant the seed for future collaborations with leaders in their fields.[105]

Finally, the Indianapolis firm assembled a "cream list" of researchers and physicians. Each month, the company sent the individuals on the list three or four "carefully chosen reprints" of Lilly research publications "as a means for acquainting outside research investigators and those interested in research with the scope of our activities in our laboratories." Lilly's cream list numbered some one thousand three hundred individuals by about 1942.[106] Lilly clearly had developed an involved network of contacts with the scientific community by the end of the period under study. The details of contact programs probably varied from company to company, but firms had to evolve some means of contact with academe to remain competitive with Lilly. By this time, discoveries in the pharmaceutical industry were rapidly becoming obsolete, and the only way to avoid obsolescence was by staying on top of the latest research in biomedical fields. A well-established in-house research program went a long way in this direction but in itself was insufficient; firms also had to keep in close contact with work in universities. The growing frequency and complexity of interactions between universities and industry reflected the needs of a competitive, research-based, rapidly changing enterprise like the prescription-drug industry.

Conclusion

As the period between the wars drew to a close, university workers were more receptive to collaborative research with industry and less censorious in their view of industrial work and were themselves pursuing certain commercial practices with respect to medical discoveries formerly decried in academe. Members of ASPET, for example, began challenging the society's policy of banning industrial pharmacologists from membership. As early as 1915 John J. Abel had begun collecting opinions from members about removing the ban. His personal opinions of cooperative work notwithstanding, Abel wondered whether interactions between academe and industry might improve the latter; membership for the better industrial workers would indicate to firms that pharmacologists were willing to help elevate the pharmaceutical industry. Four years later Abel, Arthur Loevenhart (president of the society), and five other members proposed an amendment to the ASPET constitution to eliminate the ban. They felt that the constitution already amply provided for cases of unethical conduct and that ASPET should consider membership eligibility based on individual merit alone. When the amendment came up for a vote at the 1920 meeting, the members present unanimously defeated the proposal.[107]

The issue of the ban arose again from time to time in the 1920s and 1930s; while proponents of the proposed amendment of 1919 could not secure the necessary four-fifths of the vote, they sometimes won a simple majority. The movement against the ban grew stronger during this period. Abel, among others, revealed his opinions in no uncertain terms: "I do not approve of our exclusion from membership in the Society of highly trained men like [K. K.] Chen, John Anderson, [G. H. A.] Clowes, and others just because they happen to be making their living by working in the research laboratories of some of our large firms."[108] In 1937 ASPET amended its constitution to exclude paid consultants formally from the ban, in part because several members (such as Newton Richards, Arthur Tatum, and Chauncey Leake) were collaborating with firms. In April 1941 the society finally voted to remove the ban.[109]

Once they established research programs, companies made frequent use of the patent system to protect their research investments. Squibb held only one patent as of 1920; ten years later it held 21 domestic and 33 foreign patents, and by 1940, 164 domestic and 39 foreign patents. In 1937 alone, Merck filed 27 domestic and 19 foreign patent applications. Ernest Volwiler had a hand in 27 domestic patents awarded to Abbott between 1920 and 1940. A rising number of universities, too, were using the patent system by the early 1920s. Ostensibly, schools administered patents on discoveries by their faculty for the public interest—to prevent pharmaceutical companies from monopolizing these discoveries and to maintain quality standards among firms they licensed to market the discoveries. That royalties derived from these licenses padded a university's research coffers also entered into the decision to secure patents. President Nicholas Murray Butler of Columbia admitted that one of the reasons his university pursued patents was "to enable the University itself to share in the benefits of the patents, to the end that the funds at its disposal for the promotion of research may be increased."[110]

Thus, by the mid-1920s several universities had established early precedents for the patenting of medical discoveries: Columbia, which administered the patent on T. F. Zucker's concentrated preparation of cod liver oil; Minnesota, to which Edward Calvin Kendall of the Mayo Clinic assigned his patent on thyroxin; Toronto, which administered the patent on insulin, stemming from the work of Frederick Banting, Charles Best, J. J. R. Macleod, and J. B. Collip; and Wisconsin, which benefited from Harry Steenbock's vitamin D patent, as administered by the Wisconsin Alumni Research Foundation. By the mid-1930s at least a dozen universities administered patents on medical discoveries by faculty.[111] This movement did not proceed without resistance. Pennsylvania, Johns Hopkins, and Harvard, for example, instituted policies in the early 1930s forbidding faculty to take out patents for the purpose of profiting the discoverer or the university. But in general the process of academic scientists' patenting their discoveries, a process sanctioned and even encouraged by many universities, was fairly well established by the 1930s. What once had been an impediment to cooperation between pharmaceutical firms and universities was now an important interest of academic researchers and universities.

Industry support of medical research in universities was growing at an important time. Over the period between the wars, the massive support of private foundations (Rockefeller, Carnegie, Macy) was slowly declining, particularly during the Depression, and the federal government had not yet launched its mega-support of research in academe.[112] The contact with universities helped industry too, because the former offered companies their valuable experience in research and because no matter how developed, an industrial laboratory alone could not possibly attend to all research needs in every field. Finally, collaborations between the two sides yielded important hormones, anticonvulsants, sedatives and hypnotics, chemotherapeutic agents, and other drugs between 1920 and 1940. Therapeutics and public health thus profited from cooperative research as well.

CHAPTER THREE

The Scientist as General Consultant

->>>->>>->>>->>>->>>-<<<-<<<-<<<-<<<-<<<

Pharmaceutical firms such as Squibb, Abbott, Lilly, and Merck, with their newly formed interest in developing in-house research programs, faced several problems in transforming themselves into research-based industrial organizations. For example, how would they organize, house, and staff their research programs in the various medical and pharmaceutical sciences? Once they established such programs, what research policies would they formulate to direct these new programs? They would have to decide to what extent their research personnel would be permitted to contribute to the general advance of science, which called for policy statements on attendance at scientific meetings, publications in scientific journals, and so on. What was more important, these companies would have to decide which drugs or drug groups they would explore and develop. Finally, if they were to take this course, how would they establish outside contacts to supplement their own research programs? Company executives, research directors, and research staffs solved some of these problems, but occasionally some companies turned outside, to university scientists, for counsel on such problems.

The type of academic researcher that a company would contact for advice on its internal affairs was a well-rounded, well-informed individual. He was a first-rate scientist, well respected by his peers. But he was not the type of worker who spent his life in the laboratory, like a Max Gottlieb. Rather, he formed and maintained various contacts in his field, and he developed some contacts outside of his field. If he was not aware of some recent development within or outside of his sphere of expertise, he probably knew people who were. He was persuasive and analytical and usually had some business sense. He typically had some experience in establishing a new research program at a university. His energy level was usually in overdrive; it would not be unusual for him to direct a major research program, head a professional society, and edit a major scholarly journal—

simultaneously. His experience in the planning and execution of research, his broad knowledge of research and researchers, and the universal respect and admiration that he commanded among his colleagues, all served the fledgling industrial research programs of the 1920s and 1930s well.

This type of scientist influenced not only company affairs dealing directly with his narrow sphere of expertise but many facets of the company's operations. I call this interaction between a university scientist and a pharmaceutical company a general consultantship. The cases I investigated suggest that the general consultant provided a wide range of services to the company. Moreover, he primarily served only one pharmaceutical firm in this capacity (although he might serve companies in other industries) for many years, perhaps decades. The following exemplify some of the ways in which a general consultant interacted with a pharmaceutical company, although the extent to which each of these services was emphasized varied with the individual.

First, the consultant helped the company develop its research program in one or more fields.[1] This could mean that he proposed and recruited research scientists to fill new or vacated positions, suggested designs for the laboratory facilities, supplied his graduates as staff for the program or even inculcated the necessity of industrial research programs for certain fields in the company. Second, the consultant acted as a liaison between the company and the academic community. This was an especially important service for companies that could not call upon their own reputation to engage a university scientist or group for some type of research collaboration. A consultant's long and close relationship with a company and his confidence in the company's commitment to high scientific ideals meant a lot to a prospective collaborator. Third, the consultant helped foster particularly close connections between his own university and the company. These connections might extend to other departments in the university and to the clinical units. Fourth, the consultant served as a sort of character reference for the company in any disputes with the government, in a way somewhat analogous to his connection with the academic community. In the case of the latter, however, the consultant might help bring the two parties together and assist in the cooperative research plan. The consultant's role in industry-government affairs was more of a public-relations activity. Fifth, the consultant kept the company abreast of the latest trends in pharmacology, chemistry, therapeutics, and so on. It was vital for a company in a competitive, research-oriented business like the pharmaceutical industry to know what researchers were working on so that it could be among the first to develop or apply therapeutic advances. Sixth, the consultant shared with the company practical developments emanating from his own work or from the research in his department. This arrangement potentially benefited both sides. The scientist might channel his consultantship fees or any royalties from practical discoveries back into departmental research funds, or he might pocket them. Finally, often the consultant served on the company's board of directors (the only academic scientist in such a position at the company). This gave the consultant an intimate view of the company's operations, and it afforded him the opportunity to influence the firm's research policies directly.

I have been able to identify only two bona fide examples of what I call general consultants. Perhaps this was to be expected, given the extraordinary type of person he had to be. However, this by no means indicates that no other examples exist. And although I based my generalizations on a rather substantial body of evidence, this evidence nonetheless pertains to only two consultants.

Roger Adams and Abbott Laboratories

Few twentieth-century scientists have had a career as distinguished as that of Roger Adams (1889–1971), an organic chemist at the University of Illinois. During the period that he served as a consultant to Abbott Laboratories in North Chicago, from 1917 to the late 1960s, Adams built an impressive personal research program, headed the premier chemistry department in the United States, and served in many professional, private, and governmental organizations. All of these factors figured significantly in Adams's service to Abbott (see fig. 6).

His personal interest in devising commercially useful syntheses of some therapeutic agents that had grown scarce in the United States during World War I led to his initial connections with Abbott. According to Arnold Thackray, "As Chairman of the Illinois chemistry department from 1926 to 1956, Adams was responsible for building the largest single-discipline Ph.D. machine in the world. . . . Through his Ph.D.s Adams created an ever-growing network of links with industrialists and industrial concerns."[2] Most of his Ph.D.'s that went into industry entered the chemical industry, although Adams supplied eighteen students to drug companies (including three who went to work for Abbott).[3] Adams's outside activities brought him into close contact with the national and international scientific communities. He was an active member—often occupying a powerful position—in many organizations throughout his career. Among these organizations were the American Chemical Society, the National Academy of Sciences, the American Association for the Advancement of Science, the Battelle Memorial Institute, the Sloan Foundation, the National Science Board of the National Science Foundation, and the wartime National Defense Research Committee. Despite the time that these various commitments consumed, Adams maintained his consultantship with Abbott, even during World War II.[4]

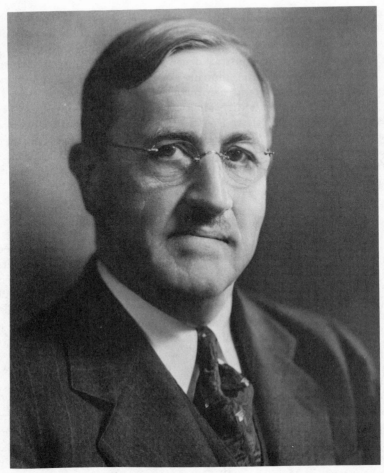

Figure 6. Roger Adams (1889–1971), professor and head of the Department of Chemistry at the University of Illinois who was a consultant to Abbott Laboratories from 1917 to the late 1960s (from the University of Illinois Archives, courtesy of Bachrach).

The connection between Adams and Abbott originated as a project collaboration, which shortly changed to a specialist-consultantship. Gradually, Adams's relationship with the company took on the character of a general consultantship. At the time Abbott first contacted Adams, in late summer 1917, the United States was suffering through a drought of many synthetic chemicals and drugs. German firms had ruled the worldwide trade in crude materials and intermediates necessary for synthetic drugs and chemicals, as well as the finished products themselves, for many years. As the war grew, European industries began shifting their focus to the war effort. Moreover, those companies still producing synthetic drugs faced closed or restricted shipping routes to the United States. U.S. industry was unprepared to meet the consequent shortages right away. However, by the time the United States declared war, in April 1917, pharmaceutical and chemical firms had begun to pick up some of the slack in synthetic crudes, intermediates, and finished products.[5] It was around this time that Adams began looking for a pharmaceutical firm to apply some small-scale methods he had devised to produce a few synthetic drugs, and Abbott was searching for a chemist to assist in manufacturing the same drugs.

Both parties had recently developed an interest in synthetic drugs and chemicals. Around 1916 or 1917 Abbott introduced several synthetic germicidal agents, chloramines, which a British researcher had developed. This was the result of the company's recent policy to deemphasize alkoloidal drugs and stress synthetics.[6] Adams's interest in the manufacture of synthetic chemicals and drugs stemmed from the organic preparations laboratory at Illinois. In the summer of 1914, C. G. Derick, the organic chemist whom Adams replaced in 1916, started a program at Illinois to prepare some key organic compounds that researchers around the country needed but could not find. The program continued for many summers thereafter, and it grew rapidly after Adams took charge. What began with a few students preparing 10 to 15 chemicals emerged, by 1917, as an $8,000 to $9,000 business employing ten students full-time during the summer. By this date, the laboratory was manufacturing about 125 chemicals—albeit in quantities generally of less than one pound each—for 30 universities, 18 government laboratories, 12 chemical distributors, and over 50 companies. Adams thought the laboratory was useful. It saved researchers the time and trouble of synthesizing these chemicals, and it provided the students with valuable training otherwise unavailable to them in a university and paid them enough to cover their living expenses.[7]

Adams first tried to convince G. Mallinckrodt and Company, of St. Louis, to collaborate with him on some synthetic drugs, but the company was not interested. Not long after this, in the summer of 1917, an Abbott representative contacted the Illinois chemistry department for a possible collaborator on synthetic drugs. Adams and Abbott soon were negotiating an agreement for the company to produce barbital, a barbiturate introduced by German researchers as Veronal in the early twentieth century. For Adams's services in helping the firm manufacture barbital, Abbott would pay him a royalty of 2.5 percent of the net sales of barbital. The royalty arrangement would continue until 1922, when the U.S. patent on Veronal expired.[8] Adams improved the patented process somewhat, but neither he nor Abbott appears to have discussed patenting any of the improvements.[9]

The Illinois chemist kept in close touch with Abbott's progress, and he visited the company intermittently. Even after he began spending much of his time in Washington with the Chemical Warfare Service, in early 1918, Adams planned to make regular monthly or semimonthly visits to Abbott. In addition, he had a student or fellow faculty member working on the project while he was away. Abbott produced its first lot of barbital in November 1917. Although the yield was less than satisfactory, Adams helped the company make the necessary adjustments, so that by about the spring of 1918 Abbott was producing barbital on a large scale, the first American firm to accomplish this.[10]

About two weeks after Adams and Abbott began negotiating a collaboration on barbital, the company solicited Adams's assistance to prepare procain, a local anesthetic introduced by a German researcher as Novocaine in 1905. By November 1917 Adams had perfected the German worker's patented process, which enabled Abbott to produce the anesthetic more inexpensively than other companies theretofore.[11] For unknown reasons, Adams originally preferred to keep his new process a secret rather than to seek a patent. Abbott urged Adams to take the latter course. The company recently had learned that a chemist at Yale, Treat Johnson, who was working with the Calco Company in New Jersey, also was on the verge of finding a new, improved process for manufacturing the anesthetic. Two weeks later the Illinois chemist submitted a patent application. Adams received letters patent on his discovery in March of the following year, and he assigned his rights to Abbott. In return, the company tentatively agreed to give Adams and a colleague a 2.5 percent royalty through most of the life of the patent.[12]

Adams continued to patent and assign to Abbott several synthetic drugs and potential therapeutic agents from the early 1920s on. For example, he helped prepare Butyn, and later Butesin, both of which were valuable additions to Abbott's growing roster of local anesthetics. Among the other numerous compounds he submitted to Abbott were antiseptic iodine preparations, antisyphilitic arsenicals, and cyclic organic acids as possible bactericides.[13]

Late in 1917, when Adams was involved in the work on barbital and procaine for Abbott, Wallace Abbott, the founder of the company, offered

Adams fifty dollars per month to "act as a consulting chemist to them, particularly in regard to the various synthetic drugs that they were starting to produce and others that they intended to produce later."[14] Dr. Abbott even went a step farther by early 1918: he invited Adams to join the company on a full-time basis. The Illinois chemist was sufficiently impressed by the company to give the offer serious consideration; however, he turned it down, probably because he feared that his colleagues might think he was selling out.[15] His refusal was fortunate for Abbott, because Adams probably accomplished much more for the company on the outside than he would have been able to as an Abbott employee. For example, simply from the standpoint of strictly chemical matters, he often sent compounds from his laboratory to North Chicago, and he advised the company on the practicality of manufacturing other drugs.[16]

Adams's services to the company had already begun to transcend the responsibilities that one would expect of a specialist-consultant before Dr. Abbott offered him the consultantship. For example, Adams helped the company establish contact with the Federal Trade Commission so that the latter would license Abbott to produce barbital, procaine, cincophen (an antipyretic and analgesic), and other drugs from abrogated patents. That a solid chemist like Adams was assisting Abbott probably enhanced the company's standing as a candidate for licenses. Abbott was among the first companies to receive licenses, and it used this advantage to take an early lead in the markets for barbital, procaine, and other synthetic pharmaceuticals after the war. Adams also served the general needs of the company by supplying some of his own students as research chemists. Ernest Volwiler was the most notable Adams-trained chemist at Abbott. Knowing the company's wish to have more in-house scientific personnel, Adams suggested that Volwiler join the firm—which he did in April 1918. By 1930 Volwiler was the firm's director of research; eventually he served over a decade as president and chairman of the board of directors.[17]

Adams consulted with Abbott personnel on all levels, from the bench scientists to the executives. It was important to him that the scientific workers and the officers understand each other. Thus, during his monthly or so visits to North Chicago, Adams typically discussed both technical problems and issues concerning general business methods with the Abbott scientists. His meetings with executive officers, such as Alfred Burdick (elected president of the firm in 1921), likewise covered a range of topics on the company's affairs: new products that Abbott might wish to consider, development of the research program, marketing and other business issues, and possible candidates—at Illinois or elsewhere—to fill new or vacated positions.[18] A postdoctoral fellow and later biographer of Adams, Dean Stanley Tarbell, characterized Adams the consultant: "Adams furnished solid benefits to his consultees. He had an encyclopedic knowledge of synthetic and structural organic chemistry, including recent developments that had not yet reached the scientific journals, such as the availability of new compounds from industrial exploratory research, and he was unusually well informed about economic and political trends that might affect a potential industrial process."[19]

Adams's involvement with Abbott as a general consultant increased considerably in the 1940s, 1950s, and 1960s, particularly as his research career declined. Alone or with the help of his many contacts in the drug and chemical industries, Adams occasionally came to Abbott's aid by solving problems in ongoing research projects at the company. He also could tap into his intelligence network to notify Abbott about the latest research of its competitors.[20] Adams used his experience as a member of official scientific delegations to postwar Germany and Japan to help broaden Abbott's research and business connections in these two countries.[21] For example, he notified the company of many German chemists who would be valuable potential consultants for Abbott. In the late 1950s, when the firm was considering branching out into Japanese markets and establishing research connections there, Adams played a vital role. He used his contacts to identify potential collaborating companies and universities for Abbott, he escorted two Abbott research directors on a reconnoitering trip to Japan, and he provided the firm with a detailed, insightful analysis of Abbott's possibilities for future joint ventures with Japanese businesses and researchers.[22]

In April 1952 Adams was elected to Abbott's board of directors; he was the only university scientist on the board until he retired as a director seven years later.[23] This directorship gave Adams the unique opportunity, as an outsider, to help formulate business and research policies at Abbott. His election to the board also reflected the company's impressions of Adams's past contributions to the firm. He maintained intimate connections with the company even after leaving the board. For example, the close contacts he had with both the bench scientists and upper-level management, coupled with his vantage point as someone not in Abbott's permanent employ, put him in a position as mediator when conflicts arose between the two. Consider one occasion when George Cain, president and general manager of Abbott, sought Adams's advice to rectify an internal problem at the company: "Certainly, everything that I have done personally, as well as with the cooperation of my associates, has been to strengthen by both word and deed our research setup. . . . the next time you are at North Chicago I would appreciate it if you would take the time to come into the office and explore this matter of the feeling on the part of some individuals in the research group that they are being used as 'whipping boys.' Since that is simply not true I am anxious to get to the root of the matter and correct it."[24]

It should not be surprising, given his long and close associations with Abbott and other companies, that Adams was a strong advocate of the development of ties between universities and companies. Cooperative ties, he believed, would strengthen research programs of both academe and industry. In an address he delivered in the mid-1930s, Adams reflected on the growing emphasis in the United States on applied research at the expense of basic research in universities. University workers did not have the time, personnel, or equipment to carry out their fundamental investigations. Industry, he argued, could help solve this problem in American universities by reinvesting in basic research at these institutions, especially since it would amount to an investment in industry's own future: "The chemical companies in the United States, progressive, efficient, well-managed, have now reached that level of success where they must consider not merely the building of powerful research and production units, but must give equal consideration to the conditions of those organizations in which the technical leaders of the future are to be trained; they must take their equitable share of the responsibility for the proper progress of pure science, which is the foundation of applied science." Adams must have been pleased when he noted about fifteen years later that industry had begun to assume much more responsibility for the welfare of science departments in universities.[25]

He believed that universities had much to offer industry (in addition to manpower), a good example being consultantships. With his broad knowledge, the consultant could provide a fresh perspective on an industrial problem—and much more:

His presence convinces the industrial chemist that the company has a real interest in science per se. He is usually a stimulus to the men in the laboratory. A teacher-student relationship often exists between consultant and chemist and provides a means for discussion of personal problems whether they be private or professional. Chemists will often mention to the consultant minor or more serious complaints about the laboratory or its management when he would not do so to his official superior. Consultants can keep the higher level executives informed of any lowering of morale so that it may promptly be corrected. An opinion by consultants of the qualifications of its employees may at times be sought. Executives may acquire information of scientific trends in this country and abroad.[26]

As a consultant to Abbott Adams contributed in all these ways.

Alfred Newton Richards and Merck and Company

Alfred Newton Richards (1876–1966), a pharmacologist at the School of Medicine of the University of Pennsylvania, served as a general consultant to Merck and Company, in Rahway, New Jersey, for over thirty years, beginning in the early 1930s. Richards was a respected researcher, teacher, editor, and administrator, and all of these roles came into play during his association with Merck. Although the company first approached him to help it establish a pharmacological research laboratory, it soon became apparent to the people at Merck that Richards had much more to offer. Richards was an expert in kidney physiology, but his overall value to Merck as a general consultant rested more in his perspicacious approach to the organization and administration of scientific research, his effectiveness as a diplomat in a variety of scientific matters, and his willingness to commit his strong opinions about the value of university-industry cooperative research to action. His progress in the worlds of scientific research and administration, both before and after he began his association with Merck, bears witness to these qualities.

Richards's training was in physiological chemistry rather than pharmacology, first under the renowned physiological chemist Russell Chittenden at the Sheffield Scientific School at Yale and later under William Gies at the College of Physicians and Surgeons at Columbia, where Richards received his Ph.D. in 1901. Over the following years, he developed a course in pharmacology at the College of Physicians and Surgeons, in part by familiarizing himself with the literature in the field and also by assisting in a pharmacology course at a neighboring institution. In 1908 he accepted an offer to establish a pharmacology department at the medical school of Northwestern University. Richards moved to the University of Pennsylvania School of Medicine two years later to head a similar department (see fig. 7).

The research that earned Richards such a high reputation among his peers, on renal physiology, began shortly after he arrived at Pennsylvania. His studies on the kidney continued until the late 1930s, when his administrative duties for the university and for the U.S. government began to occupy more of his time. Through years of painstaking research, Richards and his associates in the Department of Pharmacology provided compelling evidence to support a hypothesis dating back to the mid-nineteenth century: that the kidney filters and reabsorbs vital substances, such as glucose, amino acids, and salts, and then passes on various waste products as urine. Richards's laboratory used several pinoeering techniques, such as kidney micropuncture and ultramicrochemical analysis of the kidney contents, to localize these functions of filtration and reabsorption within specific parts of the nephron.[27]

During the period that he served as a consultant to Merck, most of Richards's duties at Pennsylvania shifted away from research and teaching and towards administration. The dean of the School of Medicine had already begun seeking Richards's advice on administrative issues by the mid-1920s. His influence among the medical faculty at Pennsylvania grew

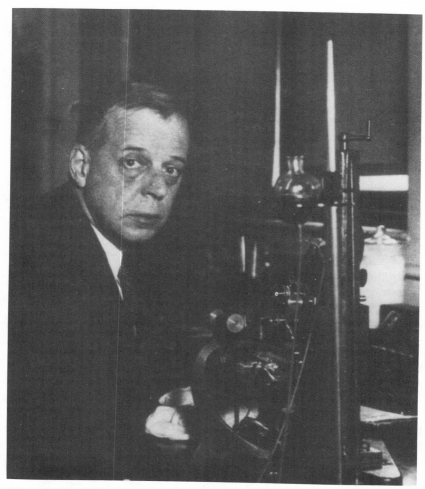

Figure 7. Alfred Newton Richards (1876–1966), professor of pharmacology and vice-president in charge of medical affairs at the University of Pennsylvania, who consulted with Merck and Company from 1930 to 1959 (from Marion, *The Fine Old House*, courtesy of SmithKline Beckman).

quickly, and in 1939 Richards became vice-president in charge of medical affairs at Pennsylvania. He took this opportunity to ensure that medical research continued to have a solid foothold at the University of Pennsylvania. However, he also was a strong advocate of the clinical utility of the medical sciences; Richards's clinical pharmacology program was one of the earliest of its kind.[28]

In 1941 President Roosevelt appointed Richards chairman of the Committee on Medical Research (CMR). This committee was created to meet the country's wartime medical needs by advising its parent body, the Office of Scientific Research and Development (OSRD), on medical research and development vital to the war effort. Among its duties, the CMR mobilized medical researchers from universities, industry, government, and private foundations, and it recommended projects to the OSRD that it believed merited the highest priority from the standpoint of national defense.[29] The government terminated the CMR in January 1947, but in the same year Richards was elected to the presidency of another major scientific organization, the National Academy of Sciences. He remained in that position until 1950. These appointments brought Richards into contact with many researchers from the different estates of science, and he became familiar with many research projects over a wide range of fields.[30] His background as a skilled and successful researcher by itself made Richards a valuable connection for Merck to have. But far more valuable to Merck was his rich experience in dealing with research and researchers on a national, and even an international, level. Merck tapped this resource in a variety of ways.

By the early 1930s Merck began to assemble a chemical research staff headed by the former Princeton chemist Randolph Major. Merck wished to establish a pharmacological laboratory as well, partially to evaluate products from the chemical group but also to generate its own fundamental contributions to pharmacological science. So George W. Merck, president of the firm, George Perkins, executive vice-president, and Major decided to seek Richards's counsel on the establishment of a pharmacological laboratory. The company approached Richards for several reasons. First, he was well known and well respected in his field. Second, he had experience in organizing the pharmacology departments at Northwestern and Pennsylvania, and he had introduced the subject into the curriculum at the College of Physicians and Surgeons of Columbia University. Third, Merck had established indirect connections with the University of Pennsylvania when it merged with the Philadelphia firm Powers-Weightman-Rosengarten in 1927. Frederic Rosengarten, whose family had long supported the University of Pennsylvania, became chairman of the board of Merck after the merger. The Rosengarten connection favorably impressed Richards when he was considering the Merck offer.[31]

Finally, Richards was a pharmacologist who favored strong ties between industry and universities—at a time when the national society of pharmacologists banned industrial researchers from membership. For example, at the time he was considering the offer from Merck, Richards expressed his opinions about academic and industrial connections: "I have long thought that the sentiment—so strong in this country—that university people should have nothing to do with commercial firms engaged in the manufacture of drugs was overdone. [Such a sentiment] works an injustice to businessmen who may have just as high ideals as do educators and research men, [and when] carried to extreme, defeats the aim of a university to be useful to its community."[32] A grant that a Philadelphia pharmaceutical firm, Smith Kline and French, awarded to one of Richards's colleagues around 1929 may have strengthened his views about the importance of university-industry links. "Certainly the liberality of the terms with which that grant was made and the spirit with which it was made gave me a changed idea of the attitude of industrial administrators to academic investigations."[33]

Merck approached Richards with an offer of a pharmacology consultantship in the late summer of 1930. Richards's responsibilities would be "to prepare opinions on various pharmacological problems which confront the company"; for the immediate future this meant that he would help Merck establish and staff a laboratory of pharmacology. While how much total time Richards was expected to devote to the consultantship is not clear, the company managers felt that he would have to spend one day per month in Rahway. Richards received a yearly honorarium for his services. The company proposed to pay him five thousand dollars annually, but Richards was unsure, at least during the initial negotiations, whether he would be able to devote the time and attention to this arrangement commensurate with such a payment.[34] He was also unsure of what his peers would think of the consultantship. Thus, Richards wrote to John J. Abel to see whether the Johns Hopkins pharmacologist would share his opinions of the consultantship. He explained to Abel that he was confident of the scientific integrity of Merck and its officers and that the company was considering the consultantship as a way to improve its products, although he felt that "it would be idle to think that the element of prospective profit does not enter in." He also informed Abel that he had to consider the feelings of the president of the University, Thomas S. Gates, and the dean of the medical school, William Pepper III, both of whom recommended that he accept the consultantship, and the feelings of his wife, who felt they needed the extra income.[35]

Abel was understanding. He agreed that the Merck firm maintained high standards; that the time had come for the American Society for Pharmacology and Experimental Therapeutics (ASPET) to admit the good pharmacologists from the better firms; that the pharmaceutical industry should develop research laboratories; and that the better firms had learned to understand the special concerns of the academic medical researcher over the past four decades. Abel avoided making any personal evaluations of industrial consultants; he merely said that some university scientists (such as Abel himself) were not compelled to serve as consultants, because they simply could not take part in a project that did not originate in their own laboratories. Other academics, such as many German pharmacologists, did not share this approach to research. But the former group, according to Abel, should not look upon consultants disparagingly, because good work could come out of consultantships.[36]

While this was not exactly a blessing from the father of American pharmacology (not that Richards was seeking such from Abel), Richards knew that whatever he decided to do, Abel's high opinion of him would not change. The opportunity to influence, in a major way, the development of a pharmacology laboratory in an institution altogether different from what he was accustomed to was too much for Richards to pass up, so Richards agreed to serve as a consultant to Merck beginning in 1931.

Richards as Liaison between Merck and the Academic Community

As a general consultant, Richards served Merck in a number of ways, but the company relied more on his service as a mediator in its transactions with the academic world than on any other service he provided. For example, he helped to identify and recruit candidates, especially those from universities, for research positions at the firm. He also established contacts for the company among (sometimes distinguished) university researchers for purposes ranging from research associations to speaking engagements. Finally, Richards attracted scientific and medical advisers from universities, who played an important part in the company's operations.

The first order of business for Merck's new consultant was to lay the groundwork for the company's pharmacology laboratory. Merck's most immediate need was a well-trained experimental pharmacologist. By 1930 America possessed a small but growing pool of experimental pharmacologists. As one indication of this growth, between 1908 and 1930 membership in ASPET increased from the charter membership of eighteen to over 140. Also, some excellent pharmacologists, such as K. K. Chen of Eli Lilly and Company and David Macht of the Baltimore drug firm Hynson, Westcott and Dunning, had recently departed universities for permanent industrial positions. The ASPET promulgation on industrial pharmacologists, while it did not prevent any academic pharmacologist from working full-time for industry, certainly did not create the kind of atmosphere that John Abel encouraged, in which "our great firms should establish extensive research laboratories of their own and preach this doctrine at every possible opportunity."[37] To fill Merck's position, Richards turned to Europe because of this situation in America but also because (1) pharmacology was a more established discipline there, which meant that there was a larger pool of good experimental pharmacologists to choose from, and (2) at least in Germany pharmacologists working in industry did not suffer the same stricture that the ASPET ban posed to industrial pharmacologists in America. Unlike academic pharmacologists in America at this time, academic pharmacologists in Germany simply did not have an inbred negative reaction to the thought of working full-time for a company.

In December 1931 Richards wrote to a colleague in the Pharmakologischer Institut of the University of Vienna asking whether he could recommend anyone for the position at Merck. The colleague suggested that Hans Molitor, an assistant professor at the Institut, was the best candidate: "an experienced researcher and a self-reliant critical scholar who has an understanding for the pharmacological problems of such a firm [as Merck]." Richards had met Molitor in 1927, and the latter had impressed Richards as much as he had impressed Richards's colleague at the Institut, so Richards recommended Molitor to Merck.[38]

Anticipating immigration problems in bringing Molitor to the United States, Merck was not enthusiastic about hiring him. While Molitor would have no problem entering this country under the Austrian quota, the pharmaceutical firm feared that "if we engage him this would involve some subterfuge on his and also on our part."[39] Merck was under the assumption that Molitor could not come to this country for the sole purpose of accepting a specific job that had been offered to him. Actually, the legislation that prohibited the immigration of contract labor, the Foran Act of 1885, applied primarily to unskilled labor. "Skilled labor needed for new industries" was exempt. Another reason why Merck was not interested in Molitor was that it was planning to hire, at least on a part-time basis, Peter Knoefel, a postdoctoral research fellow in pharmacology at the University of California, in addition to using the facilities and personnel in Richards's department.[40]

It took Merck only two weeks to change its mind about Molitor, a change in which Richards very likely played a major role. Aside from the questions concerning the feasibility of Molitor's immigration (which were probably secondary in importance at most), the firm's bottom-line concern was whether it should establish the foundations for an in-house pharmacological research program or rely on farming out its research needs. Writing to Abel a year and a half earlier, Richards had preferred to see the company rely on university connections,[41] but that was before he knew that a pharmacologist of the high caliber of Molitor might be available for Merck. Also, the thought probably occurred to Richards that Merck might want to saddle its university connections, including the Department of Pharmacology at Pennsylvania, with routine work, such as bioassays on different compounds that the Merck chemical staff produced. Richards recognized the necessity of such work, but he also realized that the bulk of this kind of work was the province of a company laboratory rather than a university pharmacology department.

In late February 1932 Richards contacted Molitor to let him know that Merck was interested in hiring him and to relate some general information about the company and the pharmacology position. Merck's decision to have Richards make the initial contact paid off. Considering that Molitor was happy with his position in Vienna and that he was not familiar with the foreign company seeking to hire him (although he must have known of the highly respected firm E. Merck-Darmstadt, formerly the parent firm of Merck and Company), it is difficult to believe that this was a job that could sell itself. Richards's role as the initial contact person was important; Molitor himself indicated that "one of the first arguments which led me to a 'yes' was the fact that the offer came from you." Richards's part in the affair did not cease when he finally put Molitor in touch with Merck; indeed, he maintained an active interest in negotiating the conditions on which Molitor would accept the industrial position, and he helped Molitor establish himself as a new member of the American pharmacological community.[42]

Molitor and Richards discussed many details of the Merck position, such as the type of job security that the firm would be willing to concede to Molitor, the layout of the new pharmacological laboratory, and the assignment to Molitor of research and development problems. Typically, Richards discussed Molitor's concerns with Merck executives and then presented Merck's counterproposals to the Viennese pharmacologist. For example, Molitor wanted a five-year contract upon the expiration of a mutually satisfactory trial year, plus a guaranteed annual salary for the full five years if the agreement had to be terminated through no fault of Molitor's. Richards suggested that Molitor accept Merck's counterproposal, namely, that the guaranteed compensation, if Molitor departed the company, be one-half the annual salary for each of the remaining five years. The consultant reminded Molitor how one-half of his Merck salary would compare with his present and future salary at Vienna. This arrangement apparently satisfied Molitor.[43]

The latter also discussed with Richards the possible make-up of the laboratory (e.g., sterile surgical facilities, sufficient space for animals, and an adequate library) and the process used for the selection of research and development assignments. Molitor felt that only a fellow researcher like

Richards, rather than the businessmen at Merck, could fully appreciate such concerns. Richards reiterated his confidence in Merck's willingness to accommodate the new pharmacologist in every way possible, and he promised that additional facilities at the University of Pennsylvania School of Medicine (such as sterile operating rooms) would be available to Molitor if needed. Richard's assurance that Molitor himself would play a large role in the selection of research problems and that the company would consult the Pennsylvania pharmacologist on difficult research decisions helped quell Molitor's fear of becoming a slave to the commercial interests of the firm.[44]

The details above show Richards's strong personal involvement in recruiting Molitor for the pharmacology post at Merck. Even after Molitor arrived in America, in the late summer of 1932, Richards helped smooth the way. For example, he introduced Molitor to several major figures in pharmacology, physiology, and medicine, such as Abel, Torald Sollmann, and Cecil Drinker.[45] As a charter member of ASPET, Richards also acted as an introducer when Molitor wished to present some of the results of his research to ASPET. Molitor was not permitted to join that organization until 1941, when ASPET removed its ban on industrial pharmacologists.[46]

Under Molitor's leadership, Merck's pharmacological laboratory—the Merck Institute for Therapeutic Research—became one of the leading industrial research centers for pharmacology. The company again called upon Richards's services early in 1933, when it was planning a dedication for its new research laboratories (of which the institute would be a vital part) before a distinguished assembly of physicians and scientists from academe, government, and industry. Richards played an important part in attracting the eminent pharmacologist Sir Henry Hallet Dale to Rahway to address the notables at the dedication. The hiring of Molitor, of course, had a much greater impact on the development of research at Merck than Dale's appearance, but the latter was also of great value to the company.

Richards apparently conceived the idea of inviting Dale after learning that the British pharmacologist planned to be in the United States in April 1933 to present a series of lectures at Johns Hopkins. Richards knew Dale well, having worked with him in London in 1917 and from 1926 to 1927.[47] President George W. Merck liked Richards's idea and sent an invitation to Dale early in February suggesting that Dale consider presenting a lecture on the relationship between academic and industrial research. Richards sent a letter to Dale at the same time, expressing his attachment to and high regard for the company and urging Dale to accept Merck's invitation: "I am convinced as a result of close acquaintance for two years past with the fashion in which Merck and Company have been managing their pharmacological research projects that the standards—scientific and ethical—which they have adopted are quite as idealistic, if not more so, than those which obtain in most of our universities. . . . I should not be writing this if I did not think this projected extension of Merck and Company's plans was worthy of the help which you could give."[48]

Dale accepted Merck's offer,[49] probably for several reasons: the opportunity to take part, at least in an honorary way, in a company's effort to develop a university-grade research program; Richards's personal recommendation of the company; and certainly to some extent, that he had already planned to be in this country and Merck offered him the then rather generous honorarium of six hundred dollars. Dale's address per se was not nearly as important to Merck as the message conveyed by his presence at the opening of its research laboratories. His appearance lent considerable credibility to Merck's efforts to cast itself as a research-oriented company in the eyes of the medical and scientific communities, particularly among those physicians and scientists in universities.[50]

Another way Richards used his contacts in the academic world for Merck's benefit was in trying to find a chief of medical affairs. The chief's responsibilities as outlined by both Merck personnel and Richards would be (1) to apprise the executive officers of developments in the general area of medicine on which Merck could have an impact; (2) to organize clinical trials of promising drugs that the company research laboratories produced; (3) to analyze the clinical results on new drugs and counsel Merck as to how to present these to the medical community; (4) to submit research proposals to Merck chemists and pharmacologists; and (5) to conduct his own research in the Merck laboratories (if he had the proper training and the desire).[51] Although the type of person Merck was interested in would have a medical rather than a pharmacological or physiological background, the company's consultant had a more than adequate familiarity with the clinical community. Richards knew of physicians who would be good candidates for this position, and he knew others who could recommend strong candidates. Richards approached several candidates for the position of chief of medical affairs at Merck, directly and indirectly.[52] Dickinson W. Richards, an associate professor at Columbia's College of Physicians and Surgeons, accepted the medical affairs post (on a part-time basis) around 1935.[53] Here we see again how Richards had a major hand in staffing a position—one outside of pharmacology—of great importance to the company.

Richards and Pennsylvania-Merck Research Connections

The University of Pennsylvania was a logical site for Merck to establish connections for biomedical research and clinical investigation of its drugs. Pennsylvania was a major research institution with access to extensive clinical facilities; the university was conveniently located not far from

Rahway; and most important, Merck had close contact with one of the faculty whom the university community esteemed—Newton Richards.

Richards began working with Merck before he was hired as a consultant. Beginning late in 1930, Merck sponsored a fellowship in Richards's department. André Simonart, of the University of Louvain, came to Pennsylvania to work on a problem of mutual interest to him, Merck, and Richards.[54] Simonart's research at Pennsylvania involved a pharmacological study of compounds synthesized at Merck that were similar to acetylcholine. Reid Hunt, of the Hygienic Laboratory of the United States Public Health Service, and especially Henry Dale (among others) shed much light on the pharmacological properties of acetylcholine in the early twentieth century. They found that this chemical, which occurred naturally in plants and animals, elicited pronounced cardiovascular, respiratory, glandular, and gastrointestinal responses. However, acetylocholine's pharmacological action was variable and what was more important, evanescent—because an enzyme in the body deactivated the chemical. Hence, acetylcholine had little therapeutic potential. Researchers then began synthesizing many compounds similar to acetylcholine but with a more promising clinical future.[55]

Merck chemists were among those searching for a useful acetylcholine homologue. They probably began their work on such compounds shortly before Simonart arrived at Pennsylvania, sometime in 1930. They developed a unique and commercially applicable synthesis for a variety of chemicals similar to acetylcholine,[56] but the company did not yet possess the pharmacological facilities to test these products. They therefore contacted Richards, who arranged for Simonart to work on the Merck products in his department. The company established a fellowship of four thousand dollars per year at Pennsylvania to support Simonart's work. Simonart's research at Pennsylvania lasted from 1930 to 1932, but Merck continued the fellowship until 1934 so that Richards and his colleagues could conduct more extensive pharmacological and clinical tests on the more promising Merck products.[57]

Simonart tested several compounds for Merck. Two of these were far better than the rest, and one of the two—the acetyl ester of beta-methylcholine—was particularly valuable when compared with acetylcholine. Workers at Pennsylvania conducted an in-depth pharmacological study of acetyl-beta-methylcholine, and they carried out the first clinical evaluations of the compound. The latter revealed the methylcholine's "spectacular action" in attacks of paroxysmal tachycardia (an excessive heart rate that begins and ends abruptly), its "striking relief" in some cases of abdominal distention, and its superior vasodilating power relative to acetylcholine.[58]

On the basis of the generally successful results with Mecholyl Chloride (Merck's trade name for this chemical) at Pennsylvania, the company arranged for about fifteen clinicians to evaluate Mecholyl on a large scale early in 1933. Richards helped Merck considerably in these arrangements. He suggested the clinics that the firm attempted to engage, and he wrote the letter of proposal—signed by President Merck—that the company sent to each of the clinicians. In those cases where the company did not receive replies from a few clinicians, it turned to Richards for advice on how to deal with these physicians. Richards also helped Merck prepare the informational booklets on Mecholyl that the company sent to clinicians.[59] These were the types of services for which Merck's chief of medical affairs was responsible, but Dickinson Richards did not assume this position until 1935; until then, apparently, it was another of the services that Richards provided as a general consultant. Richards maintained a close personal involvement in the development of Mecholyl. A visiting scholar, medical student assistants, and others carried out the initial pharmacological tests on Mecholyl Chloride in Richards's department, and Pennsylvania medical faculty with a joint appointment in the pharmacology department conducted the early clinical investigations. Later, Richards played a key role in organizing the expanded clinical testing of Mecholyl.[60]

At the same time that the Mecholyl work was in progress, Richards had a hand in another joint Merck-Pennsylvania project. In this case, the collaborators were investigating an anesthetic called Vinethene (divinyl ether). The credit for postulating that divinyl ether might be a useful anesthetic must go to Chauncey Leake, a pharmacologist at the University of California Medical School. Leake believed that compounds combining the chemical characteristics of two useful anesthetics, ethylene ($CH_2{=}CH_2$) and diethyl ether ($CH_3CH_2OCH_2CH_3$), would be worth studying, so he asked chemists at Princeton—including Randolph Major—to synthesize several possible anesthetics, among them divinyl ether ($CH_2{=}CHOCH{=}CH_2$). His preliminary tests revealed that divinyl ether was superior to the other compounds with respect to the short time required to induce anesthesia, the time for recovery, and toxicity.[61]

Major left Princeton to work at Merck in 1930, and soon thereafter he and his colleagues developed a manufacturing process that yielded Vinethene virtually free of impurities.[62] (Leake's promising results notwithstanding, the samples Major had sent to California were quite impure.) For further pharmacological tests and preliminary clinical evaluations of Vinethene, Merck turned, not to Leake and the University of California Medical School, but to Richards and Pennsylvania. In February 1932 Leake notified Merck that he and his associates would be unable to spend any time on Vinethene for several months because of their heavy teaching load and lack of funds to purchase the animals and equipment necessary for the Vinethene work. Whether or not Leake intended the latter as an informal request for some financial support, the company "did not feel that it would be advantageous to spend a great deal of money for the pharmacological study of vinyl ether in California. The distance was so great that a true cooperation could not be obtained."[63]

Around this time, Richards and Samuel Goldschmidt, a professor of physiology at the University of Pennsylvania School of Medicine, arranged with Merck to conduct further pharmacological work on Vinethene at Pennsylvania. Later, some of the clinical faculty entered the Vinethene project; they were the first to test Merck's new anesthetic. While Richards probably was not personally involved in the Vinethene research, he did help mediate some of the arrangements between the university and Merck. The firm did not engage Pennsylvania arbitrarily for the follow-up pharmacological research and the initial clinical work. As in the case with Mecholyl, Merck had a very useful contact at Pennsylvania in Richards. Vinethene was not among Richards's personal research interests, but he kept abreast of the progress on both the experimental and clinical work on this anesthetic. Among his mediations connected with this project, he helped Goldschmidt negotiate a suitable reimbursement from Merck for his contributions to the project. Also, Richards assisted in the arrangements for a Merck-sponsored anesthesia research fellowship (worth forty-five hundred dollars for the academic year 1934–35) in Pennsylvania's physiology and research surgery departments.[64] Within a few years, the Pennsylvania clinicians collected substantial evidence—more, in fact, than that assembled by any of the other two dozen or so clinics involved in the testing program—of Vinethene's value in most short-term surgical procedures and in dental use. Their results were instrumental in the establishment of Vinethene as a most useful anesthetic.[65]

Around the time that Pennsylvania was concluding its work on Mecholyl Chloride and Vinethene for Merck, Richards, in conjunction with the vice-president in charge of medical affairs at Pennsylvania and Merck, drew up a guideline for future Pennsylvania-Merck collaborations. Although couched without reference to any specific firm, this nine-point policy statement definitely intended to address Pennsylvania's connections with the Rahway firm. Richards acted as an intermediary between the representatives of Merck and Pennsylvania during negotiations over the few disputed clauses. The plan covered three areas: Pennsylvania's wish to collaborate with industry on medical research and the university personnel who would authorize such collaborations; policies on publication of the results of cooperative research, and the company's right to publicize research in which Pennsylvania took part; and Pennsylvania's right to accept or reject any outsiders that the company wanted to include in the cooperative project.

First, the plan explicitly stated that "authorities of the University of Pennsylvania regard it as desirable that members of the faculty of the Medical School should on occasion collaborate with reputable commercial firms" on therapeutic investigations. The head of the relevant department and the dean of the medical school, or the vice-president in charge of medical affairs, had the power to approve such work and thereby determine which firms were "reputable." The reference to occasional collaboration was important, because the university did not wish to see so much work of this type undertaken that it might "give a commercial aspect to the activities of [its] departments."[66] Pennsylvania, like some of its peer institutions (e.g., Johns Hopkins and Harvard), had recently instituted an official ban on the patenting of health-related discoveries for the purpose of garnering profit for the faculty member or the university. The Executive Committee of the university made an exception to this ban on those occasions when they decided that patenting was the only way to protect a discovery from monopolization by others.[67] The point is that the environment at Pennsylvania in the early 1930s was very unreceptive to any blatantly commercial activities within its medical school, and the guideline on cooperative research reflected this environment.

Second, the research guideline defended the university's right to publish any research it deemed fit for publication. Also, with the exception of literature references, the guideline prohibited Merck from using the names of Pennsylvania researchers or the university in any advertising. To these stipulations, the company had no apparent objections, but others led to some complaints from Merck personnel. Pennsylvania's wish to avoid having the company distribute reprints of university scientists prompted Hans Molitor to lament the university's failure to appreciate the needs of the company. This was just another indication, according to Molitor, of how the university had been safeguarded, while "not the slightest intention is given to the interests of the commercial concern; [the agreement] should protect both parties."[68] Molitor probably was right; not once did the agreement refer to the rights of the company. The Merck pharmacologist also objected to a clause that gave Pennsylvania the right to approve "all advertising or publicity matter based on an investigation at the University of Pennsylvania . . . insofar as the advertising or publicity material refers to or is an interpretation of the work done at the University." Molitor felt that this was too restrictive; he felt that it was the company's duty to relate as much information as possible about therapeutic products in the informational circulars that it sent to health professionals.[69]

Finally, the research agreement gave Pennsylvania at least some control over Merck's selection of other groups it wished to invite to work on the collaborative project.[70] There probably were two reasons why Pennsylvania wanted to maintain such control. First, if a group joined the collaboration to work on an aspect of the project in which Pennsylvania was not involved (for example, if Pennsylvania pharmacologists were working with Merck, and the latter sought outside chemists for assistance), Pennsylvania wanted to be sure that its researchers could work with the outsiders. The university's motive here may have been professional or even personal. Second, and more important, this clause was a source of security for the academic workers. Merck, no matter how good its intentions, was a business that had to stay close to the cutting edge of research to maintain its position in the pharmaceuticals market. For example, the firm might find itself in a situation where it had to replace the collaborating Pennsylvania pharmacologists with another group that could produce results. With this stipulation in the agreement, Pennsylvania medical researchers guaranteed themselves a quasimonopoly on any collaboration they entered into with Merck. The firm perhaps did not realize how it was potentially shackling itself; if this did occur to the company, it probably did not pay much heed to this clause. Certainly, I have not seen any evidence suggesting that Merck put up much, if any, resistance to it. A similar issue came up several years later between Parke-Davis and Arthur Tatum, a pharmacologist at Wisconsin who had been collaborating on organic arsenicals with the Detroit firm for over fifteen years (see chap. 4). Parke-Davis wanted to support a scientist who seemed on the verge of a useful discovery in the arsenical field; however, its contract with Tatum gave him the power to veto any outside involvement. Nevertheless, Tatum agreed to allow the company to bring outside workers into the arsenical project.[71]

Newton Richards often stimulated research connections between his university and Merck. He offered the company a site where it could have some of its products tested at a time when Merck did not yet possess the pharmacological facilities and personnel, much less the clinical capacity, to evaluate these products itself. What was more significant, Richards engineered a formal agreement between Pennsylvania and Merck. Despite its slant towards the rights of the university, this agreement essentially granted Merck access to one of the leading research institutions in the United States. This was particularly important to Merck in the light of the firm's still fledgling research programs in the early 1930s.

Richards's Later Services for Merck

Beginning in the mid-1930s, Richards occupied various posts within Merck; this gave him an opportunity to take a close look at Merck's operations and to influence the company's research policies directly. Richards served on the Scientific Advisory Board of the Merck Institute of Therapeutic Research, the Merck Fellowship Committee (as chairman), the Merck board of directors, the Scientific Committee of the board (as chairman), and the company's Scientific Policy Council. While he held all but the first of these positions after World War II, they all merit some attention as logical extensions of Richards's growing influence in the pharmaceutical firm during the 1930s. No academic scientist was as extensively and intensively involved in Merck's affairs as Richards.

Hans Molitor, director of the Merck Institute of Therapeutic Research, complained that two of the three original scientific advisers to the institute were Merck employees. He preferred to have as his advisers at least one clinician and one biomedical scientist, and from different universities, most likely because they would facilitate outside contacts for the institute. Molitor's wish was granted the next year, 1936, when the company engaged Richards, William Castle (a professor of medicine at Harvard Medical School), and Henry Dakin (a biochemist in a private New York laboratory) to serve as the institute's scientific advisers.[72] Richards agreed to serve on the Scientific Advisory Board, and he recruited at least one of the other members.[73]

Richards and the other advisers discussed "all principal problems of current or contemplated research" of the Merck Institute. The advisers met with Molitor, other institute staff, and Merck executive officers and researchers about three times a year. In addition, Molitor occasionally visited the advisers and corresponded with them about various research projects at the institute. It was an arrangement that called upon the "experience, judgement, and wisdom" of Richards and the others without taxing their other responsibilities. For their services Merck paid each of them one thousand dollars annually. The Scientific Advisory Board counseled Molitor and other Merck personnel with an interest in the institute on various research-related issues, often dealing with drug research and development: new directions for research on old drugs, new drugs or classes of drugs for the institute to investigate, diseases for which no useful drug existed, and so on. Richards, Castle, and Dakin also discussed less research-oriented issues concerning the institute. For example, they evaluated ways to publicize the institute to the medical and scientific communities, as well as how the institute could arrange with local universities to train some institute employees for higher degrees while they worked on institute-related projects.[74]

Richards served on the Scientific Advisory Board of the Merck Institute into the 1950s, with a brief hiatus during the war when he headed the Committee on Medical Research. Despite the tripartite (and later, quadripartite) nature of the board, Richards usually had his way on policy decisions. His way, according to Merck president John T. Connor, whose career at the pharmaceutical firm overlapped that of Richards for several years, translated into "tremendous research progress" for the institute and the firm: "Dr. A. N. Richards became the keystone of the Institute's Board of Advisors. In that capacity he always pressed for emphasis on basic research, insisting on adequate facilities for it which meant, inevitably, an adequate budget. He was a minority of one on more than one occasion, but his persistence usually brought the rest of the Board around to his way of thinking. Merck's tremendous progress through research is more than adequate testimony for the validity of his farsighted proposals."[75]

Richards also provided a useful service for Merck by helping to plan and administer the Merck Fellowships in Natural Sciences, which began in 1947 and lasted many years thereafter. Merck, of course, had supported numerous outside studies through fellowships and grants for many years prior to this. The Merck Fellowships in Natural Sciences, however, were more benevolent than directly strategic in character; they did not have a direct bearing on Merck's own research and development programs, although they surely had at least some value for public relations. A request from the Committee on the Chemistry of Proteins of the NRC late in 1945 for Merck to fund a few fellowships in protein chemistry of four thousand to five thousand dollars each prompted the firm to devise an alternative fellowship plan. Merck budgeted one hundred thousand dollars for the awards, which would range from fifteen hundred to five thousand dollars annually each. An independent Merck Fellowship Board chosen by Frank B. Jewett (then president of the National Academy of Sciences) selected the graduate and postdoctoral fellows. Rather than focus on protein chemistry, Merck opened the awards to all fields of chemistry and biology. [76]

Richards contributed to the Merck Fellowships in two ways. First, he helped the company design the fellowships program. President Merck's early draft of the fellowship plan incorporated many ideas that he and Richards had discussed in earlier years on how industry could support fundamental work in outside institutions. The final fellowship arrangements included several of Richards's recommendations, such as restricting awards to U.S. citizens, suitably reimbursing the members of the Merck Award Committee for their work (five hundred dollars), and establishing policies on the distribution of patent rights in the event that a fellow made a patentable discovery. Second, Richards served as the chairman of the Merck Award Committee.[77] In itself, this position was not a great burden; however, he was also a scientific adviser for the Merck Institute and a general consultant to the company at large. In addition, he was vice-president in charge of medical affairs at Pennsylvania (until 1948) and president of the National Academy of Sciences (1947–50). Richards had good reason to turn down the invitation to serve on this committee; instead, he accepted the chairmanship—a good example of Richards's willingness to assist the company in whatever way he could.

Richards developed a particularly intimate contact with the company after 1948, the year he was elected to the Merck board of directors. He remained on the board for ten years, during which time he was the only academic medical researcher (albeit retired) among the Merck directors.[78] His unanimous election to the board, a position that paid ten thousand dollars a year, reflected what George Merck called Richards's "broad experience in and knowledge of the problems in medical research and its related sciences that are common to our educational institutions, the government, and industry"[79] (see fig. 8).

Soon after Richards became a director, President Merck appointed Richards chairman of the board's new Scientific Committee, a post he held for the duration of the committee (1948–56). During his chairmanship Richards was thrown into a battle between the legal division and the research and development division over Merck's scientific publication policy. The former preferred that publication of patentable research be delayed from two to five years after application for the patent, whereas the research personnel wanted to preserve the established policy of publishing soon after filing letters patent.[80] Richards, of course, favored a liberal publication policy:

I believe that any substantial change from the present policy would work harm to the Company to a degree which would not be balanced by the advantages over competitors which could possibly be obtained by long-postponed disclosure. In my opinion the research staff of Merck and Co. have a unique position among those of other chemical manufacturing companies in the country. The members of our staff are looked upon as participating in the general advance of chemical and medical science on equal footing with their colleagues in academic institutions and they are held in correspondingly high respect. I regard this fact as responsible in large degree for the morale of the scientific staff and for the pride which they take in the achievements of the organization.[81]

It is difficult to imagine that anyone else involved in this dispute could so authoritatively have argued the problem from the standpoint of universities' impressions of the Merck research programs.

After the company disbanded the Scientific Committee, Richards still had the opportunity to influence Merck's research policies as a member of the Scientific Policy Council. This group, which began meeting in 1953, evaluated all aspects of research policies at Merck. It focused primarily on the exploration and development of specific drugs and classes of drugs, for example, whether to concentrate on a microbial or a synthetic means of producing a certain drug. It also addressed such topics as leaves of absence for Merck scientists to study elsewhere, fellowship programs, and scientific publication policies.[82]

I have deliberately given short shrift to Richards's later roles in the company, because they extend well beyond the period under investigation. But the examples in this section are important, because they show that his close contact with Merck during the 1930s grew even closer later on.

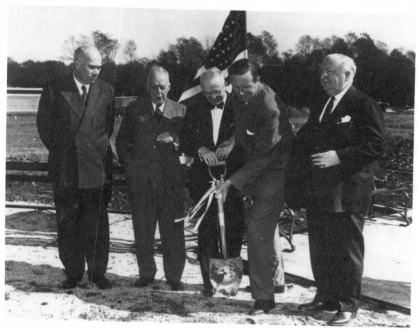

Figure 8. A. N. Richards with Merck and Company personnel at a groundbreaking ceremony for a new Merck Institute in 1951. Participants are *left to right:* Randolph Major, vice-president and scientific director; Richards; Hans Molitor, director of the Merck Institute for Therapeutic Research; George W. Merck, chairman of the board; and James J. Kerrigan, president (from *Merck Review* 19, no. 5 [1958], courtesy of Merck and Company).

There are two basic reasons for his burst of activities at Merck by the late 1940s. First, despite his commitment to the National Academy of Sciences in the late 1940s, Richards had more time to devote to the pharmaceutical firm after the war. Second, and more significant, Richards was able to rise to the highest levels of management at Merck because of his great breadth of understanding of medical research and medical researchers, which he readily shared with the company from the early years of his consultantship.

Conclusion

The company called on Richards for many services besides those discussed above. For example, it sought his advice on directions it should take in the research and development of different drugs and drug groups. In the mid-1930s Richards urged Merck to make at least a modest investment in hormone research. The company did just that, developing a hormone research program at Rahway and linking up with chemists at Princeton. The investment eventually paid off, as Merck became one of the early industrial leaders in the synthetic hormone field.[83]

Around the same time, Richards also counseled Merck on the development of the first of its host of vitamin successes, vitamin B_1. George Merck set out to "lay the whole matter before Dr. Richards and get his wise head to work on this difficult snarl." The snarl involved, among other things, a dispute between the Carnegie Institution and Robert Williams, a chemist at Bell Laboratories, over the patenting of Williams's discovery of a method to produce B_1 from rice polishings. The Carnegie Institution, which had supported much of Williams's work, opted to dedicate the patent to the public, whereas Williams disagreed, hoping to maintain some control over B_1 production. Merck supplied the vitamin in bulk to Williams for his chemical studies, and the company hoped to be one of the first licensees to produce B_1.[84] The various parties gradually worked out their differences, and Merck became an early leader in the B_1 market. What Richards contributed to the solution of this specific problem is not entirely clear, but the point is that many at Merck, from the president to the bench scientists, valued and frequently tapped Richards's keen analytical sense and his broad familiarity with biomedical research and researchers.

In the late 1930s, Richards helped connect Merck with another drug discovery. René Dubos, of the Rockefeller Institute, isolated an antibiotic from a soil microorganism called tyrothricin (later identified as a mixture of two microorganisms) in 1939. Dubos was willing to accede to Merck's request for a sample of the antibiotic, but the Rockefeller Institute was not as cooperative. After the company approached him for advice, Richards recommended that the company frame a proposal that would complement the Rockefeller Institute's own plan for tyrothricin; for example, a plan as to how Merck chemists could assist the Rockefeller Institute in developing this drug. Richards even wrote a letter of introduction for Merck to Herbert Spencer Gasser, the director of the institute, with whom Richards was well acquainted. The company received not only tyrothricin but Dubos as well—as a consultant.[85]

Richards's assistance was not always directly related to Merck research programs or specific research projects. For example, when President George Merck agreed to address the Medicinal Chemistry Division at the April 1935 meeting of the American Chemical Society, Richards lent his hand in outlining and writing the speech. Not that George Merck did not agree with the ideas, but the topic and the tone of this address—on the relationship between industry and universities in medical research—was vintage Richards.[86] After the New Jersey State Department of Health refused to grant Merck a permit to conduct vivisection experiments, Richards petitioned the president of the Department of Health to reverse this decision. He emphasized both the necessity of animal experiments for therapeutic advances and his conviction that the Merck pharmacology laboratory could become one of the great centers in the United States to further scientific medicine. Richards's arguments no doubt helped convince the department to reconsider its earlier action and issue a permit to Merck.[87]

Richards obviously was closely associated with Merck during the years when the firm became one of the research giants in the pharmaceutical industry. Merck's research personnel and expenditures for research grew tremendously from 1930 to 1940. The company had only a handful of chemists in 1930 but over seventy chemists, pharmacologists, bacteriologists, and other researchers by 1940. Merck's research budget grew nearly tenfold during the 1930s.[88] Richards was not necessarily the driving force behind this growth, but he certainly helped propel Merck research in this era of initial growth. Merck research staff, consultants, advisers, general in-house and collaborative research policies, research and development of numerous drugs, Merck prestige in the eyes of academic scientists and others—Richards influenced all of these in one way or another. He was a general consultant *par excellence*. President Merck's future plans for Richards, as expressed in a 1935 memorandum to executive officers and research heads in the company, clearly expressed Richards's value to Merck and Company:

[Richards and I] spent considerable time discussing various contacts [that] members and divisions of our organization have with him. I shall insist that a definite program be laid down to provide informal and leisurely talks with Dr. Richards by Mr. Perkins, Dr. Major, Dr. Molitor—each at least four times this year, without reference to whatever number of other conversations they may have with him accompanied by others of the organization. It is my firm belief, confirmed by experience, that in this way we will get the most from Dr. Richards, and it is essential that we get all we can.[89]

The consultantship very likely meant just as much to Richards as it did to the company. The pay was substantial; he received one thousand dollars a year as a scientific adviser to the Merck Institute, perhaps five thousand dollars annually for his general consulting work, and ten thousand dollars a year as a Merck director. How often he received these payments is unknown. As considerable as these sums may have been, they probably did not mean nearly as much to Richards as did the opportunity to take part in and help shape the evolution of the research programs at Merck. Few academic scientists connected with other pharmaceutical companies had such an opportunity. At Merck Richards had a chance to prove his conviction that industry had the potential to foster biomedical science on an equal footing with universities. Richards personally contributed a great deal towards effecting this goal at Merck.

I have tried to convey in this chapter a sense of Newton Richards' service to Merck and Roger Adams's service to Abbott as general consultants. Richards functioned in a variety of ways as a liaison, both between the company and the academic world and between the company and the University of Pennsylvania. Also, the various positions he occupied within the firm from the mid-1930s to 1959 (when his association with Merck formally ended) afforded Richards the opportunity to influence the research policies at Merck. This is not to say that the pharmacologist had to be on the inside to have an impact, for "during the difficult early years," John T. Connor reflected, "Dr. Richards participated in the formulation of Merck's whole new research plan. Even more important, he helped to attract to Rahway some of the finest research men, either as consultants or as regular staff members."[90]

Roger Adams was no less valuable to Abbott as a general consultant. As with Richards's connections with Merck, the interactions between Adams and Abbott displayed some elements of all three typologies of cooperative research. Certainly, Adams began his relationship with the pharmaceutical firm through his marketable processes for producing specific therapeutic agents, and his expertise in the chemistry of particular natural products also entered into his interactions with Abbott. Yet, Adams's service to Abbott extended well beyond those sorts of interactions to achieve the same degree of intimacy as that manifested in Richards's consultantship with Merck. In fact Adams, unlike Richards, supplied key personnel to Abbott from his own laboratory, Ernest Volwiler being the most outstanding example. Both Roger Adams and Alfred Newton Richards played crucial roles in transforming two pharmaceutical companies into research giants in the industry.

CHAPTER FOUR

The Scientist as Specialist-Consultant

＞＞＞-＞＞＞-＞＞＞-＞＞＞-＞＞＞- ＜＜＜-＜＜＜-＜＜＜-＜＜＜-＜＜＜

During the early era of cooperative research pharmaceutical companies engaged two types of consultants: the general consultant, who had a rather broad impact on a firm's research program, and what I call the specialist-consultant. The latter had an influence on industrial research that was much more intensive than extensive, because companies engaged these researchers for their expertise in a particular field of pharmacology, chemistry, microbiology, and so on. The specialist-consultant served the pharmaceutical firm in two ways. First, he was a research source who filled deficiencies in the company's own research organization. For example, in a discipline like pharmacology, in which the American labor pool was fairly low compared with that in other, more established scientific disciplines, industry suffered a manpower shortage. Thus, until companies could rely on in-house personnel, they had to search outside for trained pharmacologists to evaluate their drugs. Second, the specialist-consultant, regardless of the manpower situation within a firm, was always useful as a well-informed source for, and an active participant in, the latest developments in a field. A firm could not possibly hire experts in all fields of all scientific disciplines. It had to maintain contact with experts on certain chemical compounds, classes of drugs, or types of drug-yielding microorganisms in order to remain competitive in an increasingly research-based enterprise like the pharmaceutical industry.

This type of consultantship was a valuable source of continuing support for the university scientist of the 1920s and 1930s. It was not unusual for a scientist to consult with several firms on many topics over a number of years. The compensation he derived from these connections, in the form of graduate fellowships, consulting fees, or whatever form of compensation the collaborators agreed upon, was a vital source of support for his research program. Consultants fortunate enough to take part in a practical therapeutic discovery in the course of the collaboration enjoyed, if they made prior arrangements for such an event, the additional benefit of royalties from the sale of a drug. Depending upon the significance of the discovery, these royalties could support a major laboratory for years or significantly supplement a scientist's personal income, or both. Clearly, the specialist-consultant benefited research programs in both industry and universities.

The specialist-consultantship could contain some elements of the general consultantship and the specific project collaboration. For example, companies turned to specialist-consultants for recommendations to fill research positions in the consultant's field and possibly for assistance in dealing with the United States Patent Office or the Council on Pharmacy and Chemistry of the American Medical Association. Also, these consultantships quite often yielded specific therapeutic agents, which the consultant helped develop as part of his responsibilities as an adviser on the chemistry or pharmacology of that class of therapeutic agents. From the standpoint of the company, of course, a specific drug was the ideal product of a specialist-consultantship. While the specialist-consultantship could bear some characteristics of the other two types of collaboration, this type of university-industry interaction generally did not trespass beyond the academic scientist's sphere of expertise, and the collaborators typically initiated the specialist-consultantship to investigate a group or class of drugs rather than an individual therapeutic agent.

Examples of the specialist-consultant abound. For example, Chauncey Leake, a pharmacologist who held positions at four universities during his career, worked with several drug companies between the two world wars. Leake evaluated barbiturates in cooperation with Abbott beginning about 1929. He investigated arsenicals in amoebic dysentery and infections involving the *Trichomonas* parasite for Parke-Davis during the 1930s. Leake also worked with Lilly on the chemotherapy of amebiosis and on antileprotic agents. He collaborated with Merck on a study of derivatives of prostigmine, a synthetic drug similar in structure and action to the Calabar bean alkaloid, physostigmine.[1]

Microbiologist Selman Waksman's consultantship with Merck on industrial fermentations and antibiotics demonstrates the impact this type of collaboration could have on an entire university's research program as well as on the consultant's own laboratory. Merck established a fellowship for an investigation of industrial fermentations in Waksman's laboratory at the College of Agriculture at Rutgers in 1938. Among his other contributions to the firm in this field, Waksman helped launch submerged fermentation production of lactic, citric, and fumaric acids at Merck. Merck established another fellowship in Waksman's laboratory, for the investigation of antibiotics, in 1939, shortly after a former student of Waksman's, René Dubos, had discovered an antibiotic-producing soil microorganism.

Waksman and Merck drew up an agreement at this time whereby the firm supplied chemical, pharmacological, and mass-production assistance for any promising antibiotics the Rutgers microbiologist developed. Waksman agreed to assign Merck exclusively any patentable discoveries in his laboratory for a royalty of 2.5 percent of the sales of these discoveries, to be paid to Rutgers.[2] Such exclusive arrangements between academic scientists and drug companies were by no means unusual by this time.

Beginning with actinomycetes, Waksman isolated a host of antibiotics from soil microorganisms, including actinomycin (1940), clavacin (1941), and streptothricin (1942). Typically, once Waksman and his coworkers had isolated and conducted preliminary tests on a new antibiotic, Merck chemists tried to purify the drug and solve its chemical structure, Merck pharmacologists investigated its toxicity and therapeutic value in animals, and Merck bacteriologists and engineers developed methods to produce the antibiotic on a large scale.[3] All of the antibiotics listed above were too toxic to receive serious consideration for clinical tests. But in 1943 Waksman isolated an antibiotic from *Streptomyces griseus*—streptomycin—which was much less toxic than its predecessors and active against some bacteria that neither the sulfonamides nor penicillin could touch, most notably *Mycobacterium tuberculosis*.[4]

Fearful of criticism that they had permitted the monopolization of a very promising therapeutic agent and suspecting that Merck alone could not fill the demand for streptomycin, in 1945 Waksman and Rutgers petitioned Merck to rescind part of their earlier agreement so that other companies would be able to produce streptomycin and any other useful drugs developed in Waksman's laboratory. According to Waksman, "The response was magnanimous; the company accepted all our recommendations, thus saving me personally and the university in particular considerable embarrassment and possible ill will on the part of the public as a whole for trying to establish absolute control of a process that was to save human lives."[5] Subsequently, Merck assigned its patents on Waksman's discoveries to the Rutgers Research and Endowment Foundation around 1946, and within two years eight companies were producing streptomycin in the United States.[6]

Waksman's specialist-consultantship with Merck illustrates the potential of such interactions for long-term support of academic research programs. The royalties from sales of any Waksman antibiotics, according to the 1938 agreement, went entirely to Rutgers. After the Research and Endowment Foundation assumed control of the patents, Waksman eventually received 10 percent of the royalties, half of which he applied to the establishment of a foundation for microbiology "to promote microbiology throughout the world." In a settlement out of court, 3 percent of the royalties plus $125,000 went to Albert Schatz, Waksman's graduate student, who had brought suit against Waksman and Rutgers to achieve recognition of his part in the discovery of streptomycin. A small part of the royalties went to others who shared in the antibiotic work in Waksman's laboratory. The Research and Endowment Foundation applied the remaining 80 percent of the royalties towards the construction and endowment of the Waksman Institute of Microbiology at Rutgers. What began in 1938 as a modest specialist-consultantship on antibiotics yielded $12 million over the next forty years, the bulk of which supported research and related activities in microbiology at Rutgers and around the world.[7]

Waksman stressed the importance of the consultantship with Merck for the success of his antibiotics research program. He received "meager" assistance from Rutgers and "limited" support from two philanthropic sources, the Commonwealth Fund and the Lasker Foundation; his work received "no support whatsoever" from government sources. But the Merck connection, he felt, was responsible for the practical turn his research took: "Without the help . . . of an industrial organization that took over a major part of the pharmacological evaluation of the antibiotic [streptomycin] and large-scale production our contribution would have never attained its goal."[8] That Waksman's products would have been little more than "bibliographical curiosities" without the cooperation of Merck seems doubtful, particularly in the light of the rising interest in antibiotics in the 1940s and afterwards. But it is likely that the introduction of streptomycin to therapeutics would have been considerably delayed without this university-industry interaction.

Despite the change in the exclusive nature of their agreement, Merck maintained close contact with Waksman's group. In 1949 Merck established a Waksman-Merck Fellowship in Natural Science at Rutgers worth thirty-six hundred dollars annually; soon thereafter Merck increased the value of the fellowship to forty-five hundred dollars. The fellowship lasted until the mid-1950s and probably beyond, because "the grant is very valuable since it assures us [Merck] contact with Waksman's laboratory and early information on new developments there." Waksman also worked with Ciba Pharmaceutical Products, the New Jersey branch of the Swiss pharmaceutical firm, as a "classification consultant," but the records are too sparse to permit a characterization of his relationship with that company.[9]

During the 1930s Lyndon Small, an organic chemist at the University of Virginia, engaged in specialist-consultantships with three pharmaceutical firms—Merck, Squibb, and Mallinckrodt, of St. Louis—on the preparation of morphine derivatives. These consultantships were part of a broader program on the study of drug addiction, involving representatives from federal and state governments and private foundations in addition to universities and the pharmaceutical industry. Beginning in 1929 the

Bureau of Social Hygiene—and later the Rockefeller Foundation—offered to subsidize an investigation to alleviate drug addition under the direction of the NRC. The council appointed a Committee on Drug Addiction within its Division of Medical Sciences to organize this program.

The committee focused on nonnarcotic substances for addictive drugs. In 1929 it established a chemical unit under the direction of Small at Virginia for analytical work on opium alkaloids and preparation of synthetic compounds similar to these alkaloids. The following year, the committee set up a unit for the study of the pharmacology of these compounds under Nathan Eddy at the University of Michigan. The Division of Mental Health of the United States Public Health Service conducted clinical investigations of Small's compounds at two locations: the Federal Penitentiary in Leavenworth, Kansas, and the United States Public Health Service Hospital in Lexington, Kentucky (one of the service's "narcotic farms"). The Department of Health of the State of Massachusetts and the Departments of Medicine and Surgery at the University of Michigan also tested drugs clinically for the committee. While drug companies had connections with all phases of this program, I will focus here on their interactions with Small.[10]

Small and his group of chemists concentrated on modifications of the host of alkaloids in opium. They were especially interested in synthesizing derivatives of phenanthrene, the compound of which morphine and other opium alkaloids are derivatives. Some of the compounds produced in Small's laboratory were unrelated to opium alkaloids, and others were already known. Most of the compounds he submitted to Michigan were derivatives of phenanthrene and modifications of morphine. Eddy and his group at Michigan used mice, rabbits, and cats to conduct several pharmacological tests on Small's drugs: toxicity, analgesia, respiratory effect, general depression, and effect on the gastrointestinal tract. On the basis of these tests, which employed morphine as a standard of reference, the more promising drugs entered the next phase—evaluation in humans. Out of several hundred compounds prepared at Virginia, by the late 1930s physicians had tested sixteen in clinics, all of which were morphine derivatives.[11]

Small's earliest contact with a drug company occurred in 1930 when Merck offered to supply him with about half a dozen alkaloids, mostly from opium. Merck and other firms were an important source of alkaloids for Small. While he had nearly an "unlimited supply" of morphine through his connections with the Public Health Service, he had to depend on firms for most other opium alkaloids. A year later, to support Small's research on opium alkaloids, Merck initiated the Merck Fellowship in Alkaloid Chemistry, at seven hundred dollars each year, which the firm maintained through the 1930s. The Rahway company assisted Small's group in another way—by purifying crude alkaloids and other compounds in bulk and processing these to intermediates for further elaboration at Virginia.[12] The Virginia group prepared a particularly promising derivative of morphine (dihydrodesoxy-morphine-D) around 1933; Eddy and his associates at Michigan found that it was lower in some manifestations of toxicity relative to morphine and about ten times more effective than the latter as an analgesic. The Committee on Drug Addiction arranged for Merck to begin large-scale production, and this derivative was one of the earliest compounds tested clinically. Tests in humans demonstrated that it was addictive.[13] Harry J. Anslinger, commissioner of narcotics in the Treasury Department and a member of the committee, urged that Small's derivative be patented, "in the interest of control of narcotics." Small received a patent on this compound in 1934 and assigned it to the Treasury Department.[14]

Squibb also supported Small's research on morphine derivatives with a seven-hundred-dollar annual fellowship that had been in effect at least since 1933. The firm subsidized a similar fellowship for pharmacological work at Michigan, the only pharmaceutical firm to extend such support there. In 1936 Squibb offered to fund a special fellowship at Virginia under Small's direction on derivatives of phenanthrene, with the provision that the firm could retain exclusive rights to any patentable develoments. Neither the president of the University of Virginia nor the chairman of the Committee on Drug Addiction objected, so the Squibb Fellowship in Phenanthrene Chemistry, worth twenty-five hundred dollars annually, began in 1936. Thus, by the late 1930s Squibb was investing thirty-nine hundred dollars each year towards the support of research related to phenanthrene derivatives and modified opiate and other alkaloids.[15] Considering the magnitude of the Small-Eddy project and the potential of capitalizing on this group of important drugs, Squibb's rather hefty investment in this field was not surprising.

In the 1930s Small's laboratory obtained support in the form of alkaloids and a fellowship from another firm—the St. Louis firm Mallinckrodt. Like Merck, Mallinckrodt supplied Small with several alkaloids, and the firm assisted him by converting bulk morphine into codeine. Mallinckrodt instituted a one-thousand-dollar fellowship at Virginia in 1933, under the direction of Small, to assist the chemist in his work for the Committee on Drug Addiction. Mallinckrodt also mass-produced a codeine derivative that Small had synthesized (and later patented in 1939), a derivative with which clinicians had promising results in the relief of tubercular cough.[16]

Sharp and Dohme and the Barrett Company of New York did not offer fellowships, but they did contribute phenanthrene and other raw materials for the committee's investigation. For example, Barrett donated over one hundred kilograms of phenanthrene to Small, worth several hundred dollars, from about 1929 to 1932.[17] In all, five firms supported research on substitutes for addictive drugs in Small's laboratory between the two world wars. By the late 1930s Small and his group of chemists were receiving almost five thousand dollars each year in fellowships from industry for this work. In addition, the companies contributed many bulk chemicals, and they processed these compounds to intermediates for the Virginia group. The Bureau of Social Hygiene and the Rockefeller Foundation provided a majority of the funds for the work at Virginia,[18] but the Committee on Drug Addiction would have been forced to reduce the scale of its project considerably without the support of industry.

The industrial ties of Leake in pharmacology, Waksman in microbiology, and Small in medicinal chemistry illustrate several characteristics of the specialist-consultant. For example, their ambitious research programs necessitated appropriate support; they derived assistance in the form of raw materials, technical expertise, and funding from several firms in some cases. All three researchers were experts in their fields, fields that had great promise for drug development (e.g., barbiturates, antibiotics, and analgesics). Thus, it was incumbent upon firms like Merck, Squibb, and Abbott to maintain their position in the industry by maintaining contact with experts like Leake, Waksman, and Small.

Wisconsin Pharmacologists and the Drug Industry: Arthur Salomon Loevenhart

Arthur Salomon Loevenhart (1878–1929) received his bachelor's (1898) and master's (1899) degress from Kentucky State College and spent the next decade at Johns Hopkins. After graduating from the medical school in 1903, he began working in John J. Abel's Department of Pharmacology and Physiological Chemistry. Loevenhart left Hopkins in 1908 to establish a pharmacology department at the University of Wisconsin School of Medicine, where he remained until his death. One of Loevenhart's earliest interests, beginning when he was an undergraduate at Kentucky, concerned biological oxidations. His investigation of the effects of different compounds on biological oxidations led Loevenhart to identify benzoyl peroxide and salts of iodoxy-benzoic acid as useful therapeutic agents. The latter remained in therapeutic favor as an antiarthritic drug for several years, and the former is still a widely used antibacterial agent (see fig. 9).[19]

Loevenhart's research experience in antisyphilitic organic arsenicals led to his association with two companies—separately—on this topic. Eventually his colleague in the Department of Pharmacology and Toxicology at Wisconsin inherited the arsenical collaboration with one of the drug companies. Loevenhart developed an interest in this field during his

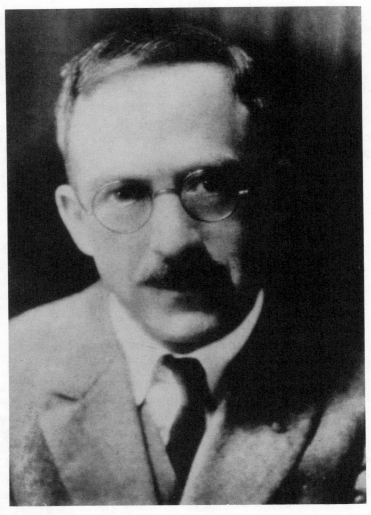

Figure 9. Arthur Salomon Loevenhart (1878–1929), professor of pharmacology and toxicology at the University of Wisconsin School of Medicine from 1908 to 1929 (from *Journal of Pharmacology and Experimental Therapeutics* 36 [1929], courtesy of Williams and Wilkins).

work as head of the Pharmacological and Toxicological Section of the Chemical Warfare Service from 1917 to 1918. The section evaluated a number of war gases developed by chemists, including several arsenicals (e.g., Adamsite and Lewisite).[20] Soon after the war, Loevenhart organized a cooperative study of arsenicals and mercurials for the treatment of neurosyphilis, a form of the disease in which arsphenamine and neoarsphenamine had little or no efficacy. The chemistry department at Northwestern prepared the compounds, Loevenhart's department conducted the experimental evaluations of the drugs, and the Wisconsin Psychiatric Institute of the Mendota State Hospital in Madison carried out the clinical tests. This project, which lasted from 1919 to the mid-1920s, received most of its funds from the United States Interdepartmental Social Hygiene Board and the Public Health Institute of Chicago.[21]

The most successful drug the Wisconsin workers tested came, not from Northwestern, but from the Rockefeller Institute for Medical Research. Tryparsamide, an organic arsenical that researchers at the Rockefeller Institute had prepared in 1915, was one of the first drugs Loevenhart and his colleagues in Madison investigated. At Loevenhart's request, the Rockefeller Institute sent tryparsamide and some other drugs to Madison in 1919 for possible applications in neurosyphilis. The Rockefeller Institute had tested tryparsamide in syphilitic laboratory animals and in some clinical forms of the disease, but the Wisconsin group was the first to establish the value of tryparsamide in neurosyphilis.[22] This major success, coupled with its efforts to organize a systematic cooperative study of a large group of drugs, targeted the Wisconsin group as a desirable potential collaborator in the eyes of some pharmaceutical firms.

Another research interest of Loevenhart's that had a significant impact on his collaborations with industry concerned local anesthetics. Loevenhart had a strong background in chemistry before he began focusing on pharmacology (his graduate degree from Kentucky State College was in chemistry). This facilitated his work on the relationship between the chemical structure and the pharmacological activity of drugs, such as antisyphilitic arsenicals and anesthetics. In the early 1920s, for example, Loevenhart and a graduate student reported their results on an extensive study of the structure-activity relationships of several local anesthetics.[23]

Loevenhart's Connections with Abbott, Commercial Solvents, and Parke-Davis

There is relatively little information documenting the interactions between Loevenhart and Abbott Laboatories. Moreover, the extant sources on this consultantship document only the negotiations between the Wisconsin pharmacologist and the firm on two different projects; it is not clear how or even if Loevenhart and Abbott worked together on these research problems. Nevertheless, this consultantship merits at least a summary. In the first place, it is the earliest known contact between Loevenhart and a pharmaceutical company for the purpose of cooperative research. Second, the proposed organization of one of the two cooperative projects between the academic researcher and Abbott appears to be the basis upon which Loevenhart organized a later, similar project with another company. Late in 1926 Loevenhart learned through a former student then at Abbott that the company was planning to market the ammonium salt of iodoxy benzoate. Loevenhart informed the company that he had been working on this compound for over fifteen years and that he was prepared to share with the firm a new, efficient method of producing the benzoate that a Wisconsin colleague had developed. At the same time, he asked whether the company would be willing to supply his department with the compound for Loevenhart's continuing pharmacological studies of the benzoate. Although Abbott felt its own process was more economical than Loevenhart's, it promised to supply Loevenhart with some of the drug.[24]

Abbott was much more interested in a collaborative project with Loevenhart on antisyphilitic organic arsenicals. Loevenhart had not only an established track record with arsenicals (tryparsamide) but a well-organized, cooperative research program between Northwestern, his own department, and the Wisconsin Psychiatric Institute. Abbott wanted to plug into this program because it was a likely source of future therapeutic innovations. Loevenhart, Abbott, and Frank C. Whitmore, a chemist at Northwestern, began drafting an agreement for collaborative research on antisyphilitic arsenicals around the fall of 1926. The three parties drew up a fairly complete contract for cooperation, but they did not sign it. The available evidence is too sparse to suggest why the agreement never came to fruition; however, Wisconsin and Northwestern came to terms on a similar agreement with a different pharmaceutical company, Parke-Davis, in 1927.[25]

Not all of Loevenhart's consulting work dealt with drugs. He spent a year directing toxicological work in his laboratory on a series of solvents for a chemical company. Commercial Solvents Corporation, of Terre Haute, Indiana, approached Loevenhart in February 1928 to study the toxicity of two of its products—butyl alcohol and butyl acetate—in relation to the toxicity of some competing compounds—Cellosolve, butyl Cellosolve, and Cellosolve acetate. Shortly after World War I, a Du Pont chemist developed a durable, quick-drying lacquer that required solvents such as these. Spurred on by immediate industrywide application of this discovery among auto manufacturers, the lacquer industry grew enormously during the 1920s. Commercial Solvents had been producing butyl alcohol since World War I based on a discovery by Chaim Weizmann, a chemist at the University of Manchester, that certain microorganisms fermented foodstuff starch to yield butyl alcohol. Carbide and Carbon Chemicals Corporation, following methods worked out by Mellon Institute chemist George O. Curme, Jr., introduced the synthetically produced Cellosolve group of lacquer solvents in the 1920s.[26]

Commercial Solvents agreed to pay Loevenhart five hundred dollars to conduct as many tests for acute and chronic toxicity as possible with that sum. If the project proceeded satisfactorily to both parties, the company would extend its support, because Commercial Solvents eventually wanted toxicological evaluations of nineteen products. The two parties agreed that the Wisconsin workers would investigate the toxicity of these solvents for several routes of administration—orally, intravenously, by skin absorption, and via inhalation of solvent vapors. The latter two routes were particularly relevant, since these were the routes by which workers in the lacquer solvent industry came into contact with the compounds. The chemical company intended the results to be kept strictly internal and thus asked Loevenhart not to publish any of this work. Loevenhart petitioned the company to allow one of his students to do this work as part of his degree work, since "a thesis gets very little publicity; it is simply filed away in the University library," but the company would not permit this either.[27] Loevenhart probably did not make this publication policy more of an issue because of the nature of the work. Basically, this was routine work, not the kind of high-level research that Loevenhart was accustomed to publishing and not the kind of work he was accustomed to directing as the basis for a graduate degree.

Loevenhart's interactions with Commercial Solvents, which lasted until February 1929, illustrate that a company could call upon the general technical knowledge and skills of a specialist-consultant whether or not he was familiar with a specific subject. Loevenhart certainly had no special training in the toxicology of lacquer solvents, nor did Arthur Tatum have any particular background in the dye he tested for another chemical firm (see below). Loevenhart and Tatum were fundamentally solid pharmacologists, and once they established themselves as pharmacologists willing to work with companies, it was logical for a company like Commercial Solvents to turn to Loevenhart for assistance. Thus, this was a case where a company approached a specialist-consultant, not primarily for his expertise in an area the company was interested in, but because he was a sound and dependable scientist.

Loevenhart had more extensive contact with Parke, Davis and Company of Detroit than with any other company. Beginning around 1927, he collaborated with Parke-Davis on local anesthetics, ephedrine preparations, and arsenicals. The latter collaboration was the beginning of an alliance that continued for twenty years after Loevenhart's death. Early in

1926 the company assured Loevenhart that "if at any time we can cooperate with you in the matter of supplying special material, or carrying out any work for which you do not have the time or facilities, we shall be very glad indeed to be of any possible service."[28]

Their collaboration on local anesthetics stemmed from promising results Loevenhart found in his study of isocaine, which the discoverer of procaine had prepared early in the twentieth century. Researchers had paid little attention to isocaine up to the time of Loevenhart's work. He found that isocaine was as effective as cocaine for ophthalmic uses, with only a third the toxicity of cocaine. Late in 1927, about three years after publishing his isocaine work, Loevenhart asked Parke-Davis to consider manufacturing this anesthetic. He told the company that clinicians he knew had been using isocaine for urethral catheterization and in many "tonsil cases." Loevenhart did not mention their source for the drug, but he was "terribly anxious to have somebody put it on the market." He also offered to perform toxicity tests on the Parke-Davis product before the firm distributed it for clinical trials. The company agreed to produce enough isocaine for more clinical trials.[29]

Around this time William L. Ruigh, a chemist at Princeton, developed an entirely new type of local anesthetic. He combined certain parts of the structure common to the procaine series of anesthetics with carbazole, a tricyclic, amino-substituted hydrocarbon that occurs naturally in coal tar. Although Ruigh's carbazole derivatives apparently were untested, Parke-Davis was hopeful enough (on the basis of structure-activity considerations) to postpone the work on isocaine indefinitely. Loevenhart began testing the carbazole derivatives in late December 1927, and by spring 1928 he, Ruigh, and Parke-Davis concluded a contract for the development and testing of carbazole derivatives. The collaborators made little progress in the following year. Ruigh's laboratory at Princeton burned down sometime during this period, which obviously slowed the anesthetic project from the Princeton end. Also, Loevenhart began devoting more and more of his time during 1928 to the ephedrine and arsenical projects with Parke-Davis. As his health deteriorated in the early months of 1929, Loevenhart became less of a factor in the local anesthetics collaboration. It is not clear whether Parke-Davis and Ruigh continued to work together through the remainder of 1929 and thereafter, but Ruigh's carbazole derivatives never found a niche in the armamentarium of local anesthetics.[30]

Loevenhart also collaborated with Parke-Davis on preparations of ephedrine, an alkaloid isolated from an ancient Chinese medicinal herb in the 1880s and investigated pharmacologically—principally by K. K. Chen—from the 1920s on. Among its many other actions on the heart, the lungs, the gastrointestinal tract, and so on, ephedrine constricts the blood vessels that serve the mucous membranes of the nose. Thus, it is (and was known in Loevenhart's time to be) a useful drug in cases such as head colds and minor infections causing nasal congestion. In 1927 Loevenhart began helping Parke-Davis formulate a compound ephedrine spray. Also around this time, he urged the company to market an ephedrine snuff, which he had recently developed.

The collaboration between Loevenhart and Parke-Davis on ephedrine preparations, the details of which are not worth relating here, typified a project type of academic-industrial research collaboration more than a specialist-consultantship, inasmuch as it focused on a specific therapeutic agent for a disease or symptom. It was not a joint study, after all, of the group of vasoconstricting drugs useful as nasal decongestants. Loevenhart, Tatum, and the other specialist-consultants examined in this volume engaged in an occasional project type of research collaboration with industry, although they served companies primarily as specialist-consultants. As noted previously, the three categories of collaboration defined in this study rarely, if ever, existed in pure form in the case of any given individual or group. The arsenical collaboration between Loevenhart and Parke-Davis was much more representative of his relationship with industry than was the ephedrine project.

Loevenhart, Parke-Davis, and Frank Whitmore and C. S. Hamilton, of the Northwestern chemistry department, concluded an agreement on 30 September 1927 for research on organic arsenicals for the treatment of syphilis and trypanosomiasis.[31] Parke-Davis, which initiated in-house arsenical research in August 1910—shortly after Paul Ehrlich reported his success with Salvarsan (arsphenamine)—wished to collaborate with the two university groups for the reasons that Abbott had. Among the Northwestern chemists involved in the collaboration, C. S. Hamilton had a much greater interest in the chemistry of arsenicals than Whitmore. Hamilton's first systematic exposure to arsenical research probably occurred during World War I, when he was part of the Army Chemical Warfare Service at Edgewood Arsenal. Also, an expert on organic arsenicals, Winford Lee Lewis, had supervised Hamilton's doctoral work in the early 1920s. Whitmore did not have such a strong interest in arsenicals. His name appeared in this contract (and in the earlier Abbott-Wisconsin-Northwestern proposed agreement) probably as a formality, since he headed the Northwestern chemistry department. Moreover, when Hamilton moved to the University of Nebraska chemistry department in 1929 (the same year that Whitmore left Northwestern for Pennsylvania State), Northwestern was no longer involved in the collaboration.[32]

Parke-Davis agreed to support the arsenical research at Wisconsin and Northwestern with payments of three thousand dollars and four thousand dollars a year, respectively. However, the company raised its support for the Wisconsin work to four thousand dollars a year in 1928 and five thousand in 1929. Loevenhart and Hamilton would disclose the complete details of their research whenever the company requested, and Parke-Davis had the right to observe and study the ongoing work at Wisconsin and Northwestern. The university workers, moreover, were prohibited from sharing their arsenical research with any individual not involved in the arsenical program. In the event that Loevenhart or Hamilton made any patentable discoveries, Parke-Davis would have the exclusive right to apply these discoveries commercially. In return, the firm agreed to pay Loevenhart and Hamilton each a royalty of 2.5 percent of the net sales of all patented products derived from the collaboration (the retail price to be determined by Parke-Davis). The university researchers had the right to inspect the company sales records for the relevant drugs. Any royalties due the Wisconsin and Northwestern groups would be applied to Parke-Davis's earlier support of the academic workers until its subsidies were reimbursed in full. Thereafter, Loevenhart and Hamilton had to apply their royalties to future arsenical research. If the royalties failed to meet the necessary support for arsenical research at the universities, Parke-Davis would make up the difference. If the royalties exceeded the necessary support, Loevenhart and Hamilton would receive the surplus funds to disburse as they pleased.[33]

The contract failed to address some key issues. For example, it did not mention any procedure by which some or all of the collaborators could terminate the agreement, and it left unclear the rights of the academic workers if company scientists discovered a patentable drug without any assistance from the university researchers. But overall, the contract was fair to both the company and the university scientists. In the late 1920s three thousand dollars went a long way towards the support of a professor's graduate students. Thus, the agreement helped support Loevenhart's and Hamilton's research programs. Also, while the agreement restricted the sharing of information with outsiders, the collaboration nevertheless served as the basis for several publications and theses by the academic workers and their students.[34] From the standpoint of Parke-Davis, the firm managed to hook up with some very talented drug researchers, and the contract ensured that it would be the only firm to capitalize on arsenical discoveries emanating from the laboratories of Loevenhart and Hamilton.

The contract also did not address the expected functions of each party, even in a rudimentary way. Even so, the collaborators established a fairly well-defined division of labor early in the arsenical program. Loevenhart and his associates designed compounds according to chemical structure and expected pharmacological activity.[35] They also were responsible for toxicological and therapeutic evaluations of the arsenicals, in which they employed both in vitro and in vivo tests. Typically, the Wisconsin group determined (1) the toxicity of arsenicals, (2) the therapeutic value of products when administered to rats or mice infected with various trypanosomes, and (3) the therapeutic value of drugs in syphilitic rabbits. The Wisconsin Psychiatric Institute and the University of Wisconsin Hospital conducted preliminary clinical tests on the more promising drugs. If an arsenical continued to show promise, the collaborators would engage other physicians around the country for expanded clinical trials. Hamilton and his colleagues worked out practical syntheses of the compounds Loevenhart proposed; and Hamilton developed some arsenicals of his own design. Parke-Davis conducted both pharmacological and chemical work on the products and supplied arsenicals in bulk for the toxicological and therapeutic tests in animals and in humans.

Loevenhart's sudden death in April 1929 ordinarily would have terminated the arsenical program—at least as far as Wisconsin was concerned. No one else in the Wisconsin pharmacology department was nearly as experienced as Loevenhart in the chemotherapy of syphilis or other infectious diseases. But the department recently had acquired another person who, like Loevenhart, put into practice his conviction that universities and the pharmaceutical industry had much to offer one another in the way of research support for academic scientists; expert consultation for companies; and possibly advances in therapeutics. Arthur Tatum picked up where Loevenhart left off and soon discovered an antisyphilitic arsenical that superseded even the arsphenamines.

Wisconsin Pharmacologists and the Drug Industry: Arthur Lawrie Tatum

Like Loevenhart, Arthur Lawrie Tatum (1884–1955) was well trained in chemistry before he began formal work in pharmacology. He received his undergraduate degree in 1905 at a small college in Iowa and a master's degree in chemistry two years later at the University of Iowa. After three years as an instructor in chemistry at the University of Colorado, Tatum spent four years in Chicago. During this first period in Chicago, when he earned a Ph.D. in the Department of Physiology and Pharmacology at the University of Chicago (1913) and an M.D. from Rush Medical College, Tatum found time to work as an instructor in Loevenhart's department. Following brief appointments in two physiology departments, Tatum joined the Department of Pharmacology at the University of Chicago in 1918. Ten years later he accepted Loevenhart's invitation to come to Wisconsin's pharmacology and toxicology department; Tatum was chairman of that department from 1929 until his retirement in 1954 (see fig. 10).[36]

Prior to the period when he began collaborating with pharmaceutical firms (in the mid-1920s), Tatum's research interests focused on the physi-

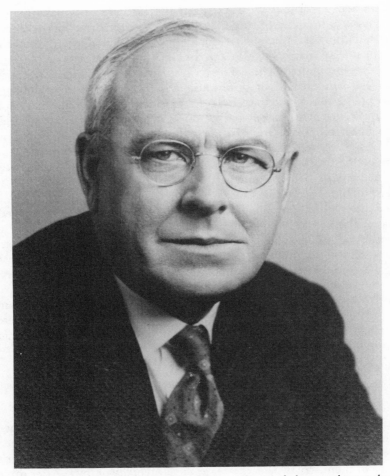

Figure 10. Arthur Lawrie Tatum (1884–1955), professor of pharmacology at the University of Wisconsin School of Medicine from 1928 to 1955 (courtesy of the National Library of Medicine).

ology of the thyroid gland and acute and chronic intoxication involving opium alkaloids, barbiturates, and local anesthetics. He did not incorporate thyroid research into any of his collaborations. Tatum emerged as an expert on the pharmacology of morphine, barbiturates, and other central nervous system depressants fairly early in his career, and this led to some important collaborations with industry. For example, Tatum contributed much to our understanding of the physiological aspects of morphine addiction.[37] On the basis of his work on drug intoxication, Tatum discovered that barbiturates were an effective antidote for cocaine overdosage. A few years later he found that picrotoxin, a central nervous system stimulant derived from a plant, was an antidote for barbiturate overdosage.[38]

In one sense, Tatum is quite atypical of specialist-consultants. Companies usually engaged a consultant for a particular series of researches because the consultant was a specialist, if not an authority, on that subject. Tatum consulted with several companies for many years on the chemotherapy of syphilis and malaria. However, his publications do not indicate any interest in this topic until *after* he began collaborating with companies on antisyphilitics and antimalarial drugs. Thus, in Tatum's case cooperative work with drug companies fostered a new research interest to which he devoted a majority of his time in the latter half of his career.

Tatum's Early Collaborations with Industry

Tatum's arsenical work with Parke-Davis was by no means his first or only collaboration with a company. The earliest research contacts between Tatum and a pharmaceutical firm began in 1925, when he was still in the pharmacology department at the University of Chicago. Cook Laboratories, a small Chicago firm, contacted Tatum in the summer of 1925 to have him conduct biological assays of some of its biological, botanical, and synthetic drugs twice a year at most. Tatum agreed, on the conditions that this work would not interfere with his research and that Cook would be willing to pay a fair amount for these services, which he estimated to be about two dollars per hour. Tatum was not an expert on any of the drugs that Cook wanted him to test, but that was not necessary, since anyone skilled in the art would be able to test these drugs. Cook probably engaged Tatum simply because of his proximity to the firm. Over the following three years, until he moved to Wisconsin, Tatum occasionally tested drugs for Cook. The total charges for his work amounted to about five hundred dollars—very little in the light of the compensation that his future collaborations produced.[39]

In 1927 another company, the National Aniline and Chemical Company, of Buffalo, hired Tatum to conduct pharmacological and toxicological tests on one of its products. His work for that firm continued through his first year at Wisconsin. National Aniline submitted a coal-tar dye to the Food, Drug, and Insecticide Administration (FDIA) of the United States Department of Agriculture in 1927 for inclusion in its list of permitted synthetic food colors. In the early 1920s the FDIA had developed criteria for evaluating submitted dyes that employed the latest techniques in chemistry and pharmacology. First, the company's method of producing the dye had to be well known so that other manufacturers could produce it if they wished. Also, the dye had to be chemically certifiable, that is, of a constant and pure composition. Finally, the dye had to be biologically certifiable. Making sure that a dye was biologically certifiable involved testing both within the FDIA and by an outside worker. The company had to file with the FDIA a "full report made by a reputable pharmacologist of the pharmacological and toxic properties of the dyes," including results of tests for acute and chronic toxicity, using approved food colors as standards. If these test results were promising, the company sent a pharmacologist to Washington to check and extend these results in cooperation with the FDIA's pharmacologists.[40]

Tatum served National Aniline as the "reputable pharmacologist" who conducted the preliminary tests on the firm's dye, alphazurine FG. National Aniline forwarded Tatum's results on the acute toxicity of the dye to the FDIA late in 1927. This work so impressed the latter that it suggested that National Aniline begin tests on the chronic toxicity of alphazurine, first on animals and later on humans. Although National Aniline arranged for Tatum to continue testing alphazurine early in 1928, he did not start this work until later in the summer of that year, probably because he was busy tying up matters in Chicago. The terms of his earlier work are unknown, but National Aniline paid Tatum five hundred dollars monthly—the total remuneration he received for three years' work for Cook Laboratories.[41]

Tatum's results with animals were sufficiently clear and promising that by November 1928 National Aniline planned "to go ahead with manufacture in the plant on the basis that results thus far indicate that the color cannot possibly be denied admission as a permitted color."[42] National Aniline could have proceeded with the manufacture and distribution of alphazurine regardless of the FDIA's decision about including it on the permitted list. Despite the widespread belief in the food industry that certification had legal backing, color certification was a voluntary enterprise. The FDIA occasionally prosecuted flagrant violaters of its certification regulations, but it could pursue legal action only within the confines of the 1906 Food and Drug Act—for example, if a manufacturer adulterated or mislabeled a food color.[43]

Tatum's work for National Aniline ended in early May 1929, when the company sent his final report on the pharmacology and toxicology of alphazurine FG to the FDIA. The FDIA's Color Certification Laboratory and Pharmacological Laboratory issued their final approval of the dye within two months. Later in the year the FDIA admitted alphazurine FG to its list of permitted synthetic food colors as brilliant blue FCF (For Coloring Food), and it remains on the list today as FD & C #1.[44] Cook Laboratories and National Aniline called upon Tatum more as a solid, reputable pharmacologist than as an expert in a particular field of pharmacology, much like the case of Loevenhart's work for Commercial Solvents. Tatum's expertise came much more actively into play in his collaboration with Abbott on barbiturates. Elements of both the project collaboration and the general consultantship would enter into Tatum's interactions with Abbott, but the overall relationship was clearly a specialist-consultantship, as characterized earlier.

Tatum and Abbott

In his first year at Wisconsin, Tatum embarked upon an investigation of the relative merits of the rather extensive series of barbiturates. Tatum approached Abbott in February 1929 to find out whether the company would subsidize part of this work. Abbott had developed an interest in barbiturates during the 1920s; by 1929 the company was marketing the high-volume barbiturates barbital and Neonal (*n*-butylethylbarbituric acid), and it had several other drugs of this class in the experimental stage. Moreover, Abbott already had formed a contact at Wisconsin through Loevenhart, who had spent a year earlier in the decade testing Butesin (*n*-butyl-para-aminobenzoate), a synthetic local anesthetic, for Abbott. The company offered to supply Tatum with various established and experimental barbiturates for his work and to subsidize a fellowship for this research. Abbott provided twelve-hundred dollars each year for the next decade for this fellowship, which covered the salary of the assistant who conducted the research under Tatum's direction and paid for animals, food, and equipment. Tatum eventually hoped to find "a substance with a wide margin of safety between the effectively depressant and the toxic or lethal dosage, one that is stable in solution (which amytal [a Lilly barbiturate] is not), whose depression period is not too long (as is barbital), and that does not produce serious late effects as does chloral hydrate. This is asking for an ideal but that is what we want." Abbott did its best to help Tatum find the ideal compound. Over the following years the Wisconsin group received over 150 hypnotics from the company, most of which were barbiturates.[45]

Abbott sent Tatum three of its more promising experimental barbiturates for comparison with established barbiturates around April 1929, but Tatum and his colleagues did not begin tests on these until the following

September.[46] At that time, Abbott workers reported their own preliminary pharmacological results with some barbiturates. One of the compounds, ethyl(1-methyl butyl)barbituric acid, known later on as Nembutal, was the "most efficient" drug compared with barbital and other well-known barbiturates.[47] This was a rather vague assessment, albeit merely a preliminary one, of the value of Nembutal. Tatum and his co-workers, on the other hand, were able to show that Nembutal offered several specific advantages relative to established barbiturates. They found that Nembutal was more toxic on a weight-for-weight basis than other barbiturates. In reality this was a benefit, since a comparatively smaller quantity of the drug could induce anesthesia and the body was therefore faced with less drug to catabolize and eliminate. In the laboratory animal this amounted to a quicker onset of anesthesia, a deeper and briefer duration of anesthesia, and a faster postanesthetic recovery. Physicians at the University of Wisconsin and the Mayo Clinic carried out the earliest clinical tests with Nembutal beginning in 1930 and confirmed the laboratory results with this barbiturate.[48]

Abbott attempted to patent Nembutal, but the patent office rejected the application, most likely because German researchers had discovered this barbituric acid derivative several years ealier. Abbott's efforts to have the Council on Pharmacy and Chemistry of the AMA include "Nembutal" in *New and Nonofficial Remedies* did not fare any better. By January 1931 Abbott requested the council to approve its proprietary name for ethyl(1-methyl butyl)barbituric acid. Lilly had been working with a similar barbituric acid at the same time and independently of Abbott, and within two months of Abbott's first publication of Nembutal, Lilly researchers also reported that this barbiturate was far more "active" than barbital and other well-known barbiturates. The publications from the two companies appeared too close together, according to the council, for it to establish priority (and thereby the right to a proprietary name) for one company's product over the other's.[49]

The council felt that if any party had priority, it was Tatum's group at Wisconsin, who clearly were the first to recognize the therapeutic contribution of Nembutal—its brief duration of action—in their publication of July 1930. Abbott and Lilly had reported merely that this barbiturate was comparatively "efficient" and "active." Since the Wisconsin article did not acknowledge any support from Abbott, the council would not consider that as a basis for the priority of the North Chicago firm even if one could argue that a fellowship somehow transferred priority for a discovery from the university workers to Abbott.[50] Ironically, two opportunities arose prior to the Wisconsin publication that could have established such priority for Abbott. First, in November 1929 Abbott sought Tatum's permission to include its pharmacology fellowship at Wisconsin in the list of industrial grants and fellowships to universities that the NRC compiled and periodically published. Tatum preferred not to have their support publicized:

My idea is this, that since we are finding your own preparation [Nembutal] to rate very high by the means of testing we are employing, it might look better if it did not appear to come from your immediate support. . . . I am inclined to think that it might be more convincing to our readers subsequently if they did not know the support you people were giving us. You know, of course, as well as others who know us personally, that we are not for sale to anyone, but those who do not know us might see in your sponsorship or subsidy, a personal interest in the matter and, consequently, a somewhat biased report.[51]

Second, Tatum composed a tentative agreement with Abbott in April 1930 whereby the company would pay him a 2.5 percent royalty on all Nembutal sales for his role in the elucidation of the therapeutic value of the barbiturate. If Abbott had agreed to this contract, the firm could have contended that there was indeed "a definite previous agreement to . . . transfer the discovery to the manufacturers," which the council charged was not the case in Abbott's claim to support Tatum's Nembutal research. There is, however, no evidence to suggest that Abbott came to such an agreement with Tatum.[52]

Abbott tried to convince the council that it had established priority on Nembutal through its early funding of Tatum's work on barbiturates. Tatum also sent a letter to the council, at Abbott's request, confirming Abbott's financial assistance. The council did not reconsider. When the council established an approved name for the barbiturate—pentobarbital—Lilly promptly agreed to market its product under that name. "In order to allow the Abbott Laboratories ample time for adjustment," the council allowed the firm to label its pentobarbital with Nembutal as a subtitle of the approved name for a year and a half—à la "Insulin (Iletin-Lilly)" of a few years earlier (see chap. 5).[53] Since Abbott refused to sell its barbiturate under the council-approved name at the end of that period, the council omitted Nembutal from *New and Nonofficial Remedies*. This precluded Abbott from advertising Nembutal in many major medical journals, although the firm continued to market the drug.

During the difficulties with the council, and the failure to patent Nembutal, Abbott did not let Tatum's contributions to the development of this drug go unrewarded. Beginning in 1933 the firm paid Tatum five hundred dollars each year as a "token of our appreciation of your pharmacological work on Nembutal." These "tokens of appreciation" continued until 1940 (two years after the collaboration on hypnotics had formally ended), when Abbott began sending Tatum payments for "consulting services." Although it is doubtful that Tatum actually was consulting with Abbott after the barbiturate collaboration ended, the consulting fees grew to one thousand dollars yearly around 1946 and continued until Tatum's death in 1955. If we assume that all of these payments were de facto rewards for Tatum's work on Nembutal, they amounted to about seventeen thousand dollars, clearly a significant sum, although most likely much less than what the royalty on Abbott's Nembutal sales would have amounted to if the company had agreed to Tatum's tentative contract of 1930.[54]

Tatum and Abbott collaborated on an even shorter-acting barbiturate beginning late in 1933. Both Abbott researchers and Tatum agreed by October 1933 that they needed a new direction in their research on hypnotics, because "the ordinary barbituric acid series has been pretty well worked over. It may be that if unusual substituents become available so that they may be used, there is a possibility of developing barbituric acid derivatives which might have somewhat different properties."[55] Ernest Volwiler and Donalee Tabern, an Abbott chemist, prepared a slightly modified version of Nembutal in which they substituted sulfur for one of the oxygens in the barbituric acid moiety of Nembutal. Abbott conducted some preliminary pharmacological tests on this and several other so-called thiobarbiturates it had prepared and then sent them to Tatum for in-depth pharmacological evaluations.

Despite very promising reports from Wisconsin on tests with sulfur-substituted Nembutal, or thionembutal, Abbott soon urged Tatum and his associates to devote more time to another of its experimental thiobarbiturates, thiosebutal (allyl secondary-butyl thiobarbituric acid). In the first place, Abbott's in-house pharmacological research on comparatve toxicities and duration of anesthesia indicated that thiosebutal was slightly better than thionembutal. Second, the former was much easier to prepare than the latter. Thus, Tabern emphasized Abbott's belief that a study of thiosebutal "may prove to be just as interesting and perhaps more important commercially" than an investigation of thionembutal. That the hypnotic project continued to focus on thionembutal despite Abbott's petitions on behalf of thiosebutal was largely because of Tatum, who knew they had something good in the sulfur analogue of Nembutal: "In regard to the virtues of #8064 [thionembutal] vs. 'Thiosebutal' we are prepared to argue the point with you . . . we feel that our own deductions are more nearly correct because of the wider spread of dosage range, which we feel gives us a better viewpoint of the comparisons."[56] Abbott, curiously, was challenging the barbiturate expert, whom the company hired for detailed investigations of its products, on the basis of preliminary data of its own pharmacological workers, who lacked any formal training. This obviously was defeating the purpose of employing a specialist-consultant. Abbott eventually accepted Tatum's counsel, and Pentothal, the firm's trade name for thiobarbital, became a successful drug for Abbott.

Abbott, having produced two successful products between 1929 and 1933, gradually lost interest in the field of hypnotics. In 1938 the firm informed Tatum that it would no longer be submitting experimental compounds to Wisconsin for testing. Towards the end of the collaboration Volwiler suggested that Abbott was considering projects with Tatum on local anesthetics and analgesics, but these projects never materialized.[57] During the ten-year collaboration Abbott provided over thirteen thousand dollars in support of research fellows under Tatum's direction, and this research served as the basis for a number of publications that came out of Tatum's laboratory. Also, the company paid the Wisconsin pharmacologist over fifteen thousand dollars in consulting fees, which Tatum could disburse as he saw fit. If Tatum and Abbott had agreed to some type of royalty settlement at the start of their collaboration, the compensation almost certainly would have exceeded these consulting fees, probably by several fold. But in the depressed economy of America in the 1930s, when salaries and research funds commonly were cut to ease pressure on academic budgets, particularly at state universities such as Wisconsin, Tatum probably was satisfied to secure whatever support he could for his laboratory.[58] Also, Tatum found an even greater source of support during these years in a collaboration with another company on an entirely different research project.

Tatum and Parke-Davis: Antisyphilitics and Antimalarials

After Arthur Loevenhart died in April 1929, neither Parke-Davis nor Cliff Hamilton appeared to question Tatum's move to supervise the Wisconsin side of the tripartite collaboration on antisyphilitic organic arsenicals, even though he had never published a single paper on the chemotherapy of infectious diseases up to that time.[59] However, within about a year he independently discovered the therapeutic value of an arsenical that superseded all other arsenicals in the treatment of syphilis, including the hallowed Ehrlichian arsphenamines.

Tatum's group examined scores of antisyphilitic drugs for Parke-Davis over two decades. The collaborators eliminated the vast majority of these pharmaceuticals as early as the preliminary laboratory investigations. Some warranted testing beyond the laboratory, but even then the clinical results typically were disappointing. In the case of some antisyphilitics, such as their so-called arsenical 142 and phemarsenol, latent toxic side effects dashed the coworkers' great expectations for these drugs. In such cases, the workers persisted in their attempts to find some molecular modification, some dosage form, or some other disease in which these compounds might be useful. Clearly, the collaborators wanted a return on their intellectual and economic investments in drugs like arsenical 142 and phemarsenol, investments that often extended over many years.

Tatum began working with the arsenical known for decades as arsenoxide—which Parke-Davis eventually introduced as Mapharsen—in January 1930.[60] Tatum was using Mapharsen as part of a theoretical investigation into the role of the host in arsenotherapy. He soon noticed that Mapharsen, the toxic oxidation product of the well-established antisyphilitic known as arsphenamine (which Ehrlich had introduced in 1910 as Salvarsan), *itself* oxidized to a much less toxic product. This was a revelation of immense potential. The oxidation of arsphenamine and its analogue known as neoarsphenamine was a vital concern for physicians. They had to be extremely careful to protect these drugs from exposure to the atmosphere because of the possibility of conversion to the toxic oxidation product—Mapharsen. If enough of a normal dose of an arsphenamine were oxidized accidentally to Mapharsen and then administered, it could kill the patient. However, this would not be a concern if one administered Mapharsen, the toxic yet active component of the arsphenamines;[61] since it was much more toxic than arsphenamine, much less drug could accomplish what a larger amount of arsphenamine could.[62]

The Wisconsin group and the pharmacological laboratory of Parke-Davis launched an intensive comparison of Mapharsen, arsphenamine, and neoarsphenamine in the summer of 1930. By March of the following year Tatum concluded that Mapharsen was as effective as arsphenamine and neoarsphenamine in experimental syphilis. Clinical tests, which began at the University of Wisconsin Hospital and the Wisconsin Psychiatric Institute in August 1931 and included nearly a dozen clinics by the mid-1930s, confirmed the laboratory results. The consensus of clinicians was that results achieved with Mapharsen were equal to the best results obtained with the arsphenamines in primary, secondary, and congenital syphilis.[63] It was not only efficacious but also safer than the arsphenamines— a great irony considering that researchers before Tatum (including Paul Ehrlich) had ignored Mapharsen as a therapeutic agent, primarily because of its toxicity.[64]

The specialist-consultantship as I have defined it did not originate for the study of a particular therapeutic agent; that was more the province of the project collaboration. But specific projects could, and often did, emerge from the specialist-consultantship. Tatum's consultantships, for example, helped produce such drugs as Nembutal and Pentothal. From the standpoint of the company, a strike such as one of these drugs was a fulfillment of the consultantship, since the aim was to find therapeutic agents. From the standpoint of the academic researcher, a therapeutic find could be a source of additional financial support for his research program. Mapharsen illustrates the impact a therapeutic discovery could have on a specialist-consultant.

Tatum received a patent on Mapharsen in 1937. In accordance with the original agreement dating back to 1927, Parke-Davis had an exclusive license to manufacture the drug, and Tatum and Hamilton each received a royalty of 2.5 percent of the net sales of the drug. Parke-Davis withheld 60 percent of each royalty payment until the firm was fully reimbursed for its past investment in arsenical research at Wisconsin and Nebraska. Once the company was fully compensated, Tatum and Hamilton fully subsidized their arsenical research with the royalties.[65]

Tatum collected royalties from 1937 until the Mapharsen patent expired in 1954. The initial payments were fairly modest, but they grew tremendously in the 1940s, especially during the war. The royalties fully compensated Parke-Davis's past support by mid-1942; thereafter Tatum received his full complement of royalties, part of which he applied to cover the arsenical research at Wisconsin.[66] Consider the period from 1937 to 1947, for which there is fairly complete financial data. Parke-Davis estimated the total cost of the research at Wisconsin from mid-1942 through 1947 at $4,800 per year, or about $26,000. Tatum's royalties through 1947, consisting of the 40 percent payments up to mid-1942 and the full payments from then through 1947, amounted to about $240,000, exceeding the expenses of the arsenical research at Wisconsin by $215,000. Whether Tatum channeled these surplus royalties back into the Department of Pharmacology, pocketed them, or both is not clear. But the point is that Tatum, whose salary did not exceed $6,000 until 1942, had incoming funds that averaged over $21,000 a year from 1937 to 1947 to spend as he pleased.[67] It is worth mentioning again that this period of plenty overlapped several years of retrenchment on the Madison campus.

Late in 1947, twenty years after the original agreement, Parke-Davis informed Tatum of its intention to terminate the Wisconsin side of the arsenical collaboration. The company felt that it had sufficient pharmacological personnel and facilities to carry out this work on its own.[68] In one sense this was a surprising decision, since the connection with Wisconsin was basically gratis; the Mapharsen royalties fully subsidized Wisconsin's research expenses at this time. However, with the rise of penicillin after the war the organic arsenicals were rapidly approaching obsolescence. In this respect, the dissolution of the collaboration was not such a surprise.

Tatum, Hamilton, and representatives of Parke-Davis held a conference in June 1936 to discuss the arsenical work and new lines of collaborative research. E. A. Sharp, the director of clinical investigation at Parke-Davis, suggested that a project on therapy for malaria would be a worthwhile endeavor, given the prevalence of the disease and the strong possibility of finding a useful antimalarial drug. The company general manager, A. W. Lescohier, disagreed. He felt that a long-term study of antimalarials would be impractical, requiring too much time to produce any tangible results. Tatum sided with Sharp: "Dr. Tatum argued strongly against limiting our cooperative work to one or two problems. He feels that we should not risk having all our eggs in one basket. He is quite enthusiastic about the malaria problem because he feels that it fits in well with our cooperative arsenical work, that methods of testing are already available and that the hope of some practical outcome is reasonable."[69] Others argued that notwithstanding available therapeutic and public health procedures, the incidence of and mortality from malaria remained shockingly high.[70] As late as 1930 India alone had 100 million cases of malaria, of which 2 −3 million died. According to Macfarlane Burnet, "If we take as our standard of importance the greatest harm to the greatest number, then there is no question that malaria is the most important of all infectious diseases." Lescohier decided that it would be advisable after all to enter the malaria field. The collaborators, he felt, could plan the pharmacological work at a later date, after they established a chemical program.[71]

Tatum began testing some old arsenicals and new compounds as antimalarials in 1937, but Parke-Davis did not start subsidizing the malaria work at Wisconsin until 1940. Perhaps, as Lescohier urged, Tatum spent most of his time during this period "cleaning up" the antisyphilitic arsenical research. Also, Tatum wanted to set up his laboratory for the malaria work before taking on research assistants for the program.[72] Parke-Davis supported both Hamilton's group and Tatum and his associates. The firm funded the pharmacological work under Tatum at a rate of two thousand dollars annually from 1940 to 1944, three thousand dollars annually from 1944 to 1946, and four thousand dollars annually from 1946 until the termination of the project in 1948.[73]

Knowing that some investigators had some success with neoarsphenamine in malaria, Tatum started with Mapharsen and a few other arsenicals. Since these lacked any activity, Parke-Davis, Hamilton, and Tatum abandoned arsenicals and focused instead on derivatives of the bicyclic compound quinoline, which made up half of the molecule of quinine. Also, one of the two major synthetic antimalarials known at this time, pamaquine (Plasmochin), was a derivative of quinoline. By 1941 Tatum's group had tested about fifty compounds from Parke-Davis and Nebraska; less than ten of these had any appreciable activity. The collaborating chemists thus decided to concentrate on different series of compounds, including sulfonamides.[74]

The complexion of the collaboration on antimalarials changed significantly in 1942. At that time a plethora of panels, conferences, committees, subcommittees, and surveys of the NRC, in association with the Committee on Medical Research of the OSRD, consolidated all phases of antimalarial research in the United States. Over a dozen other nations contributed to this wartime work as well. The planning for this project had begun two years earlier, in anticipation of quinine shortages during the war. After Pearl Harbor, the needs of American troops in the Pacific and the Mediterranean for treatment and protection against malaria became especially urgent. Participants in the national malaria program sent chemical, pharmacological, and other data on antimalarials to a central CMR-NRC clearing house for circulation among other participants, although contributors had the right to restrict whatever information they wished. The clearing house also arranged for pharmacological and clinical testing of all submitted products.[75]

Strategically, according to Oliver Kamm, director of research, Parke-Davis could not avoid taking part in the program: "Presumably the research divisions of practically all competing pharmaceutical houses have been asked to collaborate and so it turns out that, although we have expended more effort in the past than others in the direction of antimalarial research, our competitors may be securing a real advantage unless we also take part in the work sponsored by the Government through the National Research Council."[76] The company joined the national program, but it also developed its own scaled-down version of a crash antimalarial program. It engaged an additional six outside chemists and three pharmacologists; Parke-Davis communicated the results of this group to the CMR-NRC clearing house.[77] Meanwhile, Tatum's laboratory streamlined its work such that by early 1943 it alone was prepared to evaluate thirty antimalarials per month, while the chemical group was planning to produce one hundred compounds monthly.[78] Within just a few years, the Parke-Davis cooperative group processed hundreds of antimalarials; the national clearing house arranged further pharmacological evaluations and clinical tests for many of these.

Parke-Davis produced a compound later during the national malaria project that was as much as thirty times as active as quinine in pharmacological tests. The company introduced this drug in 1950 as Camoquine (amodiaquine).[79] After twelve years collaborating on a project that started out as a modest tripartite arrangement and eventually plugged into an international research network, Parke-Davis broke off the cooperative antimalarial research program with Tatum in 1948. Just a year earlier the company had terminated the syphilis project with Wisconsin. Even if Parke-Davis had not lost interest in malaria,[80] it probably would have ended the connections with Wisconsin for the same reason that it ended the arsenical project: its own pharmacology department was far enough advanced to carry out most of the company's needs in that area, including innovation. Yet the university scientist and the pharmaceutical firm did not part empty-handed. Parke-Davis at least could point to Camoquine to justify its investments in the program, and Tatum had found an additional twenty-two thousand dollars to support his research program at Wisconsin during the 1940s.

Tatum's Work with Other Firms

Tatum collaborated with two other companies on the chemotherapy of syphilis during his arsenical work with Parke-Davis—Charles Pfizer and Company and Upjohn. Tatum's work with Pfizer and Upjohn concerned bismuth compounds, which physicians had employed in syphilotherapy since the late nineteenth century. Bismuth grew in popularity during the first quarter of the twentieth century, and it soon replaced long-esteemed mercury as the heavy metal of choice in the treatment of syphilis. Bismuth was especially useful when administered with arsenicals, although physicians used bismuth alone as well. The bismuth research with these two companies illustrates how Tatum, sometimes to the point of frustrating the firm, incorporated company-sponsored projects into his personal research interests.

In October 1931 Pfizer engaged Tatum to investigate the clinical suitability of its bismuth preparation, bismuth mannonate. Tatum agreed to test Pfizer's product for toxicity (acute and chronic), distribution and fate in the body, and therapeutic value in experimental and clinical syphilis. Pfizer in turn would pay Tatum $250 monthly for six months, with the possibility of continuing the support beyond that time. Tatum reported on the toxicity of bismuth mannonate two months later. In his next step, however, Tatum began a comparison of the toxicities of other bismuth preparations with mannonate instead of focusing on the latter and its possible role as an antisyphilitic (as he had promised Pfizer). Thus, "in order to get a basis of comparison for the mannonate," Tatum initiated an investigation of the toxicities of bismuth citrate, tartrate, and iodide.[81]

By the end of the six-month period Tatum admitted to Pfizer that on the basis of comparative studies of its toxicity and absorption characteristics, bismuth mannonate did not seem sufficiently promising as a therapeutic agent to extend the collaboration. Bismuth citrate, on the other hand, impressed Tatum so much that he recommended extending the collaboration to study this preparation in depth. The company was not enthused, because "there are now citrates and tartrates of various makes on the market and our prime interest was in the mannonate." Still, Tatum reminded the firm, the therapeutic proof was in the pudding, and since he had not yet administered bismuth mannonate to a single syphilitic rabbit, he could not yet pass a final judgment on the preparation. Pfizer then seemed interested in extending the bismuth work. But Tatum informed the company that he would need another six to eight months to form a definite idea of the value of the bismuth preparations in experimental syphilis. Also, his arsenical collaboration took priority for whatever clinical cases of syphilis became available at Wisconsin for the next several months. Faced with the strong possibility of another long investigation that might fail to produce any marketable ideas about "the suitability for clinical purposes of our sodium bismuthyl mannonate," Pfizer finally terminated its support of Tatum's bismuth research in the summer of 1932.[82]

Tatum did not have to wait very long to find support for his bismuth research. The Upjohn Company, of Kalamazoo, Michigan, approached Tatum in December of 1932 for pharmacological and toxicological work on bismuth mannonate and other bismuth preparations. Upjohn personnel were considering marketing the mannonate, and perhaps other compounds, but they needed more pharmacological data to inform this decision. Upjohn had no spare research staff to whom it could assign this problem, much less anyone familiar with the pharmacology of bismuth preparations. In accordance with Tatum's wishes, Upjohn paid Tatum three thousand dollars per year for this investigation.[83]

Walter W. Enz, who studied under Edward Kremers at Wisconsin and joined Upjohn as a pharmaceutical chemist in 1932, prepared for Tatum new bismuth compounds as well as a few well-known preparations that Tatum was not able to acquire from other firms. (Parke-Davis and G. D. Searle and Company, of Chicago, supplied Tatum with some bismuth preparations, athough they did not provide capital support for his bismuth research.) Herbert A. Braun, another recent Wisconsin graduate whom Upjohn hired in 1933, conducted preliminary pharmacological evaluations on the experimental bismuths before sending these to Wisconsin. Despite his assurance to Pfizer in June 1932 that he was ready as early as then to begin testing bismuths in experimental syphilis, Tatum continued to focus on the chronic toxicity of these compounds during the early collaboration with Upjohn. He reported his first therapeutic results two years after the collaboration began—on a Searle product. Upjohn issued a pungent reply acknowledging Tatum's familiarity with its competitor's product and expressing disappointment that the Wisconsin worker had to "exclude our bismuth preparations from similar considerations."[84]

Upjohn ended its support of bismuth research at Wisconsin in 1938, probably because, first, the firm was by then interested primarily in bismuth ethyl camphorate alone, whereas Tatum still emphasized the rigorous, comparative approach to the investigation of bismuth compounds. Second, since Tatum provided substantial pharmacological results with the camphorate, the AMA Council on Pharmacy and Chemistry, having been approached by Upjohn to include the camphorate in its *New and*

Nonofficial Remedies, required more clinical evidence of this drug's value. Thus, in the following years Upjohn focused on the expansion of testing with humans. Shortly thereafter, Upjohn renewed its research fellowship under Tatum for "more extensive and complete studies" on camphorate and other bismuth compounds, at a lesser rate (two thousand dollars annually) than earlier. Tatum apparently applied this fellowship to continue his earlier research on the synergy of bismuth and arsenical compounds in syphilis. He also investigated the elimination of bismuth in clinical syphilis. Upjohn renewed the support for at least one year, but records of the collaboration cease after 1943.[85]

The bismuth research programs with Pfizer and Upjohn were a logical extension of Tatum's established collaboration with Parke-Davis on the chemotherapy of syphilis. The two programs complemented each other nicely, in much the same way that bismuth compounds and arsenicals complemented each other in the treatment of syphilis. Tatum did not enjoy the same kind of success in his bismuth research as he had in the arsenical work, but he did help Upjohn develop a new bismuth preparation that filled a therapeutic niche in an armamentarium replete with such compounds. The Wisconsin pharmacology department was able to supplement its research funds with over twenty-five thousand dollars from bismuth fellowships—most of this support coming during the Depression. Thus, the bismuth collaborations yielded many benefits to the principals in this consultantship—benefits to the company (in the form of a marketable drug), to the consultant (in the form of long-term support of his research program), and to therapeutics as well (in the form of an enhanced understanding of the pharmacology of a group of drugs, with the added benefit of a useful drug for the treatment of disease).

Conclusion

Both Loevenhart and Tatum were examples of very active consultants to industry. In the late 1920s Loevenhart was consulting with three companies on six different research topics. Tatum was a virtual consulting machine, at least prior to World War II. He worked with a total of six companies on a variety of topics. At one point in the late 1930s he was consulting simultaneously with Abbott on barbiturates, Parke-Davis on antisyphilitic arsenicals and antimalarials, and Upjohn on antisyphilitic bismuth compounds. By this time he even had developed standardized contracts for consultantships. Both Loevenhart and Tatum fostered these many industrial contacts without any noticeable drain on their university duties.

Loevenhart and Tatum were valuable resources for companies. While a few firms had solid pharmacologists on their staffs in the 1920s and 1930s, the majority of companies did not. Thus Abbott, Parke-Davis, and the other companies turned to Loevenhart and Tatum to sift and winnow arsenicals, antimalarials, barbiturates, bismuths, and other groups of drugs. The host of successful pharmaceuticals they helped to develop is testament to their value to these companies. In turn, the consulting arrangements provided a valuable resource for the Wisconsin pharmacologists. They derived hundreds of thousands of dollars from associations with industry, which helped support their students and their research programs.

CHAPTER FIVE

The Scientist as Project Researcher

-->>>->>>->>>->>>->>>- <<<-<<<-<<<-<<<-<<<-

The specific project collaboration had the narrowest scope of the three typologies of cooperative research discussed in this book. It was not unusual for elements of this typology to exist in the other two (as, for example, in Adams's work with Abbott on barbital, Tatum's Nembutal research for Abbott, and the joint development of streptomycin by Merck and Waksman), but we see very little of the reverse case. The object of scientists involved in specific project collaborations was to develop a particular therapeutic agent, usually to such a point of safety, efficacy, and economy that the product was ready for general distribution. This chapter describes exemplary specific task-oriented collaborations between 1920 and 1940. While there was no standard formula by which collaborations like these operated, certain common characteristics of the project type of arrangement are clear.

First, researchers from either academe or industry discovered the therapeutic agent prior to the collaboration. This contrasts markedly with the case of the scientist who, if lucky, discovered an agent, such as Mapharsen, after the start of the academic-industrial agreement. Second, it was often but not always the case that a company extended an offer of collaboration to the university scientist who made a therapeutic discovery. It was a fact of corporate life that a company needed to be among the first to capitalize on therapeutic discoveries in order to remain competitive in the pharmaceutical industry. On the other side, university scientists who hoped to apply their discoveries to practical therapeutics required assistance too. If not already known, a suitable method of preparing the product—capable of being scaled up—had to be worked out. Also, the product had to be made available to the thousands or millions who needed the therapy. Universities did not have the facilities to manufacture drugs on a large scale, so some academic scientists turned to companies to mass produce their drug and occasionally to assist in the experimental development of the drug.

The company and the university scientist, then, required assistance from each other.

Third, at the conclusion of their negotiations a company and university usually came to some formal agreement, which was not necessarily unique to this typology. This contract typically addressed such topics as the tasks of each party, possible commercial arrangements, the sharing of research (including publication policies) with outsiders, quality control for the drug, and advertising. Fourth, the collaborators laid out plans for testing the item in the laboratory and the clinic. In the case of clinical evaluations, a few outside testing centers were needed in order to obtain a sufficient number of cases for the collaborators to be able to make a reliable estimation of the value of the drug.

Fifth, if the company could manufacture the drug adequately (without its being prohibitively expensive for the patient), and if the preliminary clinical tests were promising, the collaborators invited additional clinics to test the drug. Sixth, if the expanded clinical testing program was satisfactory, the collaborators elected to have the company begin general distribution of the product across the country. Finally, the pharmaceutical firm and the university usually terminated their active interchange of research data at this point, although the two might remain in contact for many years thereafter. For example, the academic party might arrange to receive patent royalties from the company, or it might maintain quality control over the manufacture of the product. Also, the company might give the university workers unsolicited support for a research program unrelated to the collaborative project—as a reward for the university scientists' decision to work with the company and as a means of keeping an open channel of communication should that group develop another profitable discovery.

While the cooperative developments of insulin and liver extracts may have been two of the more celebrated project collaborations during the era between the world wars, these certainly were not the only joint university-industry research projects. Sharp and Dohme, of Baltimore, for example, worked with Johns Hopkins University scientists to introduce the bactericidal chemical hexylresorcinal (Caprokol) in the mid-1920s. Also, William Murphy, of the Harvard Medical School, helped Lederle Laboratories develop a liver extract for the treatment of pernicious anemia at the same time that his colleagues at Harvard were working on a similar problem with Eli Lilly and Company. Lilly developed its popular mercurial antiseptic Merthiolate (thimerosal) in cooperation with chemist Morris Kharasch, of the University of Chicago; the company introduced this drug in 1928.

In the 1930s two faculty members at the Harvard Medical School collaborated with Parke, Davis and Company, of Detroit, on Dilantin, a drug for epilepsy that is still used today. A German chemist synthesized Dilantin (diphenyl hydantoin) in 1908 as a laboratory curiosity. Parke-Davis workers investigated Dilantin as a potential hypnotic agent in the early 1920s, most likely because it was very similar chemically to an established hypnotic—Nirvanol—but they rejected Dilantin. When two neurologists at the Harvard Medical School—Tracy J. Putnam and H. Houston Merritt—initiated a program to screen various potential anticonvulsant drugs, they contacted Parke-Davis for samples of any drugs its researchers thought might be useful. Putnam and Merritt were particularly interested in anticonvulsants without the inconvenient sedative action of phenobarbital, a drug used in epilepsy since about 1912. Dilantin was among the first lot of drugs that Parke-Davis sent to Harvard, as Merritt recently related: "We asked the pharmaceutical houses to send us some drugs which had been devised as hypnotics but had not been useful in that capacity. Parke-Davis was one of the first drug companies we asked, because the Director of Research there [Oliver Kamm] was a friend of Tracy Putnam. Parke-Davis sent about twenty-five drugs that had not worked as hypnotics. The first drug which they sent was diphenylhydantoin."[1]

On the basis of preliminary experiments in which they tested the ability of various compounds to extend a cat's convulsive threshold (by using electric shocks), Putnam and Merritt concluded that Dilantin was one of the best drugs they had investigated. Moreover, it did not manifest any soporific effect on the animals. These results, coupled with the similarly promising results that Parke-Davis scientists obtained, convinced Putnam and Merritt to launch a clinical study of the drug.[2] Their results with hundreds of patients from about 1938 to 1940 indicated that while Dilantin produced uneven results with petit mal epilepsy patients (the less severe of the two forms), the drug gave 85 percent of the grand mal patients complete or nearly complete relief from their seizures. A comparative study of Dilantin and phenobarbital in about 250 patients with grand or petit mal epilepsy conducted in the late 1930s at over a dozen medical centers revealed that over half of the patients responded better with Dilantin.[3] Not surprisingly, Dilantin was a great commercial strike for Parke-Davis.

Shortly before World War II, workers at the University of California at San Francisco and Lilly joined efforts to develop a new sulfa drug, nicotinyl sulfanilamide. Troy C. Daniels, of the College of Pharmacy at California, prepared this drug (4-nicotinyl-amino-benzenesulfonamide) in 1937 to see whether the product of a reaction between sulfanilamide and nicotinic acid would combine the pharmacological properties of each reactant. The preliminary pharmacological work on this compound, carried out by Chauncey Leake and his associates at California, suggested that nicotinyl sulfanilamide was as effective as sulfanilamide against meningococcal infections and superior to sulfanilamide in clearing some streptococcal infections.[4]

Scientists at Lilly were working with nicotinyl sulfanilamide at the same time and independently of the California group. An interference resulted late in 1939 when both sides attempted to file letters patent on this drug. However, Lilly and the Research Corporation, a private organization established in 1911 to administer patents, issue licenses, and distribute profits from patents in the form of grants throughout the United States (the Research Corporation managed Daniels's patent application), soon reached an agreement whereby Lilly withdrew its patent application.[5] By January 1940 Leake began organizing clinical evaluations of nicotinyl sulfanilamide, first among clinics in the San Francisco area and later among selected clinics elsewhere in the United States. Lilly supplied the drug in bulk for these clinical tests. Leake's occasional progress reports to the company on results in San Francisco–area clinics suggested that nicotinyl sulfanilamide might find a therapeutic niche. For example, it was considerably less toxic than sulfanilamide and yet at least as effective as the latter in some infections. But Lilly was not convinced that the results with nicotinyl sulfanilamide justified marketing this sulfa, and the firm soon lost interest in the drug.[6]

In this chapter two phenomena are apparent. First, in contrast to the general and specialist consultant, the scientist of the specific project typology of collaboration often functioned as part of a larger group of ad hoc committees and higher-level administrators on the side of the academy. For example, the fruits of the collaboration could yield tremendous dividends for the entire university, which thus required the involvement of those at higher administrative levels in addition to the collaborating biomedical scientist. Paradoxically, the implications of a nonprofit institution engaging in the development of commercial goods with a corporation necessitated certain policy statements. Such statements addressed the extent to which the university would enter the business of manufacturing, distributing, promoting, or approving drugs.

Second, again in contrast to the previous typologies of interactions, the project collaboration focused on a specific therapeutic agent rather than on a broad research program or a large class of pharmaceuticals. In other words, the drug itself was the star of this show. The following sections examine in depth how both sides contributed to the development of the drug and, in turn, how the drug affected (1) the academic scientist and his research program, (2) the university overall, and (3) the company. As we shall see, these project collaborations brought out humanitarianism, greed, solid scientific work, petty bickering, magnanimity, and subterfuge on both sides. Such a dramatic ebb and flow in the relationship between the academy and the company was inevitable when one of the estates of science lost sight of the different mission of its counterpart. However—one might say miraculously—on the whole, the collaborations accomplished what they set out to do.

The University of Toronto, Eli Lilly and Company, and Insulin

The search for the internal secretion of the pancreas to treat diabetes mellitus began three decades before Frederick Banting initiated his celebrated work at the University of Toronto. Endocrinology itself was a comparatively new field at that time.[7] The modern era of endocrinology dates from 1855, with the publication of Thomas Addison's *On the Constitutional and Local Effects of Disease of the Supra-Renal Capsules.* Although physicians and scientists knew little of the physiology of these capsules, that is, the adrenal glands, Addison was the first to identify a disease syndrome and associate it with pathological changes in the suprarenal capsules. His announcement stimulated others to investigate the physiology of the adrenal glands, including the French-American physiologist Charles Edouard Brown-Séquard. Brown-Séquard's more significant work concerned rejuvenation studies with testicular extracts, which he reported in 1889. Based on this research, he postulated the existence of various internal secretions in animals, a lack of which produced diseases. He suggested that extracts could be prepared from certain animal tissues to capture these internal secretions and that these extracts could then be employed to fight diseases connected with those particular tissues.

Brown-Séquard's work was applied much more readily in medical quackery than in scientific medicine.[8] Some discoveries during the 1890s, however, lent credibility to Brown-Séquard's theories and accelerated investigations of internal secretions. In 1891 George Redmayne Murray, of the Hospital for Sick Children in Newcastle, reported his successful treatment of myxedema, a thyroid disorder, by injecting an extract of the thyroid. Three years later an English physician from Harrogate, George Oliver, and Edward Schäfer, a physiologist from University College, London, published their discovery of an adrenal gland extract that elicited a pressor reaction. They later collaborated on the discovery of another pressor substance, vasopressin, located in the posterior pituitary gland.

William Maddock Bayliss and Ernest Henry Starling, of University College, demonstrated the nature of the mechanism involved in internal secretions. In 1902 they published their results on the triggering of pancreatic juice. They found that the pancreas secreted this juice after the stomach contents passed into the duodenum even if all nerves connecting the pancreas and intestine were cut. Next they prepared an extract from the duodenal mucous membrane and injected this into the animal's bloodstream. This triggered the secretion of pancreatic juice, thus establishing the chemical—rather than the neurological—nature of the mechanism. They named this internal secretion from the duodenum secretin. In 1905 Starling proposed the term *hormone* (from the Greek *hormōn*, present participle of *horman*, "to excite, stimulate") for substances that, like secretin, form in one organ and pass through the circulation to another organ to produce a response.

Joseph von Mering and Oscar Minkowski, at the University of Strasbourg, provided a solid link between the pancreas and diabetes in 1889. Much to their surprise, when they removed the pancreas to observe its effect on digestion, diabetes resulted. Eugene Opie, a pathologist at Johns Hopkins, localized the connection between the pancreas and diabetes even further. In 1901 he demonstrated a link between diabetes and impaired islets of Langerhans—pancreatic cells smaller than the others in this organ, discovered in the late 1860s.

Once scientists discovered which organ was most likely responsible for diabetes, it was a logical step for them to attempt to extract the active ingredient, that is, the internal secretion, from that organ.[9] Minkowski was the first of many who tried to treat diabetes with pancreatic extracts. The results, on the whole, were uneven. Attempting to isolate the internal secretion was a very difficult maneuver, because the proteolytic enzymes in the pancreatic external (digestive) secretion rapidly inactivated the internal secretion. From 1911 to 1912 a graduate student at the University of Chicago, Ernest Lyman Scott, tried to bypass this problem by tying off the pancreatic ducts. He believed that this would force the pancreatic juice-secreting cells to atrophy, leaving the islets of Langerhans intact, but he failed to induce atrophy of any part of the pancreas. Next he prepared extracts of whole pancreas with alcohol, achieving good results with a few of his diabetic dogs. But Scott abandoned this research. For one thing, the alcoholic extracts actually elevated the blood sugar in some of his animals. Also, Scott was aware that a growing number of physiologists, including his adviser, doubted that the internal secretion of the pancreas could be isolated.

Between 1915 and 1920 Israel Kleiner, at the Rockefeller Institute, and Nicolas Paulesco, in Bucharest, compiled perhaps the best results with pancreatic extracts prior to the Toronto work. Using water as an extractive agent and making use of recent advances in the technology of blood-sugar determinations, they reported impressive reductions in sugar and ketones in the blood and urine. Moreover, toxic side effects from these extracts were comparatively minor. Such untoward effects as kidney failure, vomiting, and convulsions invalidated whatever positive results earlier researchers had managed with their extracts. Unfortunately, Kleiner ceased diabetes research after leaving the Rockefeller Institute, probably because of a lack of funding, and while Paulesco continued his investigations, his results failed to generate much interest among researchers in the field.

The person responsible for initiating the research at the University of Toronto that eventually led to the discovery of insulin, Frederick Grant Banting (1891–1941), was hardly a mainstream investigator in diabetes research; in fact, his laboratory experience in general was limited at most.[10] Banting was a practicing physician in London, Ontario, when he devised an experiment late in October 1920 to ligate the pancreatic ducts of dogs, wait for the pancreatic juice-secreting cells to atrophy, and finally isolate the internal secretion from the islets. (Although this was similar to Scott's experiment several years earlier, Banting was not aware of Scott's work at the time.) Banting approached John James Rickard Macleod (1876–1935), a physiologist at the University of Toronto with a special interest in carbohydrate metabolism, about the feasibility of pursuing his research in Macleod's laboratory. Macleod was understandably hesitant at first, but eventually the determined Banting convinced Macleod. With Charles Herbert Best (1899–1978), a medical student and research assistant to Macleod, at his side, Banting began his search for the internal secretion of the pancreas on 17 May 1921.

The experimental procedure that Banting and Macleod mapped out was straightforward. In one group of dogs, Banting would ligate the pancreatic ducts, wait several weeks for degeneration to occur, and then remove what was left of the pancreas. In another group he would extirpate the pancreas and upon the onset of diabetes either graft pieces of the atrophied pancreas into the diabetic dog or inject an extract. Best had charge of the blood-sugar and glycosuria determinations. Banting operated on many dogs before he mastered the operations, but between 30 July and 7 August the pair managed to perform their first series of therapeutic tests. Their extracts lowered the blood sugar in each of three diabetic dogs; they even revived one dog from a diabetic coma. However, their data were far from complete or satisfactory. In another test, carried out through August, Banting and Best compared two diabetic dogs, only one of which they gave pancreatic extracts. The blood sugar of the dog receiving "isletin" (the name Banting and Best gave to their extracts) remained well below the control dog's blood sugar. The latter survived only four days, whereas the dog given isletin lasted over two weeks.

The lack of a steady supply of extracts impeded the progress of these experiments; it took about five to seven weeks for the pancreas to atrophy sufficiently before removal. Hence the importance of Banting and Best's observation early in December that alcoholic extracts of fresh, whole adult pancreases could significantly lower blood sugar. Earlier, Scott had made the same observations, which he may have passed along to Macleod; however, it is not clear whether Macleod later informed Banting and Best of Scott's observation.

Soon after Banting and Best's December observation, Macleod invited a biochemist on sabbatical at the University of Toronto, James Bertram Collip (1892–1965), to join Banting and Best. Banting had long been needling Macleod for more manpower; Collip had told Macleod earlier of his desire to take part in the research; and most of all, the preliminary results were promising and warranted an expansion of personnel. Collip soon made his presence felt: he significantly improved the purity of extracts by preparing each batch of whole beef pancreases with increasingly concentrated alcohol; also, he discovered that the extracts could lower the blood sugar of normal rabbits. This provided the group with a means of standardizing their preparations. Collip provided the first experimental evidence at Toronto that the pancreas extracts could eliminate ketones as well as sugar from the urine, and he compiled incontrovertible evidence that the preparations restored the liver's glycogenetic function. Both results were solid indications of the extract's antidiabetic value (see fig. 11).

The Toronto group tested their insulin clinically in late December and early January: it had little or no benefit to the patient. But in late January 1922 an extract prepared by Collip drastically reduced the patient's blood sugar and glycosuria and eliminated his ketonuria. The group soon planned an expansion of the clinical testing program in Toronto. To accommodate this expansion, the University of Toronto's Connaught Anti-Toxin Laboratories, established in 1914, set up facilities in the basement of the medical building for large-scale production of insulin, which Best directed. For unknown reasons, the ability to produce insulin escaped the Toronto researchers through March and April, but they modified their process, and in May production was on again. The publicity generated by their initial reports and publications resulted in a rising number of requests for the treatment in May.[11] This, coupled with recurrent problems in scaling up insulin production, led the group to seek outside assistance.

Negotiating an Agreement for Collaboration

The Toronto group hoped to produce as much insulin as possible, as inexpensively as possible. Their attempts to produce insulin on a large scale, however, resulted in zero yield.[12] Even if Toronto had succeeded in scaling up production, the university (including its Connaught Laboratories) simply lacked the resources necessary to satisfy the demand for this drug. What the Toronto group needed was a reliable pharmaceutical firm with the facilities, know-how, and desire to help them fulfill their aspirations for insulin. They found such an organization in Eli Lilly and Company, of Indianapolis.

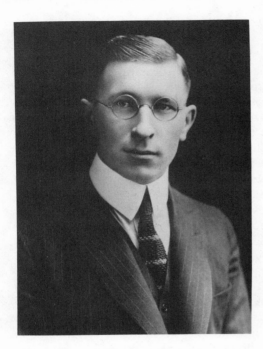

Figure 11. The principal workers who discovered insulin (1921-22) at the University of Toronto.

Frederick Grant Banting was a general practitioner from London, Ontario (courtesy of the University of Toronto Archives).

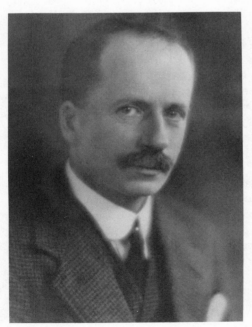

John James Rickard Macleod was professor of physiology at Toronto (courtesy of the University of Toronto Archives and Ashley and Crippen).

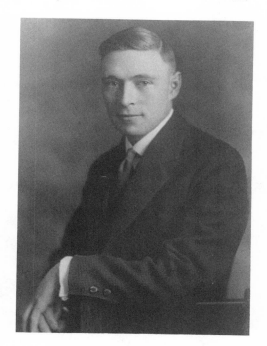

James Bertram Collip was professor of biochemistry at the University of Alberta (courtesy of the Banting-Collip Collection, Medical Museum, University Hospital, London, Canada).

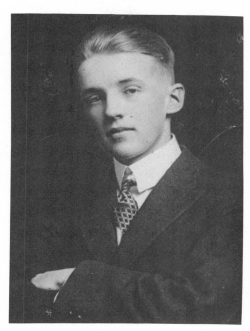

Charles Herbert Best was a medical student and an assistant in Macleod's laboratory (courtesy of the University of Toronto Archives).

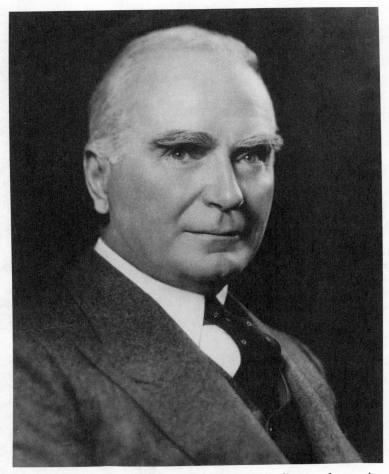

Figure 12. George Henry Alexander Clowes (1877–1958), director of research at Eli Lilly and Company from 1919 to 1946 (courtesy of Eli Lilly and Company).

The Toronto group had good reason to select Lilly as a collaborator. In the first place, Lilly recently had added several therapeutic gland products to its inventory when Banting and Best started their insulin research. The company listed many different preparations of nearly a dozen glands and gland products in its 1922 price list. The experience Lilly gained in manufacturing and physiologically standardizing such items as pituitary extract played no small part in Toronto's decision to work with the Indianapolis firm.[13] Even more important to Toronto was the company's director of research, G. H. A. Clowes, who represented Lilly in the negotiations with the university. Clowes's scientific stature and Lilly's support of his ongoing fundamental research in Indianapolis and at the Marine Biological Laboratory in Woods Hole, Massachusetts, convinced the Toronto group that this was the kind of company they wanted to work with (see fig. 12).[14]

Clowes first heard of Toronto's insulin work in October 1921, possibly from Lewellys Barker, a professor of medicine at Johns Hopkins and an alumnus of the University of Toronto. However, Clowes did not approach any of the Toronto researchers to volunteer his company as a collaborator until late December 1921. He met with Banting, Best, and Macleod immediately following the presentation of their results at the meeting of the American Physiological Society in New Haven, Connecticut. Even though the group had no clinical results and had not even attempted to scale up production, Clowes informed them that the company wanted to help in any way possible to advance the research and mass production of insulin.[15] Lilly's offer of assistance was a logical extension of both the company's recent policy emphasizing the development of specialties and Clowes's personal belief in the importance of industry-university collaborations. In addition, getting in early on a treatment for a disease for which no satisfactory treatment existed made enormous commercial sense, given the prevalence of diabetes. It was the kind of opportunity that could elevate a company to the upper echelons of the pharmaceutical industry. Thus, even though the Toronto group's work by late December 1921 was still inconclusive, Lilly was eager to collaborate.

Macleod informed Clowes that the group was not far enough along on insulin research for industrial production of the drug, but he promised to consider the offer from Lilly. Clowes contacted Macleod again three months later, reminding him of Lilly's interest in the insulin work. If Toronto would share with Lilly the details of its method for producing insulin, Clowes said, the company could supply the university with the hormone for experimental and clinical investigations. Moreover, the company would not market insulin until the University of Toronto believed the drug was ready for mass distribution. If Lilly could arrange with Toronto to market insulin, Clowes said, the university could expect to receive royalties. Lilly was prepared to begin its own research on insulin with or without Toronto's assistance, although Clowes assured Macleod that Lilly preferred the former. Macleod's position had not changed since his meeting with Clowes in New Haven. His laboratory was still working feverishly in the hopes of publishing a detailed method so that insulin production could begin "elsewhere." If Toronto's failures persisted, they would possibly engage Lilly to help find a solution.[16]

The Toronto group were not incognizant of parties that might, and probably would, profit from their discovery by taking unfair advantage of the public; indeed, the history of medicine is replete with examples of medical fraudulence.[17] Macleod and his colleagues believed, rather naively, that publishing a detailed process for making nontoxic insulin preparations would sufficiently protect the public. But such a procedure did not appear in any journals, because the Toronto scientists never found a reliable method of production to report prior to the collaboration with Lilly. Also, in April 1922 they began to move towards another means of protection, protection for both the public health and their own research—the patent. As patentees, the Toronto group could control licenses to pharmaceutical firms for the manufacture of insulin. While this would not—and in fact, did not—prevent unlicensed firms from producing pancreatic extracts, at least it would enable the scientists to ensure that there were safe, effective, and perhaps reasonably priced preparations of insulin on the market.[18] A patent would give Toronto, rather than a commercial interest, a monopoly on insulin, and thereby effect a de facto demonopolized insulin industry: "The patent would not be used for any other purpose than to prevent the taking out of a patent by other persons. When the details of the method of preparation are published anyone would be free to prepare the extract, but no one could secure a profitable monopoly."[19]

The Toronto group applied for a U.S. patent on insulin and a method of preparing it in May 1922, shortly before representatives from the university and Lilly met to arrange terms for a collaboration. The patent would have a profound bearing on later interactions between the university and Lilly. Lilly encouraged the group to patent insulin and offered them counsel on the U.S. patent application. This advice, combined with Clowes's continuing inquiries about both the status of the Toronto work and the possibility of cooperative research, and Toronto's continuing problems with large-scale production led the Toronto group to invite Lilly representatives to Toronto for a conference in late May. Clowes, company vice-president Eli Lilly (1885–1977), a chemist (probably George Walden), and a patent attorney from the Lilly Company together with personnel from the University of Toronto, forged a contract for cooperative research on insulin that was the source of more than a few disputes between the two parties over the next year.[20]

Around the time when the University of Toronto was considering the issues of the insulin patent and collaborative research, the board of governors created the Insulin Committee. The committee, composed of representatives from the board of governors, the Connaught Laboratories, and the university faculty,[21] had several functions. For example, it was responsible for licensing companies to produce insulin. The chief responsibility of the Insulin Committee was to oversee quality control for North American insulin producers. As part of this function, the Insulin Committee Laboratory was established early in 1923 to provide the necessary checks for proper standardization and uniformity on commercial products. The committee also screened advertising by Lilly and other companies producing insulin. In all dealings with the Lilly Company, the Insulin Committee represented the interests of the University of Toronto.[22]

The bulk of the agreement between Toronto and Lilly, dated 30 May 1922, addressed strategies in the exchange of information between the university and company and how the former would license the latter. The Toronto group would divulge all they knew about insulin and would send representatives (usually Best and one other scientist) to Lilly to demonstrate personally how to produce and physiologically standardize insulin. A virtual hormonal highway was beaten between Toronto and Indianapolis during 1922; Best claimed that he visited Lilly nine times in that year, and Clowes made as many as twenty-five trips to Toronto. Lilly could not share information obtained from Toronto with anyone else, although it is difficult to believe that the company would even want to divulge any of Toronto's data. Lilly also was obligated, as long as it was a licensee, to inform Toronto of any improvements it made in producing insulin. If any of these improvements were patentable, the company had to assign the patents to Toronto, with the exception of patent applications in the United States.[23]

As the sole collaborator with Toronto, Lilly would have an appreciable head start over its competitors in the nascent insulin industry. Toronto considered it inefficient to collaborate with more than one company. But despite Lilly's retention of rights in the United States, it ceded considerable ground to Toronto—not that it was in a position to offer much opposition; Toronto certainly needed assistance, but there were several capable firms the university could have approached. The Toronto group had the upper hand. The fact that they were under no obligation to keep their own or Lilly's research secret attests to this. If sensitive information fell into the hands of one of Lilly's competitors, the Indianapolis firm could find itself embattled in a U.S. patent interference.

Toronto took steps against such a possibility by circulating production details among only a minimum of outsiders. In order to keep this information away from commercial organizations, Macleod issued warnings to the few diabetes specialists who received insulin data.[24] Clowes, however, was more concerned with the fact that the Toronto workers were releasing production information to outsiders before Lilly had a chance to supply them: "Information regarding the mode of preparation of [insulin] was given by members of the Toronto group to a few individuals with the result that the procedure was widely known some months earlier than we had anticipated would be the case. . . . Information about such matters spreads rapidly and most of the men to whom we are now supplying the product have indicated their intention of making it if we could not supply them at once."[25] The licensure stipulations of the contract established a limited-term exclusive license for Lilly. During a so-called experimental period, Lilly would have the sole right to produce and sell insulin. The experimental period would last one year, and the Toronto group could extend it if they so desired. Lilly would sell insulin at cost or distribute it gratis, at its own discretion, to a select group of clinicians. Toronto was guaranteed a proportion of Lilly's output—12–28 percent, depending on whether or not the company charged for insulin.[26] This last clause was probably included because (1) production at the University of Toronto's Connaught Laboratories, which was mostly earmarked for Canadian distribution, was still uneven at best; (2) it assured the Toronto group of avoiding a potentially embarrassing situation—an insulin drought in Canada while Americans would be receiving the drug;[27] and (3) insulin was, after all, the Toronto group's discovery, and they probably felt that this warranted them certain proprietary rights in its development.

The terms of licensure also covered the years following the experimental period, when Toronto planned to institute a program of general licensing for the pharmaceutical industry. The university guaranteed Lilly an insulin license for the life of the patent, in exchange for which Lilly (and other licensees) would pay the university a 5 percent royalty. Lilly actually supported insulin research at Toronto decades after the insulin patents expired.[28]

Finally, the Toronto-Lilly contract included somewhat ambiguous statements regarding advertising and publicity. The university and the company would collaborate on how Lilly advertised the drug. Also, Toronto would decide in what way Lilly could use the names of the Toronto scientists in publicizing insulin. The university already had transgressed traditional medical ethics, at least in the eyes of some, by applying for a patent on a medicinal agent.[29] So Toronto wished to play down its own role in the marketing of insulin and thereby avoid any misconceptions that the group was personally profiting from the sale of insulin. Another issue related to advertising concerned Lilly's use of a trade name for insulin, Iletin. The relevant clause in the contract did not state explicitly that Lilly had the right to use a trade name but suggested that "upon the termination of this agreement [if Lilly cannot profitably produce insulin] the Trade

Name or Names used by [Lilly] in connection with the said extracts [i.e., insulin], shall thereupon become the property of [Toronto]."[30]

Research, Production, and Distribution

The Lilly Company organized its insulin research team and even produced its first successful lot of the hormone before signing the contract. The company heads, Josiah K. Lilly, Sr. (1861–1948), and his son Eli, were prepared to invest a quarter of a million dollars to get large-scale production rolling. George Walden headed insulin research at Lilly, and Harley W. Rhodehamel, Jasper P. Scott, and Walden's wife, Eda Bachman, all chemists, assisted in the project.[31]

The clinical evaluation of this scarce and dangerous drug required thoughtful planning. It should be remembered that the clinical trials were voluntary; the time had not yet arrived when controlled trials of experimental drugs were mandated by legislative fiat. The collaborators decided that distribution would be limited to jointly selected diabetes specialists during the experimental period. Furthermore, because of the uncertainty in production, clinicians could administer insulin in only the most severe cases.[32] Clowes organized a clinical advisory committee—the first to use insulin in the United States and Canada—who evaluated questions about the posology, forms of administration, and overall value of the hormone. They also processed all clinical data—a considerable task after 1922 as the clinical program expanded. The clinical advisory committee maintained a discreet existence in order to avoid both popularizing insulin in the press and offending clinicians not invited to join the committee.[33]

Lilly's strategy was to maintain small-scale—that is, experimental—projects and mass-production projects simultaneously in Indianapolis. The company also supported insulin research at Woods Hole under Clowes's direction during his summers away from Indianapolis. The pharmaceutical firm took quick advantage of Toronto's results and started a laboratory scale run of insulin on 2 June 1922. Best, probably accompanied by Collip, arrived in Indianapolis five days later to demonstrate personally how to make insulin. The Lilly researchers learned fast. They successfully produced their first lot of the drug by 17 June. Within a month they were able to devise several useful innovations in the extraction process. For example, Lilly workers used 5 percent of the amount of solvent (alcohol or acetone) that Toronto had employed in part of its method. The company also improved the procedure by extracting insulin under refrigeration; this helped to inhibit the catalytic deterioration of the active ingredient of the pancreas.[34]

Another problem that Lilly solved from the start involved eliminating the solvent used to capture insulin from the pancreas. Too much heat to evaporate the solvent could destroy the active ingredient. The Toronto researchers alleviated the problem by placing shallow pans containing the insulin extract beneath hot coils in a wind tunnel. The process worked, but it was inefficient and dangerous. Lilly was never satisfied with the wind-tunnel method and instead concentrated extracts in vacuum stills. These lowered pressure sufficiently to evaporate the solvent at a low temperature, thus avoiding the possibility of destroying the hormone. Vacuum stills were expensive, however, and the University of Toronto was unable to purchase a still until late in the summer of 1922.[35]

Lilly's insulin production was maintained on a small scale until the autumn of 1922; nevertheless, it increased enormously through June, July, and August. Virtually all Lilly insulin not earmarked for experimental studies went to Banting during June and July. In fact, Toronto received nearly 60 percent of Lilly's output from June through August, far above the amount the company was contractually obligated to provide. Lilly's success came at a crucial time, because Toronto's production, which had been struggling for some time, apparently broke down completely in July. During the late summer and early autumn of 1922, Lilly essentially was the sole supplier of insulin with the exception of W. D. Sansum, of the Potter Metabolic Clinic in Santa Barbara, California, and R. T. Woodyatt, of the Otho Sprague Memorial Institute Laboratory for Chemical Research and the Presbyterian Hospital, in Chicago. Both of these physicians prepared insulin for their patients according to Toronto's publications and directions provided by Macleod.[36] The collaborators expanded the clinical testing program in August by including the American members of the clinical advisory committee and four other medical centers. Thus, by the end of August, a total of twelve groups representing eight states and one Canadian province were involved in the clinical side of the insulin project. Banting, the least experienced of all the participating physicians, received the most insulin from Lilly, an average of over 550 units per week from late July through August.[37] The leading diabetes specialists—Elliott Joslin, of the Harvard Medical School and the New England Deaconess Hospital, Boston, and Frederick Allen, of the Psychiatric Institute, Morristown, New Jersey—received much more insulin from Lilly during August than any other American physicians—more than 150 units per week each—although this was still well below Banting's complement.[38]

Assembling clinical personnel to evaluate insulin led to some disagreements between Toronto and Lilly. The contract stipulated that Lilly and Toronto together would choose the clinicians to receive insulin during the experimental period. Clowes interpreted the agreement differently. Of the first one to two dozen physicians who took part in the clinical program, Clowes sought the Insulin Committee's permission to supply only those who received an appreciable amount of insulin (one hundred units or more weekly). The Insulin Committee was unaware that Lilly was supplying about a half-dozen fairly inexperienced physicians with fifty to one hundred units of insulin. When Macleod voiced his disapproval of this procedure, Clowes retorted in characteristic fashion. First, he explained that knowing the kinds of problems that confronted an inexperienced doctor using insulin therapy would be helpful later, when insulin became available to the general medical public. Second, Clowes assumed that as long as the collaborators had a solid group of investigators working on insulin (Joslin, Allen, and so on), a few more physicians in the testing program need not warrant approval from Toronto. Third, he believed the contract should not be interpreted rigidly anyway; it should "be handled as a sort of gentlemen's agreement." Finally, Clowes admitted that Lilly feared that physicians would start manufacturing their own insulin or would collaborate with other firms to produce the drug if Lilly could not supply them. (The company's motivation here, to inundate the market during the experimental period, will be discussed later in this chapter.) Clowes's arguments may have explained the company's procedure, but after September 1922 Lilly made sure to obtain the Insulin Committee's approval before adding new names to the list of clinical investigators.[39]

Lilly continued to increase its insulin output during September, almost doubling its production in June and July. Qualitatively, however, Lilly already had begun to experience difficulties. By mid-September clinical results revealed that Lilly's insulin lots produced in late August were less than half the strength of earlier lots. Clowes attributed the loss in potency to errors in standardization, since Lilly workers diluted the extract to the desired strength on the basis of bioassay results. Impurities began to creep into the Lilly product at the same time. Clowes believed that this was due to a reagent too weak to precipitate unwanted proteins and other substances out of the insulin solution. He could not settle the problems unequivocally until he returned to Indianapolis from Woods Hole, but he was confident enough in September to inform Toronto that his company was ready to swing into mass production around 1 October: "You may rest assured that the industrial problem has virtually been solved and that we shall be able to produce [insulin] in very large amounts in the near future" (see fig. 13).[40]

The problem was far from solved. Although Clowes felt that the manufacturing process was not the source of the loss in potency, he really had little on which to base this assumption. The company ceased performing stability tests on insulin lots in August. To account for this, Clowes argued that the clinical demand for insulin was too great to withhold samples for experimental work or to pull employees off production work, especially after the breakdown in production at the Connaught Laboratories. Also, he continued, even if there were a chance of deterioration, physicians would use the drug soon. Clowes learned in mid-October, upon analyzing a

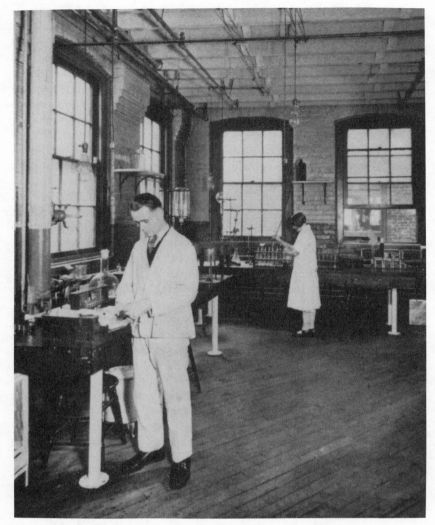

Figure 13. Eli Lilly and Company employees testing the potency of insulin (from *The Lilly Laboratories,* 1930, courtesy of Eli Lilly and Company).

sample from an early lot produced by a scaled-up method, that the problem with diminishing strength of insulin was indeed due to the manufacturing process. The insulin deteriorated even before it left the plant. Thus,
Lilly switched to a different large-scale method, one that produced a stable
product but had a small yield.[41]

That physicians would be using insulin soon was an unacceptable ex-
cuse for Lilly's abandoning stability testing. Clowes knew very well that
stability considerations were an important part of quality control. But the
question of demand for the drug was a more complex issue. Late summer
and early fall were chaotic for Toronto and Lilly. To some extent the chaos
was self-imposed. Both were overextending themselves, expanding the
clinical program at a rate beyond their capacity to fulfill the demand for
insulin. Toronto's production was struggling, and Lilly was hard-pressed
to pick up the slack. The company was trying to fill Banting's complement
of the drug and maintain the other clinicians' supplies as well while
strapped to either a small-scale process or a poor industrial-scale method
of producing insulin. The ethical dilemma in this issue—whether or not
the collaborators should distribute a product of undetermined stability—
is too tangential to address here. Certainly this was a decision that Toronto
and Lilly should have made together, in the spirit of a true collaboration.
In any case, the issue soon became academic: during the fall of 1922 Lilly
was working out a method that drastically improved insulin production.

The person most responsible for turning Lilly's production around was
George B. Walden. Walden joined the company in 1917, the same year that
he received the bachelor of science degree from Franklin College in Indiana. At Woods Hole, Clowes introduced Walden to studies that the latter
would use to refashion insulin manufacture.[42]

The renowned physiologist Jacques Loeb recently had carried out important fundamental work at Woods Hole on the nature and importance
of isoelectric points of proteins. Proteins and their constituent parts,
amino acids, have the ability to behave as either acids or bases, depending
on the circumstances. The isoelectric point of an amino acid or protein is
that pH (a measure of hydrogen ion concentration) of the solvent at which
the amino acid or protein has a balanced positive and negative charge. For
example, the substance will not move to a positive or negative cathode in
an electrical field. At the isoelectric point, proteins are "less soluble [than
at any other pH] and more readily coagulated and more readily salted out."
Loeb showed that one could determine the isoelectric point of a protein in
solution by plotting certain physicochemical properties of the protein,
such as osmotic pressure, as a function of the pH of the solvent. The isoelectric point occurred at the pH corresponding to the minimum values of
any of these properties. For example, the osmotic pressure of a protein
solution will decrease as the pH is increased, but beyond a particular pH

the osmotic pressure will increase; that particular pH is the isoelectric point of the protein. By examining several physicochemical properties, one can arrive at a fairly narrow range on the pH scale within which the isoelectric point lies.[43]

Walden applied the method of isoelectric precipitation to ipecac, squill, and some other medicinals at least a year before he began working on the isoelectric point of insulin. It took him a few months to perfect the process for insulin production, but by November Lilly was ready to apply isoelectric precipitation on a mass scale. Walden discovered that the problems with deterioration of the insulin solutions and impurities had resulted from the slow formation of an insulin-bearing precipitate from the solution, leaving some of the hormone and impurities in the latter. The aim of Walden's process was to stimulate as much precipitation as possible. Starting with the old process—extracting insulin directly from the pancreas with some solvent, continuing the extraction with a more concentrated solvent, and evaporating the solvent so that insulin could be transferred to an aqueous solvent for delivery to the patient—Walden adjusted the pH of the insulin solution to what he determined to be the isoelectric point—between 4.5 and 5.3—and he let the solution stand for about a week. After collecting the precipitate, he readjusted the pH of the solution to the isoelectric point, obtaining as much additional precipitate as possible. He dissolved the precipitates in water and adjusted the pH of the aqueous insulin solution so that it fell outside of the isoelectric point.[44]

Walden's method markedly bettered the yield and the purity of insulin, in addition to the stability. Theretofore, workers customarily had discarded the insulin-containing precipitate during extraction, believing that all of the insulin was in solution. Isoelectric precipitation also solved the difficulties with manufacturing pure insulin: "This purity is so great that out of several hundred patients to whom [insulin] has so far been administered, including some who exhibited sensitization effects with the best product previously obtainable, not a single instance of sensitization or any other deleterious effect has been reported."[45]

Walden was not the only person working on the isoelectric precipitation of insulin in the early 1920s. Collip apparently investigated this subject for a time, but without success. A biochemist at Washington University School of Medicine in St. Louis, Philip Shaffer, developed the isoelectric precipitation of insulin independently of Walden. Shaffer's interest in diabetes arose from his research, begun around 1910, on blood and urine analysis. When Banting and his associates announced their discovery, Shaffer tried unsuccessfully to obtain some of the hormone from Toronto for testing. Consequently, Shaffer's group started to produce insulin themselves and in the course of their research discovered what Walden had found at about the same time. Shaffer and a colleague announced their discovery at the annual meeting of the American Society of Biological Chemists in Toronto in late December 1922. Shaffer's discovery was especially important to Toronto as a means of blocking Lilly's attempt to monopolize the insulin market in the United States (see below).[46]

The improved process began to manifest a dramatic impact on insulin output late in the fall of 1922. Also at this time, the University of Toronto Insulin Committee and the informal clinical advisory committee met in Toronto to work out a strategy for an efficient clinical study of insulin in the least possible time. The participants charged certain clinics to examine particular problems associated with insulin therapy. They also decided to publish the first extensive clinical results with insulin together in a special issue of the *Journal of Metabolic Research*.[47]

Lilly was at the point where it could easily furnish more than enough insulin for the investigators in the clinical program, so the Insulin Committee asked the company to increase the allotments to the cooperating clinics. For example, in December 1922 Lilly was prepared to supply Toronto alone with 8,000–10,000 units weekly. By January the Connaught Laboratories were able to exploit Lilly's manufacturing advances, and the two were supplying insulin to about 250 physicians in sixty clinics. Two months later Lilly alone supplied at least one hundred clinics, producing nearly 300,000 units weekly for American and Canadian consumption. Clowes's declaration in March 1923 spoke as much for his hard-sell approach for a Lilly insulin monopoly as it did for his company's technical accomplishments in the past few months: "Our over-production is now so tremendous that you can assure the Toronto Committee that there is not the remotest chance of our having any difficulty in supplying any amount that may be required, not only in the United States and Canada, but throughout the entire civilized world."[48]

The number of clinical groups increased from the fall of 1922 to the spring of 1923, but the increase in distribution was not nearly as rapid as Lilly wanted. According to the contract of 30 May, Toronto and Lilly were supposed to collaborate on the selection of physicians for the clinical testing program. But the Insulin Committee continually rebuffed the pharmaceutical firm's requests for a much more extensive distribution of insulin during the experimental period. Toronto was waiting for the preliminary clinical reports to appear in print and for the establishment of a sufficient number of insulin instructional centers in major diabetes clinics to educate the medical community about this new and potentially dangerous drug.[49]

Lilly abided by Toronto's decision, holding its sales force at bay with circulars that cautioned against volunteering information on insulin to physicians.[50] The most important criterion employed for the expansion of the clinical program was the physician's access to adequate clinical and laboratory facilities for metabolic disorders. Hence, most of the cooperating physicians chosen early in the program were attached to university clinics or well-established hospitals. The collaborators also had to supply the drug to the family physicians of patients discharged from distant diabetes clinics. Independent group clinics began to play an active part in the testing of insulin by the late winter and/or early spring of 1923. However, fearing that many of these clinics existed primarily for business reasons, and not for the sake of efficiency, Macleod wanted to be absolutely sure that such clinics had proper facilities.[51]

The clinical results with insulin by the end of the experimental period mirrored Henry Dale and H. W. Dudley's preliminary assessment of the drug's therapeutic application seven months earlier: "These practical difficulties being clearly recognized as compromising the value of the treatment, we are left with the impression that the clinical application of insulin has, nevertheless, been brilliantly successful in its general result."[52] Toronto maintained restrictions on the distribution of insulin through the summer and early fall of 1923. Finally, the Insulin Committee permitted Lilly to offer the drug through general distribution beginning on 15 October.[53]

Confrontations during the Experimental Period

Lilly desperately wanted to distribute insulin on a much wider scale than Toronto had planned. To some extent, Lilly's motivations had an altruistic component—to supply dying diabetics with this drug. President J. K. Lilly's proclamation on finding his company in the middle of this historic research illustrates this sense of humanitarianism: "I am almost overwhelmed with this tremendous situation, and experience some difficulty in keeping my feet on the ground and my brain in normal operation." But profit clearly was the driving force for Lilly to spread insulin. Toronto guaranteed Lilly's exclusive license for only one year; having a short-term monopoly on a drug with a restricted distribution was hardly an ideal commercial situation, but Lilly made the best of it. The basic strategy, according to J. K. Lilly, was to "create [insulin] centers in every possible place, thus securing priority and cementing the doctors to us."[54]

Lilly cemented the doctors in two ways. The contract of 30 May 1922 left it entirely up to Lilly whether to offer insulin free to the participating clinics or to charge cost for the drug. The company circulated insulin gratis from June through most of January 1923. It considered switching to distribution at cost as early as September 1922 but decided otherwise. Of course, this approach put Lilly deep into debt during the early months of the collaboration, but the company was planning for supremacy in the insulin market after the experimental period. Judging from Joslin's reaction, Lilly's decision paid off. Joslin affirmed his allegiance to Lilly insulin in an address at the company's dedication of its new research laboratories; he specifically mentioned that he routinely reminded salesmen of competing companies that his clinic had received free insulin from Lilly for several months.[55]

The second way Lilly tried to assure itself of superiority in the future insulin market was by establishing a trade name for its product—Iletin— early in the collaboration. The available evidence suggests that Toronto not only consented to Lilly's use of a trade name but recommended Iletin, based on *isletin*, a term Banting and Best originally coined for insulin. The Toronto workers themselves referred to insulin as Iletin on occasion. Lilly had been labeling its shipments to Toronto as Iletin for over three months when, in September of 1922, Henry Dale finally enlightened the Insulin Committee as to the real implications of the trade name: "The Lilly name, which these people [i.e., the Insulin Committee] could not understand, seems to me now perfectly obvious. If they can make use of their start [i.e., the experimental period] to get the name 'Iletin' used by all the clinicians as the name for the hormone they will easily upset the patent, get clear of control, and snap their fingers at competition."[56] Dale, unlike the Toronto workers, was very familiar with the tactics of a pharmaceutical firm. Burroughs Wellcome and Company had hired him in 1904, where he remained for a decade, mostly as director of the Wellcome Physiological Research Laboratories.[57]

In a 30 September 1922 meeting between Banting, Best, Macleod, R. D. Defries (of the Connaught Laboratories), Dale, and Clowes, the participants agreed only as to how the name Iletin would be used in the upcoming clinical reports. The authors would use *insulin* in the titles of their papers and in the text when referring to the hormone," 'Iletin' being used only when details of case histories was [*sic*] given." The meeting closed with no decision on Lilly's use of the trade name as a means of curbing competition from other firms. The issue did not reappear until 29 December when the Insulin Committee apparently had to remind Clowes of their earlier agreement. Presumably, clinicians had sent reports to Toronto using the name Iletin where they should have used *insulin*. What is more important, on the following day the Insulin Committee and Clowes reached a wider understanding on usage of the name Iletin; Clowes agreed that Lilly would stop using it altogether. Within a week J. K. Lilly fired off a memorandum to Clowes informing him of the fundamental necessity of a trade name wherever competition existed. Clowes passed the memorandum on to the Insulin Committee, saying that he had little influence in the issue since the trade name was a business matter. The company had no plans to relinquish its trademark; what it would do, however, was label its product "Iletin (Insulin, Lilly)."[58]

Legally, Toronto was on shaky ground. Lilly could have pointed to the contract as its right to establish a trade name for insulin. (I have not seen any evidence suggesting that Lilly did this.) The company did not take a more active stance on Iletin because it was pushing hard for an extension of its exclusive license, and Iletin could become an academic issue, since Lilly was in the process of filing a patent on its isoelectric precipitation method. If granted, it would essentially make the Toronto patent obsolete in the United States, giving Lilly a monopoly on American production.

Clowes petitioned Toronto to extend the experimental period as early as September. He argued, first, that Toronto should extend the exclusive license beyond 30 May 1928 so that Lilly could recoup its research and development expenses. That Lilly insisted on offering insulin free did not help Clowes's argument. Second, Clowes claimed that the problems in production at Toronto forced Lilly to pick up the slack, which in turn delayed its experimental work by about two weeks. Clowes felt that this put his company at a considerable disadvantage, because Lilly "knew that others were working on the problem [of insulin manufacture]" and because Macleod disclosed Toronto's method "to a few individuals with the result that the procedure was widely known" sooner than Lilly would have wanted.[59] As mentioned above, Toronto was not obligated under the contract to withold information from others. But Macleod nonetheless cautioned those to whom he sent the process to keep the information away from other drug companies. Clowes may have had some reason for concern but his concerns were exaggerated.

Four months later J. K. Lilly made a bid, not just for an extension of the experimental period, but for a permanent exclusive license for his company. This, Lilly argued, would be in the best interest of Toronto and the diabetics, because without competition his company could "produce at lowest cost, test at lowest cost, sell at lowest price, and be able to give, without charge, much larger quantities for indigent cases." With their strong stance against allowing their discovery to be monopolized, the Toronto group were not about to entertain an offer of anything more than a temporary extension of the exclusive license. However, Lilly's argument that Toronto would only have to oversee one company in the case of a permanent exclusive license probably had some appeal to the Insulin Committee. Harvard refused to supervise any manufacturers of liver extracts other than Lilly for this very reason.[60]

As the end of the experimental period crept closer, Clowes's arguments for an extension grew increasingly frank and involved. First, he urged Toronto to continue the experimental period and not issue additional licenses, because Lilly could meet any demand for insulin. The university was not likely to pay much attention to this argument. Second, he advocated restricting insulin distribution through the remainder of 1923, which "would mean that during the current year no additonal licenses would be issued in the United States." He believed such a restriction to be necessary because of the possibility that the public might obtain insulin directly from the pharmacist without a doctor's prescription and because the company was not yet certain of the stability of its product. Third, the company needed an extension to recover its expenditures on insulin research and development; it would not be possible to accomplish this goal by 30 May, the last day of the experimental period. The collaborators had agreed earlier that general distribution could not begin until the clinical reports appeared in print, tentatively in November and December of 1922. But by March of the following year the reports still had not appeared. This delay, according to Clowes, made it impossible for the company to "saturate" the United States with its product. So Clowes argued that Lilly needed a six-month monopoly on insulin to recover its investment.[61]

Clowes also claimed that it would simply be unfair to Lilly if Toronto refused to extend the experimental period and issued licenses to other firms. Those firms could take advantage of Lilly's improvements without having to make the same investments. Finally, Clowes reminded the Insulin Committee of how much his company had contributed to the project. He said Lilly was entitled to an advantage in the insulin market.[62]

Even though Clowes's arguments may have had some validity, they must have been confusing to the Insulin Committee, because they contained several inconsistencies. For example, Clowes mentioned the need to continue restricting the distribution of insulin (at cost), yet he complained that the delay in publishing the reports (and in initiating a widespread distribution of insulin) prevented Lilly from recovering its expenditures. Also, Clowes cited the need for more data on the stability of the Lilly product as a reason for continuing the experimental period, but his letters earlier in the year claimed that the isoelectric precipitation process had solved the stability problems.

But there was a deeper problem. Even if Clowes's arguments had been more lucid, it is doubtful that he could have convinced the university to extend the exclusive license, because Toronto and Lilly had inherently different conceptions of what the experimental period was and what it was supposed to accomplish. For Toronto, the experimental period was primarily a time to perfect the manufacture of insulin and to collect all the clinical data possible within about a year. The clinical work obviously depended on the success of the manufacturing process. I have already mentioned Toronto's strong feelings against monopolies and against the commercialization of medical discoveries. These kinds of feelings were not at all unusual among academic biomedical researchers in North America at this time. Yet the Insulin Committee made a major error, because they naively assumed that Lilly, too, had the diabetic in mind above all else. Given Lilly's long history as a respectable drug manufacturer and its recent hiring of a major scientist who was given at least some free time for fundamental research, one can perhaps appreciate how the academics could have misconstrued Lilly's intentions. On the other hand, the university workers did not exercise much prudence in the matter of the trade name; the Toronto group not only affirmed Lilly's right to a trade name, they encouraged it. It was difficult, however, for Toronto to discern Lilly's long-term commercial goals when it signed the pact.

The pharmaceutical firm informed the University of Toronto very early in the collaboration that it wanted, perhaps even expected, a head start (in the form of a trade name) on the competition in the insulin market. Eli Lilly and Clowes emphasized that Toronto was aware of this and even consented to it prior to concluding the contract.[63] The appearance of a clause in the contract specifically addressing the company's use of a trade name supports this contention. Moreover, Toronto should have realized that Eli Lilly and Company depended on the sale of pharmaceuticals for its livelihood. It is true that Lilly was one of the more scientifically oriented firms, but bottom-line reasoning rested in business interests, and the company expected a return on its investments. So from Lilly's standpoint, the experimental period provided an opportunity to fulfill all possible demand with its brand of insulin, to "cement" doctors to the house brand, and to head off competition before the race even started. Unfortunately for Lilly, the firm was beginning to lose sight of the fact that the experimental period represented another opportunity: the chance to show that it could collaborate well with a university. If the insulin collaboration went smoothly and productively, it would establish a precedent for other academic workers to turn to Lilly for assistance in the development of new and profitable drugs. By March and April of 1923, neither Toronto nor Lilly was acting in a spirit conducive to future collaborations of this sort.

Macleod telegraphed Clowes on 16 March to inform him that the Insulin Committee had rejected Clowes's petitions for an extension of the experimental period, for several reasons. The University of Toronto had already published statements that it would license additional firms once the manufacturing process was perfected,[64] and once it felt that the latter was finally effected. The Insulin Committee had received "insistent requests" for licenses from some pharmaceutical firms. Also, the Medical Research Council, whom the Toronto group had licensed to supervise insulin production in Britain, had already granted licenses to several firms there. The belief that competition, rather than a monopoly, would witness as much insulin as possible produced in the shortest possible time at the lowest possible price also influenced the group's decision. Finally, the Insulin Committee feared criticism from many sides that they were favoring one company over others if they extended the license.[65]

What ensued were several turbulent weeks of moves and countermoves involving the "collaborators," Shaffer of Washington University, and the Council on Pharmacy and Chemistry of the AMA. Walden filed a patent application in the United States on his isoelectric precipitation process two weeks prior to Macleod's telegram. Under the terms of the agreement of 30 May 1922 this was perfectly acceptable. The Insulin Committee requested several changes in the application, even though they had no contractual right to do this. They felt that the application was so broad in its claims that, if granted, it would essentially defeat the Toronto patent application and give Lilly an American monopoly on insulin. A comparison of the patent of Banting, Best, and Collip with that of Walden confirms the Insulin Committee's fears.[66] The Toronto patent, which runs two and one half pages, briefly describes the steps used to extract insulin from the pancreas. It makes eight claims for the pancreatic extract and the method used to collect it. Walden's patent, covering more than six pages, makes thirty product and process claims. He repeatedly mentions the superiority of his process, in terms of yielding a pure and stable pancreatic extract, over all previous methods.

The Lilly Company, despite Clowes's promise to the contrary, did not revise its patent application according to the wishes of the Insulin Committee. The Toronto group then faced the problem of protecting themselves. This was not the first time Toronto felt threatened by a Lilly patent application. The company had drawn up an application around late August 1922 to cover its developmental work in the three previous months and to protect itself against American competition. When some of the Toronto workers began to grumble, Clowes tried to explain away that patent application as nothing more than a formality, although he thought the Lilly counsel may have gone a bit too far: "It was drawn up by one of our patent attorneys who apparently was anxious to get everything possible into it and whose zeal was superior to his discretion. It is really a purely technical procedure and in my opinion has little or no value especially in the light of recent developments." Not convinced that the application was next to worthless, the Insulin Committee asked Lilly to reword its patent application so that it would not appear to threaten Toronto's application. The conflict subsided as Lilly's patent application fell into desuetude, probably because the "recent developments" Clowes referred to dealt with the isoelectric process.[67]

In April, Toronto launched an attack on both Iletin and the isoelectric precipitation patent. Representatives of the Insulin Committee conferred with Philip Shaffer, the biochemist at Washington University in St. Louis who had independently discovered the isoelectric precipitation procedure. Shaffer agreed to file a patent on his discovery, which the Insulin Committee hoped would interfere with Lilly's patent application. Meanwhile, the Committee informed the Council on Pharmacy and Chemistry of the

AMA that they did not approve of Lilly's use of the name Iletin.[68] This step, like a patent interference from Shaffer, presented potentially damaging consequences to the pharmaceutical firm's anticipated marketing advantage.

The AMA had established the Council on Pharmacy and Chemistry in 1905 as part of its war against the proliferation of questionable ethical and patent drugs. The function of the council was to evaluate drugs on the basis of several rules concerning composition, brand name, advertising, therapeutic claims, and so on, for the benefit of physicians and the public. The council compiled a list of drugs it accepted in *New and Nonofficial Remedies*, although it published information on unacceptable drugs too. Many state and regional medical and pharmaceutical journals, and some popular lay journals as well, followed the example of the *Journal of the American Medical Association* by refusing to advertise drugs not approved by the council.[69]

According to rule 8 of the official rules of the Council on Pharmacy and Chemistry, the Toronto scientists, as discoverers of insulin, had the right to object to any name a firm used for the hormone.[70] Clowes's reaction to the whole affair, mixing lamentations with a sense of braggadocio, was typical of the Lilly scientist:

If we are compelled to withdraw the product after having submitted it to the Council, it will be extremely detrimental to us and to everybody concerned. . . . We shall be prevented from advertising our preparation in the A.M.A. and the large majority of State Journals throughout the country. This would, of course, represent a great loss to us, but rather than expose ourselves and the public to the risk of confusion which is already arising over the name Insulin, our management is prepared to forgo all commercial advantage that may accrue to them as a result of approval of the product by the Council.[71]

Lilly had already given in to Toronto just a few days earlier on the matter of the isoelectric precipitation patent, so the company's resolve to preserve its trade name was by no means surprising. Lilly probably was also aware that Toronto violated the contract by (1) working to overturn the company's U.S. patent application and (2) refusing to approve Lilly's trade name for insulin. The Insulin Committee's primary objective was to persuade Lilly to assign them the isoelectric patent; thus the fight against Iletin probably was more for the sake of leverage. Once Lilly assigned the isoelectric patent to Toronto, the committee allowed Lilly the use of a brand name: "Iletin (Insulin, Lilly)."[72] The Insulin Committee accomplished what they felt was necessary to prevent an outright American monopoly, and Lilly maintained what it regarded as a fundamental commercial necessity.

The events during the spring of 1923 led to several safeguards in the new contract between Toronto and Lilly, of 30 June 1923, wherein Toronto issued a nonexclusive license to Lilly. Toronto's contracts with other firms bore almost the same provisions as the Toronto-Lilly pact. The only major difference between the two agreements was Lilly's right to use a trade name; other licensees could use only the name Insulin on their products. The licensing and cross-licensing stipulations were framed in such a way as to avoid the isoelectric patent fiasco. Lilly, as well as any other company Toronto licensed to produce and sell insulin, could retain any patents it received on insulin-related product or process discoveries as long as these discoveries were "beyond the scope" of all present and future Toronto patents. Otherwise, if there were a potential conflict with the Toronto patents, the company would have to assign its patent to the university. It was not clear who would decide whether a patent was "beyond the scope" of the Canadians' patents, but the intentions of the Insulin Committee surely were to thwart any possible commercial monopolies on the hormone. The Insulin Committee would license any patents acquired from other companies to all firms included in the agreement.[73]

The new contracts allowed Lilly and other companies to reap some dividends from patents that fell outside the realm of Toronto's patents. A patented synthetic insulin substitute, for example, would meet this criterion. The company had to put its discovery into a patent pool by licensing the Toronto group (royalty-free) and the firms operating on a license from the university. These firms paid the patentee a royalty not exceeding that which the patentee had been paying Toronto for the right to produce and sell insulin. That is, 5 percent of the net sales from insulin. Certain provisions from the 1922 agreement between Toronto and Lilly continued under these nonexclusive licensing pacts. For example, companies had to keep the university informed of their latest researches, patentable or not, and Toronto maintained control over companies' advertising. The cost of insulin treatment was an important consideration for the Insulin Committee, so this also received attention in the 1923 contracts. If the Insulin Committee and the company could not agree on a fair price for insulin, a board of three arbitrators (two selected by the concerned parties and a third chosen by the first two) decided the issue.[74]

Ironically, after all the controversy surrounding the extension of the experimental period and the efforts of Toronto to avert a monopoly on insulin, Lilly remained the only American producer for a year after the experimental period ended. Problems in standardizing insulin accounted for part of this delay, as did the time required for other firms to set up mass-production facilities. Toronto and Lilly had difficulties agreeing on an insulin unit from the beginning of their collaboration, and the Insulin Committee wanted to resolve these differences before putting insulin on the market and issuing additional licenses. Two international conferences of the Health Organisation of the League of Nations, which met in 1923 and 1925 under the direction of Henry Dale, addressed the unitage problems. The conferences established an international standard of reference for the insulin unit.[75] In any case, Lilly had a considerable jump by the time its American competition began marketing insulin—Frederick Stearns and Company in June 1924, E. R. Squibb and Sons in January 1925, and Sharp and Dohme around April 1925.[76] Lilly never relinquished this lead.

The Impact of the Collaboration on Toronto and Lilly

Each of the collaborators reflected on their association with hearty thanks for the other's assistance. Banting lauded the "intimate reciprocation of all results" between the university and Lilly, and the Insulin Committee measured their plaudits in terms of diabetics saved:

The Insulin Committee desires to express its appreciation of the whole hearted manner in which the Lilly research laboratories have cooperated in working out the problems of large scale production of insulin. Without this collaboration it is unlikely that a non-irritating product of such satisfactory potency and durability could have been produced in adequate amounts to meet the demand of the medical profession, in this comparatively short time.[77]

Clowes not only referred to the "unselfish co-operation" and "best endeavors" of Toronto and Lilly but also saluted the contributions of Philip Shaffer—a bit ironic given the leverage with which the Insulin Committee used Shaffer's work in April of 1923.[78] Notwithstanding the confrontations over the experimental period, the trade name, and the isoelectric precipitation patent, the insulin collaboration accomplished what it set out to do. Lilly and Toronto shared their research faithfully, and by the end of the experimental period diabetics had a mass-produced, safe, effective, and fairly well standardized product. Insulin was expensive, even at cost, but it was far preferable to alternative treatments.[79]

Their insulin research and associated work benefited Toronto and Lilly in many different ways. The Toronto scientists were showered with numerous individual accolades. Most notably, Banting and Macleod received the 1923 Nobel Prize for Medicine or Physiology, the money from which they shared with Best and Collip, respectively. On the other side, the American Diabetes Association honored Clowes with the Banting Medal in 1947. Insulin royalties and the sale of the Connaught Laboratories added considerably to the research funds of the University of Toronto. The university collected around $8 million in royalties from various patents that expired in the late 1950s. A small proportion of the royalties covered the modest expenses of the Insulin Committee, which continued to test insulin samples from manufacturers. Half of the remaining royalties went towards research funds for Banting, Best, and Collip, while the general research funds of the University of Toronto received the other half. The University's Connaught Laboratories grew rapidly as the insulin supplier to Canada, so rapidly that the university's sale of the Connaught Laboratories in 1972 swelled their general research funds by $24 million.[80]

When the insulin royalties began tailing off, Best approached the Lilly Company for funds to support diabetes research at the University's Banting and Best Department of Medical Research. Lilly responded by initiating a number of grants and consultantships in 1957 that totaled fifty thousand dollars annually: twenty-five thousand dollars to the Insulin Committee for their work; twelve thousand five hundred dollars to the Banting and Best Department; five thousand dollars to the Collip Research Foundation Laboratory of the University of Western Ontario (where Collip was a long-time faculty member); and consultantships for Best (five thousand dollars) and Collip (two thousand five hundred dollars). The grants and consultantships, as the president of the Lilly Company explained, were a goodwill gesture; they were "not based upon any legal obligation but would be given merely as evidence of our high regard for the friendly relations which have existed for so many years with these individuals and groups." The aid continued for many years. Collip's consultantship did not cease until the scientist died, in 1965; the grants to the Collip Research Foundation Laboratories ended three years later. Lilly terminated its support of the Insulin Committee in 1970, by mutual agreement. Best's consultantship, which had grown to ten thousand dollars by the late 1960s, remained in effect at least until the mid-1970s and probably lasted until Best's death in 1978. The grant to the Banting and Best Department also continued at least until the mid-1970s.[81]

Insulin had an immediate impact on Lilly. Despite the fact that the Insulin Committee did not release the product for general distribution until mid-October, insulin was by far the highest-selling specialty (in dollars) in the company's history. The restricted 1923 sales exceeded $1.1 million—over 14 percent of Lilly's total sales for that year. Insulin also accounted for half of the firm's profits of over $1.3 million for 1923. Iletin sales increased, even when the first three American competitors began marketing insulin. From the standpoint of cooperative research, the successful collaboration on insulin helped put the company in touch with the research of groups from over a dozen different universities by 1925. Five years after Lilly signed its first pact with Toronto, the company engaged in another major collaborative venture, with two university groups on the development of liver extracts for anemias. J. K. Lilly, president of the firm during the early insulin years, reflected in 1941 on the importance of this drug to the company: "Insulin revolutionized our place in the industry and put us on the way to present and future greatness."[82]

Harvard University, the University of Rochester, Eli Lilly and Company, and Liver Extracts

Like the insulin project, the collaborations on liver extracts focused on the development of an organ extract useful against a deadly disease. However, these two projects differed in many ways. The most obvious difference was that Lilly worked with two university medical schools to isolate different extracts from the same organ for two related illnesses. Lilly worked with Harvard University scientists to produce an extract from mammalian livers useful against pernicious anemia; this collaboration lasted from about the spring of 1927 to the autumn of 1928. Lilly engaged researchers at the University of Rochester in 1929 to test various liver fractions for activity against secondary anemia; this collaboration remained in effect for a quarter of a century.

Thomas Addison presented the first clinical picture of pernicious anemia. In the preface to *On the Constitutional and Local Effects of Disease of the Supra-Renal Capsules* (1855), the same work that marked the birth of modern endocrinology, Addison described this disease in detail, from its "slow and insidious" onset to its relatively painless and fatal termination.[83] Pernicious anemia, like other anemias, is a symptom complex rather than a disease per se. Blood actually is destroyed, and the body's blood-producing ability is diminished. This is the type of anemia that the Harvard workers investigated, an anemia resulting from an abnormality in blood production. Lilly's other collaborators, the Rochester group, were interested in simple posthemorrhagic anemia, an anemia, as the name indicates, resulting from a loss of blood. General recognition of pernicious anemia as a deficiency illness lagged until well into the twentieth century, primarily because of the unitary nature of the germ theory of disease. However, once scientists—particularly F. G. Hopkins at Cambridge, the Polish biochemist Casimir Funk, and a group of agricultural chemists at the University of Wisconsin—established the importance of trace nutrients in certain diseases in the early twentieth century, the medical community began to take a more open view of dietary treatment of pernicious anemia.[84] The results of extensive studies at the University of California and the University of Rochester provided an even more compelling reason to investigate dietary therapy in pernicious and chronic anemia.

George H. Whipple (1878–1976) was an associate professor in pathology at the Johns Hopkins Medical School when he accepted an invitation in 1914 to head the new George Williams Hooper Foundation for Medical Research at the University of California Medical School in San Francisco. Whipple continued his research on the function of the liver in the conversion of hemoglobin to bile pigments when he arrived at the Hooper Foundation. Whipple and his assistant, medical student Charles W. Hooper, reported in 1916 that the production of bile pigments (and thus the production of hemoglobin, which contributes most of these pigments) varied according to the diet. Fresh pig's liver or sheep's liver was much more productive than any other foodstuff, including blood and bile itself. Whipple's results, published as a series in 1920, were far from conclusive, but he indicated that liver was particularly promising as a means of returning the anemic dogs to their normal state.[85]

Whipple left California in 1921 to become professor of pathology and dean of the new University of Rochester Medical School. The Whipple group resumed their experiments a year later, this time correcting their investigations for the possibility of spontaneous recovery from anemia. First, they devised a special basal diet that maintained the dogs in their severe anemic condition; in addition, the diet did not contribute to the production of hemoglobin and red blood cells. Second, Whipple and his colleagues at Rochester bled the animals continuously during the feeding experiments to assure a constant low hemoglobin level; this was in contrast to his procedure at the Hooper Foundation, where he and his assistants had bled the dogs only at the beginning of the experiment. Through this changed procedure they could measure the blood-regenerating capacity of the test foodstuff by the volume of blood they had to remove to preserve the original hemoglobin level. Whipple and his colleagues reported in 1925 that liver was by far the most potent producer of hemoglobin and red blood cells in sustained severe anemia. Even inorganic iron, which was a fairly standard remedy for this type of anemia, gave results significantly below those achieved with liver. The latter results, according to the Rochester group, suggested that physicians should give more consideration to dietary treatment in the management of anemia.[86]

Charles Hooper was the first to apply his colleague's ideas to the clinic—even before the original feeding experiments had begun. Based on his bile-pigment work with Whipple, Hooper and an instructor at the California Medical School treated eight patients with subcutaneous injections of liver tinctures during the summer of 1916. Even though at least some of the patients began to recover, Hooper abandoned the clinical work. Apparently the clinicians drove away the young and timid laboratory scientist, since they believed that the hopeful results were merely spontaneous remissions. Shortly after Whipple published a summary of his California work in 1922—"Pigment Metabolism and Regeneration of Hemoglobin in the Body"—a biochemist and a physician at the University of Iowa found beneficial results with a diet of liver and meat for a few of their patients with pernicious anemia. The Iowa work had little impact, however, probably because most specialists attributed the improvements to spontaneous remission.[87]

George R. Minot (1885–1950) and William P. Murphy (b. 1892), who spent most of their careers at the Harvard Medical School, applied Whipple's laboratory results in the clinic and compiled unequivocal evidence that liver feeding remitted pernicious anemia indefinitely. Minot had begun to manifest his acumen in hematology while a medical student at Harvard. He spent most of 1914 working with physiologist William Henry Howell at Johns Hopkins, where he honed his skills in hematology. Minot returned to Massachusetts General Hospital the next year, about the time when Whipple was starting his anemia work at California. When he returned to Boston, Minot resumed recording copious dietary histories of his patients, including those with pernicious anemia patients—as he had as an intern at Massachusetts General. Thus, by the time Whipple published his results on the effect of liver on blood regeneration, Minot was more than prepared to apply these findings to his patients.[88]

In 1922, following the reports of Whipple's research at the Hooper Foundation, Minot and Murphy began treating pernicious anemia patients with a diet that included liver. Several of their outpatients responded well on diets that featured liver. This evidence, coupled with the recent appearance of the Whipple group's first substantial report of their research at Rochester, led Minot and Murphy to initiate a controlled study of the effect of liver feeding on hospitalized anemia victims in 1925. Minot and Murphy made a quick and accurate determination of the efficacy of liver by measuring the increase of reticulocytes, which are nascent red blood cells. Convincing their patients to ingest one-quarter to a half-pound of lightly cooked or, preferably, raw liver daily was not easy. One of their patients actually died because he could not tolerate the nauseating diet. The patients had to take raw-liver cocktails, raw-liver soup, or very lightly cooked liver steak, without onions or any other dressings; pâté, Braunschweiger, and liver tartare were out of the question. It was difficult, but on the whole the patients cooperated.[89]

The treatment was enormously successful. The patients' elevated reticulocyte count usually fell back to a normally low level within two weeks, and the diet sustained this level. In the spring of 1926 Minot and Murphy addressed the meeting of the prestigious Association of American Physicians. The two physicians made the rather conservative announcement that based on a study of forty-five patients who had taken the liver and a high-protein diet for six weeks to two years, "the dietetic treatment of pernicious anemia may be of more importance than hitherto generally recognized." They did not state explicitly that liver was the key to remission of the disease until the following year.[90]

They must have had liver in mind, though, because in 1926 Minot's group began a cooperative research project with Edwin J. Cohn (1892–1953), professor of physical chemistry at the Harvard Medical School, to test different fractions of liver in pernicious anemia. It is not surprising that the Harvard team started a search for the active fraction of liver: in the first place, whole liver was entirely unsatisfactory from the patient's standpoint; in the second place, the liver work came in the wake of discoveries by others of trace nutrients in different foods, such as milk, used to treat disease or promote health maintenance.[91] Cohn, a protein chemist, isolated different extracts of liver through an array of physico-chemical manipulations. Minot, Murphy, and their associates tested these extracts in theretofore untreated pernicious anemia patients. An appropriate bioassay was not yet available, but the method of measuring reticulocyte increase furnished results in less than two weeks. Whipple's group, too, was searching for the active ingredient of liver at this time; however, the Rochester scientists tested fractions in their chronically anemic dogs instead of in humans.[92] This was the situation when Lilly launched its joint investigations with Harvard and with Rochester.

The Birth of the Harvard-Lilly Collaboration

The Lilly Company had been collecting different liver fractions for some time prior to Minot and Murphy's announcement of their liver-feeding success but for an entirely different pharmacological reason. Sometime between 1923 and 1925, Lilly began extracting portions of liver effective against high blood pressure, based on the results of some Canadian and American workers. The available evidence suggests that the research of biochemists A. A. James and W. J. MacDonald and physiologist N. B. Laughton, all of the University of Western Ontario, and Ralph Major, of the University of Kansas, attracted Lilly to antihypertensive liver fractions.[93] By the spring of 1925 Lilly was supplying Major with fractions for laboratory testing, and the company had begun negotiations to test its extracts in the clinic at Western.[94] But Lilly's interests in antihypertensive fractions changed sharply over the following year.

Leon Zerfas, the person most responsible for the establishment of the Lilly Clinical Research Laboratories at the Indianapolis City Hospital, joined the company in 1925. Zerfas had acquired a strong interest in pernicious anemia during his tenure as chief resident physician at the Thorndike Memorial Laboratory of Boston City Hospital, which was affiliated with Harvard. He was working on antihypertensive liver fractions with Edward Campbell, a company biochemist, when the wife of the company president, Lilly Lilly, came down with pernicious anemia in 1926. Zerfas, who probably was more familiar with pernicious anemia than any other physician in the Indianapolis area, contacted his former chief at the Thorndike Laboratory, Francis Peabody, to ask him to come to Indianapolis to confirm Zerfas's diagnosis. Peabody, in the throes of stomach cancer at the time, suggested that Minot go in his place. Minot arrived in Indianapolis sometime between January and April 1927, but by that time Mrs. Lilly was already beginning to recover. In any case, this visit established an important future contact for the firm.[95]

Even before Minot's visit, once his and Murphy's first publication on the liver treatment of pernicious anemia appeared in August 1926, J. K. Lilly approached Campbell and Zerfas to see whether they could extract from liver the component that was active against pernicious anemia. Zerfas directed Campbell to save some of the alcoholic extracts that the latter had been discarding in his antihypertensive extract work. Mrs. Lilly responded well to these fractions, and Zerfas also treated at least two other pernicious anemia patients at Indianapolis City Hospital with these liver extracts. Lilly carried out all of this experimental and clinical work, not knowing that Harvard was working on the same problem. The two groups were not aware of their similar interest in liver fractions effective against pernicious anemia until early November 1926. It is very likely that they were not aware that each had isolated and clinically tested specific liver fractions until Minot visited Indianapolis early in 1927.[96]

Although there is some difference of opinion about who approached whom, most of the evidence indicates that Lilly contacted Harvard about a possible cooperative project.[97] Harvard chose to work with Lilly, even though several reputable firms with research staffs, such as Squibb, Stearns, Parke-Davis, Abbott, and Mulford, offered to collaborate with the university.[98] The Lilly Company was an attractive potential collaborator, because it was already working on liver extracts and, what was more important, because Lilly could point to its overall successful experience with the University of Toronto on insulin. Like the Canadians, Harvard chose to work with only one firm, for the sake of efficiency. The two parties probably began exchanging information on their liver extract research in April 1927. The initial negotiations more than likely transpired during Minot's visit to Indianapolis. The basic strategy was that Lilly would "manufacture under the direction of the [Committee on Pernicious Anemia] one of the extracts developed in the laboratory of physical chemistry" at Harvard Medical School.[99] While it might appear that Lilly was not to be much more than a mass-producing servant of the university, with Harvard assuming all laboratory-scale investigations, this certainly was not the case.

Upon the recommendation of A. Lawrence Lowell, president of Harvard, and David Linn Edsall, dean of the Medical School, Harvard formed a committee to organize and direct the development of liver extract research. This was much like the University of Toronto's Insulin Committee which is not surprising, given Harvard's stated wish to follow the example of Toronto's experience in the development of insulin as a therapeutic agent. In addition to Minot and Cohn, the Committee on Pernicious Anemia included Walter Bradford Cannon (chairman), William B. Castle, El-liott Joslin, and Edwin A. Locke. From its inception in May 1927 the com-mittee exercised several functions, including (1) securing and supervising a manufacturer to produce a liver extract according to Cohn's direction; (2) arranging for clinical evaluations (an especially important function, since clinical, as opposed to pharmacological, tests were the only available means of estimating the value of liver extracts); and (3) collecting and analyzing the clinical data.[100]

By the time the collaboration began, Harvard already had isolated and clinically tested the fraction of liver containing the active ingredient against pernicious anemia, just as the Toronto group had isolated and tested their pancreatic extract prior to their original agreement with Lilly. But in the case of the liver extract program, Lilly also had a tested liver fraction in hand when the company began working with Harvard. Lilly's extract represented the company's understanding of the physicochemical problems involved in research on the pernicious anemia principle from liver, an understanding that Harvard did not fully appreciate at first.

Progress on Extracts and Clinical Evaluation

Cohn's laboratory prepared an extract effective against pernicious anemia, the so-called G fraction, within two months of starting the search for a useful extract. Cohn undertook a "chemical dissection" of the liver, that is, a procedure "to divide the liver into the smallest possible number of fractions to discover which of these fractions was most active and to continue by subdividing the active fraction."[101] Cohn's group em-ployed five steps to collect fraction G:

1. extracting raw minced beef liver in an alkaline aqueous solution, pro-ducing a residue (fraction A);
2. adjusting the pH of the solution to acid, yielding a precipitate (frac-tion B);
3. heating the solution to 70°C, giving the heat-coagulable fraction C, and then concentrating the solution to produce fraction D;
4. extracting with ether, removing only a small part of D and producing fraction E; and
5. extracting with strong alcohol, yielding the alcohol-soluble fraction F and the insoluble fraction G.

The Boston clinicians tested all but the C fraction in patients; they did not test fraction C, because they believed that it was derived from blood in the liver rather than from the liver tissue itself. Fractions D and E caused a regeneration of reticulocytes in the anemia patients. The alcohol-soluble F fraction contained the antihypertensive principle that Lilly had been interested in. The remaining fraction, G, promoted rapid recovery from pernicious anemia.[102] The Harvard group continued to work on additional fractions,[103] but during the collaboration the workers focused on fraction G.

The process Lilly used to produce its so-called fraction L, which the company championed during the early months of the collaboration, is unknown; however, it was probably not very unlike Harvard's G fraction. Lilly was working for some time with the blood-pressure-lowering extract of liver (similar to Harvard's F fraction), and its L fraction was an alcoholic extract of the antihypertensive fraction. Also, Minot counseled Lilly on its pernicious anemia extractives when he was in Indianapolis. The company had good results with the L extract, on the basis of its effect on Mrs. Lilly and a few other patients.[104]

The immediate plans of the Committee on Pernicious Anemia were (1) to have Lilly manufacture as much as the G fraction as possible in the least possible time and (2) to organize a small clinical trial of the liver fraction among a few scattered medical centers, similar to the early setup during the insulin project. Although several area hospitals cooperated with the committee, Boston alone possessed an insufficient number of cases for an adequate assessment of the liver extract. So the committee engaged physicians familiar with the treatment of pernicious anemia at several medical centers to assist them in evaluating the liver extract: Johns Hopkins, Stanford, Bellevue Hospital (New York), Albany (New York) Hospital, the University of Michigan, the University of Wisconsin, the University of Chicago, Presbyterian Hospital (New York), Indianapolis City Hospital, and a private practice in Atlanta. In addition, St. Bartholomew's Hospital in London and the University of Toronto tested the liver extract for the committee.[105]

During the summer of 1927 Harvard had considerable difficulty convincing Lilly to manufacture its liver fraction G. The Pernicious Anemia committee wanted fraction G, as crude as it was, to be made available to the cooperating medical centers as soon as possible. The collaborators could refine this preparation later, according to the committee, when the patients would already have a tested extract (G) if needed. Thus, Minot firmly stated this view to Clowes early in the collaboration:

Of course it would be nice to give [a liver extract] in very concentrated form. Undoubtedly the time will come when that can be done, but I frankly believe we are wasting time both of your company and of patients suffering from the disease by trying now to obtain a fraction that is efficient in but a few grams a day. I feel convinced we should not send material to other clinics until we have a preparation known to be effective that you have prepared. I likewise feel that it will be a great mistake to send to other clinics at this time material that only *may be* effective.[106]

Minot was taking issue with some of Lilly's recent practices namely, trying to create an elegant extract, favoring its own L fraction, and pursuing research in its own laboratory when Lilly's prime task supposedly was to scale up Cohn's findings (see fig. 14). Lilly was trying to refine *both* the L and the G fractions. Harvard knew the G fraction worked, but Lilly's L fraction was comparatively untested—only a handful of cases in Indianapolis had received this extract—so the committee must have wondered why Lilly was emphasizing L rather than G. Henry Dale could have told them. Lilly certainly was more familiar with the L fraction, but what was more important, the company could file a patent application on L. If Lilly could circulate its extract among the cooperating clinicians and get good results, this would solidify fractions L's place in the market.

The mere fact that Lilly was devoting time to the study of extracts—investigations unrelated to the mass production of these extracts—seems to have annoyed some members of the committee, as witnessed by Minot's letter to Clowes above. It was not as if Cohn's laboratory were struggling to isolate the antianemic fraction; it was a very different situation than what Macleod's laboratory faced at the time it started working with Lilly. The Harvard group underestimated the research capabilities and the ambitions of Lilly. They simply wanted the firm to follow their directions, but that was about as likely as Cohn dedicating his life to industrial problems. It is worth mentioning that George Walden, who had so much success in isolating the pancreatic extract, joined Campbell and Zerfas in their liver extract research at the start of the collaboration.

The Pernicious Anemia Committee, after waiting weeks for Lilly to send enough G extract to initiate the clinical program, received a rather ironic letter from president J. K. Lilly. This time it was President Lilly who charged that the collaborators were stalling, because the company had extensive evidence that its L extract produced "uniform improvement" in pernicious anemia. As seen in the case of President Lilly's effort to increase distribution of insulin, he had both humanitarian and business motivations here. On the one hand, he emphasized that "my principal concern, however, is to save a lot of lives." Yet he also called attention to the fact that the Armour Company and possibly another firm (who perhaps also wanted just to save lives) already were distributing liver extracts for pernicious anemia, which could threaten his firm's position in the market. That other companies could be producing extracts was a surprise to the Pernicious Anemia Committee. Armour and the Wilson Company, meat packers with pharmaceutical divisions, were indeed marketing liver preparations. Armour's product, which the company claimed they did not promote as a pernicious anemia treatment per se, was a concentrate of whole liver. Wilson's preparation was an encapsulated extract marketed

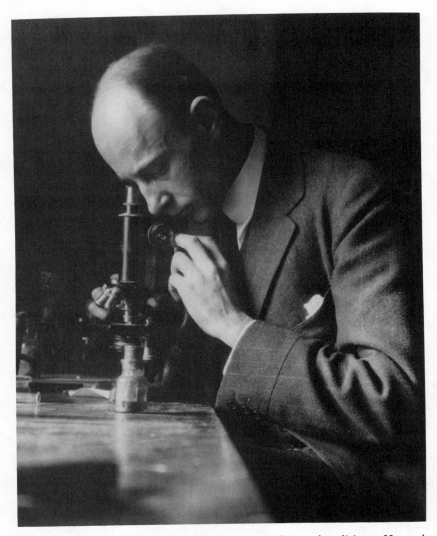

Figure 14. George Richards Minot (1885–1950), professor of medicine at Harvard Medical School from 1918 to 1950 (courtesy of the Harvard Medical Archives in the Francis A. Countway Library of Medicine).

as a treatment for this anemia. It is not clear whether the committee attempted to take any action against these companies. The committee had little if any legal recourse at this time, since there still were no federal laws dictating that a remedy be either tested or effective.[107]

President Lilly's claim about the value of the L fraction had some serious problems. In the first place, it was based largely on the evaluations of Zerfas, who was a Lilly employee.[108] There was no reason for the committee to question Zerfas's integrity, but this was simply not in the realm of proper protocol, at least as far as the Harvard Pernicious Anemia Committee was concerned. The committee also had doubts about the L extract on the basis of their own experiences with the preparation. In fact, the committee had had poor results with both Lilly's G fraction and its L fraction, perhaps because the products deteriorated or perhaps because Lilly's alcoholic extractions did not adequately remove the proteolytic enzymes in liver tissue. Lilly apparently did not heat its extracts the way Cohn had, which could explain why Cohn's extracts were more successful. Elliott Joslin, Lilly's former associate on the insulin project and a member of the Pernicious Anemia Committee, tried to explain to the company why a restricted distribution of extracts was still necessary: "If a product were widely distributed with the name of the P.A. Committee and the Lilly Company attached to it, and if such a product should deteriorate or prove in any way unsatisfactory, it would be very unfortunate for both the P.A. Committee and Company."[109]

The rest of the committee also thought it would be unfortunate. In early August they informed President Lilly that they could no longer consider the L fraction a feasible liver extract for widespread distribution; that it would require some time for the cooperating clinical group to assess the value of an extract prior to general distribution; and that the collaboration could be dissolved if Mr. Lilly were not satisfied with these arrangements. Lilly was beginning to push itself out of a collaboration again. While the company had not gone as far to threaten its good relations with Harvard as it earlier had with the University of Toronto and the insulin collaboration, it was approaching a point at which termination of the agreement was possible. From the start of the collaboration the Pernicious Anemia Committee seemed to be on its guard against any attempt by Lilly to turn the collaboration in the firm's favor. In April 1927, upon receiving an attractive offer for cooperative work from John Anderson of Squibb, Minot wrote Cohn that "should it come to pass that the Eli Lilly Co. played some game we do not expect I should think Anderson might be a very good man to deal with." Charles Best's revelations of Toronto's difficulties with Lilly could only have made Harvard more cautious about its connections with the Indianapolis company.[110]

Lilly genuinely felt that it had a solid product in fraction L. The company had too much at stake to market a questionable product and thereby run the risk of damaging its good reputation among the medical community. But Harvard believed, quite reasonably, that Lilly had come to this conclusion about fraction L on the basis of inadequate testing. Fraction G, unlike fraction L, was "tried and true." Thus, "by bringing steady pressure to bear" on the pharmaceutical firm, the committee finally convinced Lilly to manufacture a "reliable" extract, which the company produced through a slight modification of Cohn's fraction G process. Following successful preliminary tests of this preparation in Indianapolis and Boston, beginning in September 1927 the committee distributed the extract to the clinical group. Two months earlier, Clowes had told J. K. Lilly that the committee most likely would permit the company to submit other fractions for testing as long as a fully potent extract based on the G fraction were available to the clinical group. The committee agreed to have additional fractions tested, although they warned at least one member of the group to test only material that he and the committee deemed worthy of evaluation.[111] The company's search for a reliable testing center for its antianemic liver extracts eventually led Lilly to George Whipple.

Since the results with the G-modified fraction were "invariably good," beginning in December the Pernicious Anemia Committee significantly widened the distribution of the fraction. In the same month, they introduced the fraction to the Council on Pharmacy and Chemistry of the AMA as liver extract no. 343.[112] The council promptly reported their approval of the extract in February 1928.[113] Many of the problems concerning patenting, trade names, AMA Council approval, and so on, that emerged between Lilly and the University of Toronto simply did not exist in the collaboration with Harvard.

Monopoly on Liver Extract 343

According to personnel on both sides of the liver extract collaboration, Lilly patented liver extract no. 343 and proceeded to give the patent to Harvard. The university then dedicated the patent to the public so that anyone having the inclination could manufacture the product.[114] Harvard considered applying for a patent on Cohn's extract by early 1927 but temporarily waived that idea because it believed that such a patent would conflict with a patent application on the antihypertensive liver extract. As mentioned above, the methods for extracting the liver principles active against high blood pressure and those active against pernicious anemia were similar. Lilly already had applied for a patent on the blood pressure principle and the process to prepare it by the spring of 1927. The university wanted to see whether Cohn could resolve the pernicious anemia principle sufficiently to justify a patent application. Actually, scientists did not reduce this principle to its essence until 1948, when a group at the Merck Company under Karl Folkers isolated vitamin B_{12} in crystalline form.[115]

Recall that Lilly battled Toronto over the Walden patent and the trade name Iletin. In the case of the liver extract collaboration, the company apparently voiced no objections to handing over its patent and did not push for a trade name. The differences here rest in the very different ways that the Insulin Committee and the Pernicious Anemia Committee handled the issue of the monopolization of their discoveries. The Insulin Committee took many steps to ensure that no company could control insulin; the Pernicious Anemia Committee, on the other hand, was satisfied "to provide a supply of potent liver extract adequate to the needs of those suffering from conditions which could justifiably demand treatment with this specific principle of liver" and leave their responsibility at that.[116] In other words, the committee tested the fractions that Lilly manufactured—and only Lilly's product—until they were confident of its strength, purity, and shelf life, and then they terminated the collaboration and the committee itself. It is no surprise, then, that the liver extract collaboration did not have the same kind of confrontations that the insulin collaboration had. Other companies could (and did) manufacture liver extracts, but only Lilly's preparation had the imprimatur of the committee. The pharmaceutical firm took advantage of this de facto monopoly. For example, Lilly instructed its "detailers": "You should convey to the medical profession at large the fact that Lilly Extract No. 343 is the only product that had the unqualified approval of the Harvard Pernicious Anemia Committee." The company included this "unqualified approval" in its medical journal advertisements as well.[117]

Other companies knew very well how this exclusive arrangement between Harvard and Lilly would affect their positions in the liver extract market. For example, a representative from the H. K. Mulford Company complained to William Castle that "for the Committee to test the product of one commercial laboratory and permit it to market the same with their approval, places other firms at a decided disadvantage, even though no patent, trade-mark or other restrictions enter into the question at all."[118] The committee felt that any kind of mass testing was simply beyond their means. True, the Insulin Committee managed to supervise several companies, but the Harvard Committee believed that this was an unfair comparison: "The Committee on Pernicious Anemia has decided not to collaborate directly with any other manufacturing firm for the present than Eli Lilly and Company because of the impossibility of really supervising and therefore guaranteeing the product. The difference from insulin which has involved this decision has been the impossibility of testing the potency of material except by feeding it to patients with pernicious anemia."[119] While the Insulin Committee easily maintained checks on products of various manufacturers by bioassays on rabbits at Toronto, the Pernicious Anemia Committee did not enjoy the advantage of a bioassay. Physicians had to evaluate liver extracts by administering the test extract to a patient.

Harvard's reluctance to enter into a supervisory role in the liver extract industry thus is understandable. The type of organization needed for standardizing several different brands of pernicious anemia liver extracts finally emerged in the late 1930s under the auspices of the U.S. Pharmacopoeial Convention through its Anti-Anemia Preparations Advisory Board.[120] So Lilly launched liver extract no. 343 into the market with a decided advantage. The company, with considerable experience in pernicious anemia, logically branched out into the field of secondary anemia. Soon after Harvard ceased testing Lilly's liver extract in the fall of 1928, the company approached another leader in the field, George Whipple, with an offer of collaboration

The Agreement between Rochester and Lilly

George Whipple's Department of Pathology at the University of Rochester was one of two "Special Laboratories" that Harvard's Pernicious Anemia Committee included in their early group of testing centers. Whipple reported in a September 1928 publication that liver extract no. 343 had had very little effect on his dogs suffering from severe secondary anemia. Clowes and Whipple had been acquaintances for many years, and Clowes occasionally supplied Whipple with materials when the latter was building up his anemia investigations. Whipple's recent publication gave Clowes an opportunity to remind Whipple that, "the facilities and resources of our laboratories are always at your disposal and . . . should you so desire we shall be glad to prepare any fractional products for you on a larger scale than would be possible in a purely research laboratory." Whipple promptly replied that he would be happy to cooperate with Lilly.[121]

That Whipple unhesitatingly agreed to work with Lilly can be attributed to several circumstances. Clowes's steady contact over the years certainly was important, as was Lilly's involvement with the Insulin Committee and especially with the Pernicious Anemia Committee. Successful collaborations facilitated future collaborations, as witnessed by Lilly's experience in the 1920s. Whipple's own experience during a botulism outbreak when he was at the Hooper Foundation also played no small part in stimulating future collaborations. The problem was traced to the ripe olive industry in California, among other states. Eventually foundation bacteriologist Karl Meyer designed a canning method to safeguard olives against this poisoning. Whipple was very impressed by the conduct of the industry during this crisis. The industrial representatives with whom he had personal contact were interested in more than stopgap measures; they wanted to know everything they could about botulism in order to prevent such an incident from recurring. This was an "enlightening experience" for Whipple, and he henceforth looked forward to contacts with industry (see fig. 15).[122]

Rochester and Lilly began exchanging research data around February 1929. Although their early negotiations suggested that the company would provide Whipple with different liver fractions according to Whipple's specifications, the Rochester scientist did not object when Lilly began requesting that Whipple's group test the firm's own extracts. One of the liver fractions that the Rochester group tested in 1929 and early 1930 was particularly beneficial in the anemic dogs. It had 3 percent of the weight of whole liver, yet it possessed up to 75 percent of the latter's activity in secondary anemia. Its rather simple preparation consisted of heating a preparation of ground liver in dilute sulfuric acid to about 80° C, evaporating the filtrate to a syrup, and collecting the precipitate that formed when 50–75 percent alcohol was added to the syrup. Despite the fact that the patent on this extract bears only George B. Walden's name, Whipple clearly contributed significantly to this discovery. First, Whipple simply would not allow his name to appear on any patent. Second, the contract between Rochester and Lilly referred to the University of Rochester as the discoverer of this extract. Finally, several of the fractions that Whipple and his associates mentioned in a publication of research performed prior to the Lilly-Rochester collaboration closely resembled the patented extract.[123]

Lilly put this so-called liver extract no. 55 on the market as a treatment for secondary anemia in September 1930. The following month, after finding that Whipple and the University of Rochester had no objections, the company filed a patent application on the extract.[124] Whipple had strong feelings about the commercialization of medical discoveries, feelings that his mentors at Johns Hopkins, such as William Henry Howell and William Henry Welch, inculcated in their students. Whipple refused to patent liver extract no. 55; in fact, he claimed that he never even considered a patent. He maintained an aloofness from the commercial aspects of the development of this extract. For example, Lilly marketed no. 55 largely on the basis of Whipple's excellent experimental results with his dogs, even though clinical evaluations were sparse. This generated some controversy from which Whipple kept his distance:

Some people used to say that the reaction of anemic dogs to liver extracts was all right, but it didn't necessarily prove that it would be the same with humans. We hadn't anything to do with that argument because we were not concerned with the

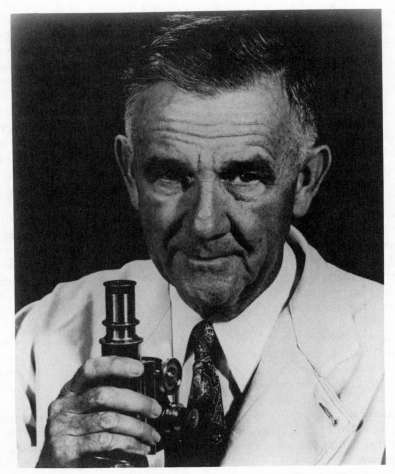

Figure 15. George Hoyt Whipple (1878–1976), professor of pathology and first dean of the University of Rochester School of Medicine and Dentistry from 1921 to 1955 (from Corner, *Whipple,* courtesy of Lippincott/Harper and Row and the National Library of Medicine).

marketing of the substance. [Lilly] used whatever they thought would be fair to the situation, always sending it to us for review. We were glad to know that sick people thought they were benefiting.[125]

Ironically, even though Whipple may not have been concerned with the marketing of no. 55, his research program and the University of Rochester Medical School profited enormously from the marketing of the extract.

Three weeks before liver extract no. 55 went on the market, Lilly offered Whipple a formal agreement. Theretofore the collaboration had operated on a handshake rather than a contract, which was the way Whipple preferred. Though the two groups had not yet signed an agreement, Lilly reimbursed Whipple's group four thousand dollars for expenses incurred in the extract project. The contract that the university and Lilly concluded on 1 January 1931 underwent some changes over the years, but it remained in force for twenty-five years. According to the contract, Rochester would continue testing extracts, which Lilly would produce and sell, and both parties were expected to recommend potential extracts for investigation. The agreement did not emphasize patent matters, as the Toronto-Lilly agreements had; rather, Rochester allowed Lilly to patent any product or process it wished. Rochester would receive a five percent royalty on no. 55 and any other patentable discoveries emanating from this agreement. As in the case of the Toronto-Lilly agreements, Rochester had the right to inspect any of Lilly's relevant records, to demand that the Lilly products meet the university's standards of quality, to approve Lilly's advertising related to any products covered by the agreement, and to call for arbitration if the company and the university could not agree on a fair price for a product. Given Whipple's predilection for an informal collaboration, on the academics' side the contract was probably more for the benefit of president Rush Rhees and other members of the university's governing board.[126]

The only significant changes in the agreement during the following years concerned the method of reimbursing Rochester. Presumably, the collaborators made these changes by mutual agreement when extract sales exceeded by far what both parties had anticipated in 1931. The royalty was reduced to 2.5 percent in 1933, and ten years later Lilly began paying Rochester a flat fee of ten thousand dollars per year for the testing work; the fee rose to eighteen thousand dollars in 1946.[127] The collaboration between Lilly and Rochester on liver extracts active against secondary anemia ended when Whipple retired in 1955.

The Impact of the Collaboration
on Harvard, Rochester, and Lilly

As in the Toronto-Lilly cooperative project, the liver extract collaborators derived benefits from their association. Harvard did not receive any compensation per se from the sale of liver extract no. 343, but Lilly supported the later research of a few members of the Pernicious Anemia Committee, Minot most notably. Minot received grants from the company of five thousand dollars per year from 1928 through 1936 and sixty-five hundred dollars annually from 1937 until his death in 1950, for a total in excess of one hundred thousand dollars during the postcollaboration period. For Minot, this money was support for research on pernicious anemia and other blood disorders. From Lilly's standpoint, this money was "part compensation for favors in [the] early days of liver extracts."[128]

The compensation Rochester received was no less impressive. The testing of liver extracts did not burden Whipple's research. Rather, the royalties and fees that Lilly paid to the university supported a broad research program in Whipple's laboratory. Whipple reflected near the end of the collaboration that "much of the money coming to this department as a result of these contracts has been used to further our research program, dealing not only with experimental anemia, but with general body pigment metabolism and the complex reactions of various proteins in the body, within the blood plasma, within the tissue fluid and within organ parenchymal cells; the whole complex problem designated as 'an equilibrium of body proteins.' "[129]

The funds also supported the University of Rochester School of Medicine overall. Over the years, Whipple had put Lilly funds above those required to support both the testing expenses and his own research program into a Lilly Research Fund. Two years before his retirement, Whipple proposed a few ways to disburse the fund, which by that time (1953) had grown to about $700,000. First $250,000 would fund the establishment of a chair in the Department of Pathology. Second, $300,000 would be spent on scholarship programs for premedical and medical students at Rochester. Finally, Whipple suggested that $75,000 be used to endow visiting lectureships in physiology, biochemistry, and pediatrics. The university trustees would use the remainder at their discretion. As he requested, the Trustees effected Whipple's proposals upon his retirement.[130]

Lilly also derived direct and indirect benefits from the liver extract collaborations. While its Harvard colleagues no longer approved Lilly's extract exclusively, the university workers were willing to test liver extract no. 343 after the collaboration. In addition, Minot assured Lilly that Harvard would keep it abreast of the latest developments at the medical school. For example, he suggested that Lilly approach Cohn about mass-producing an extract the chemist was on the verge of obtaining, a liver extract pure enough for intravenous administration. Five years later, Harvard still was updating Lilly on its progress with injectable liver extracts.[131] Lilly's extracts for both pernicious and secondary anemia sold well. In 1933 Lilly introduced Lextron, a shotgun approach to anemia therapy. This preparation included liver extract no. 55, the pernicious anemia principle,[132] iron, and, to stimulate the appetite, vitamins B_1 and B_2. Despite some criticism from the medical community for marketing such a multipurpose remedy, Lextron was a popular anemia remedy.[133]

The prestige afforded by collaborating with another pair of Nobel laureates enhanced Lilly's established image as a progressive, research-oriented company. It is no coincidence that Lilly's contacts with academic workers grew to encompass eighteen different groups by 1930. The reputation of Lilly's Clinical Research Laboratories grew as well. This was one of only a handful of medical centers that took part in the early testing of pernicious anemia liver extracts under the supervision of Harvard's Pernicious Anemia Committee.[134]

Conclusion

The cooperative research projects on liver extracts between Harvard and Lilly and between Rochester and Lilly differed in many ways from the insulin project. First, Harvard apparently carried out its work with Lilly without a formal agreement. Liver extract no. 55 was on the market before Rochester concluded an agreement with Lilly; in this case, the delay was almost certainly because of Whipple's preference for informal arrangements and his desire to remain apart from the commercial affairs of the collaboration. In contrast to Harvard and Rochester, Toronto concluded three detailed contracts with Lilly between May 1922 and December 1923. Toronto probably wanted to spell out the responsibilities of each party because the Insulin Committee was not very familiar with Lilly. Also, this sort of arrangement—on such a grand scale—was unheard of in North America at the time. This was not as much of a problem for the Pernicious Anemia Committee and for Whipple's group. However, a contract that explicitly stated the functions of both parties might have saved the Harvard Committee (and Lilly) some frustrations over the matter of Lilly's L extract.

The liver extract and insulin projects also differed with respect to the company's experience with the research problem before contacting the university. Lilly had some background in extracting substances from other glands and testing these through biological assays prior to the insulin collaboration, yet the company was not familiar with pancreatic extracts. On the other hand, Lilly had prepared and clinically tested liver extracts for pernicious and secondary anemias before negotiating agreements with

Harvard and Rochester. This definitely enhanced Lilly's image as a desirable potential collaborator. Of course, Lilly's rapid success with insulin demonstrated that prior experience with the proposed project was not crucial as long as the company was willing to invest the necessary time, funds, and personnel to make up for the lack of experience.

Another difference between the cooperative projects was that from the standpoint of therapeutics one of the collaborations really was more important than the other. Minot and Murphy, based on Whipple's research, discovered that feeding whole liver to victims of pernicious anemia could put the disease into indefinite remission. The use of the liver extract indisputably had many advantages over liver feeding, but when it came to healing the patient, as Murphy explained, "the use of liver, itself, is just as satisfactory except that it is sometimes a little more difficult to take the required amount than it is to take the extract."[135] If the liver extract work were a complete failure, there was no reason why victims of pernicious anemia should continue to die from this disease. Even for the few patients who preferred the consequences of the diseases to the treatment, they could have raw liver administered by a stomach tube. If scientists had failed to isolate and produce a pancreatic extract useful in diabetes, victims of that disease would not have been so fortunate.

Finally, the academics involved in the collaborations on insulin and antianemic liver extracts had radically different opinions about permitting monopolies on their discoveries. The Insulin Committee's position was explicitly antimonopolistic. Following the temporary exclusive arrangements with Lilly, the committee issued licenses from their patent to several manufacturers, whose insulin they periodically tested. The Harvard Pernicious Anemia Committee, by contrast, dedicated the patent on liver extract no. 343 to the public and tested only Lilly's preparation. The University of Rochester divorced itself from the marketing of liver extract no. 55, although it accepted royalties and other fees from Lilly that well exceeded its testing expenses. Rochester allowed Lilly to patent and market virtually any extract it wished to develop cooperatively. The Insulin Committee pursued their course, they said, to protect the diabetic. This by no means indicates that the Pernicious Anemia Committee or Whipple cared less about the anemic patient. The committee claimed that the pharmacological circumstances of their liver extract prevented them from pursuing a course similar to Toronto's. Whipple's personal opinion of medical patents motivated his decision to avoid having the University of Rochester exercise any kind of Torontonian controls over the liver extract market. The three universities had very different reasons for dealing with the commercial applications of their discoveries the way they did. Harvard and Rochester also may have had in mind the inconvenience and expense of supervising liver extracts of several firms, particularly Rochester, a medical school barely on its feet in the early 1930s.

The liver extract projects produced substantial rewards for the collaborators. For Minot (indirectly, through goodwill grants) and Whipple (directly, through royalties and fees for assay work), the collaborations were the source of considerable research support for the remainder of their careers. For Lilly, the collaborations satisfied both the business and the scientific interests within the company. The projects yielded drugs that fared very well in the market, and they reinforced Lilly's image among the academic community as an enlightened pharmaceutical firm. For the public health, the collaborations on liver extracts may not have been as crucial as the joint work on insulin, but the liver extracts nonetheless were an important addition to the therapeutic armamentarium.

The early university-industry collaboration on insulin obviously did not run smoothly. Two points must be realized, though. First, the problems did not prevent the overall success of the project. Second, the problems resulted more from a misunderstanding of the other's objectives than from a deliberate attempt to mislead the other collaborator. Collaboration between academe and industry on biomedical research was relatively new at this time in North America, and patterns and models needed to be worked out. The Toronto workers felt that a monopoly would eventually have a deleterious impact on the diabetic. Lilly could not understand Toronto's opposition to a monopoly, because the company believed that its business could prosper under a monopoly without gouging the diabetic. Clowes, who was new to the pharmaceutical industry, could appreciate Toronto's position. But Lilly management had the final word. The University of Toronto could not fully understand the Lilly Company's wish for a commercial advantage on insulin, because the University of Toronto was not a business institution where the bottom-line concern was revenue. Despite the misunderstandings and difficulties, the project came off well considering that it was the first long-term, large-scale case of biomedical collaborative research between a North American university and a pharmaceutical firm.

Epilogue: The Search
for the Genetic El Dorado

→>>-→>>-→>>-→>>-→>>- ‹‹‹-‹‹‹-‹‹‹-‹‹‹-‹‹‹

Research interactions between academe and industry grew rapidly during the 1920s, 1930s, and early 1940s. By the end of World War II a National Research Council survey revealed that over 300 companies representing a variety of industries were supporting research in universities through fellowships, scholarships, and direct grants-in-aid. Of these firms, nearly 50 were subsidizing over 270 biomedical research projects at about 70 universities. A few universities, such as Cornell, Harvard, Cincinnati, and New York University, led the rest of the group in total projects funded by companies, but by and large the support (which amounted to a minimum of $400,000–500,000) was spread fairly evenly among all the schools.[1]

In the decades following World War II, despite the birth of some novel forms of interaction at a handful of academic institutions, such as Stanford, MIT, and North Carolina, contacts between academe and industry slowly weakened, eventually reaching their nadir by the early 1970s. Some authorities on science and technology policy have blamed this decreasing level of collaborative research at least partially for the decline of American industrial innovation.[2] Several reasons account for this change. First, the post–World War II era witnessed the rise of mega-support for academic research by the federal government. Consequently, university researchers had less incentive to engage in work for industry. In particular, the support that federal defense and aerospace agencies offered to academic scientists led more and more of the latter to focus on the "performance improvements" of high technology rather than the "cost improvements" of other industrial research. Second, as more federal funds filled university research coffers and as higher education in general expanded in the postwar years, graduate students increasingly lost interest in careers in industrial research. Faculty appointments seemed more promising than in the past, and professors began training their students primarily for positions in academe. Finally, industry's involvement in basic research declined. Firms supported less basic research in universities after the mid-1950s, which eroded an important point of contact for academic and industrial scientists.[3]

In the late 1970s and early 1980s, however, links between academe and industry were on the rise again. Federal funding for health research was erratic throughout the 1970s, and the purchasing power of the research dollar plummeted in the inflated economy; not surprisingly, competition for federal research support intensified within academe. At the same time, growing federal regulations over experimentation challenged the flexibility and independence of the academic investigator. From the standpoint of American industry, stiffening competition from abroad and the need to satisfy environmental, health, and safety regulations called for a reinvigorated and profitable technology.[4] Both sides had strong incentives to step up research connections. Representatives from both estates of science advocated more links between universities and firms; they urged educators to facilitate interactions through industry-oriented coursework and even issued extensive guidelines for effective research agreements between academe and industry.[5]

Academe and industry have developed a wide variety of research contacts in recent years. Industrial research parks near universities, for example, are becoming a popular way to establish linkages. Nearly four dozen universities are actively engaged in or seriously considering establishing such research parks, including major research institutions such as Yale and Wisconsin. The University of Maryland is arranging a series of specialized research centers in the Baltimore-Washington corridor devoted to medicine, marine science, and agriculture that will serve as a basis for ties with industry. The National Bureau of Standards, the National Aquarium, and the Beltsville Agricultural Research Center are collaborating with Maryland in these ventures.[6] A few universities have had successful research parks for over twenty years, most notably the Stanford Research Park and a joint venture of North Carolina, North Carolina State, and Duke, the Research Triangle Park.

Typically, a number of firms representing chemical, electronics, pharmaceutical, communications, and other industries rent space in these parks for multidisciplinary research and development facilities. Research parks can contribute significantly to a university's funds. The Princeton Forrestal Center, for example, concludes fifty-year prepaid leases with its industrial tenants for an average of $250,000 per acre. Ideally, from the standpoint of industry, research parks facilitate the integration of university research into commercial products through various means of contact, such as faculty consultantships and the participation of industrial scientists in departmental seminars. In reality, few research parks so far have stimulated a transfer of technology from universities to industry.[7]

Research consortia are another popular way by which academe and industry have developed links. In this case, several firms pay a fee to support research at a single university in an area in which the university excels. The participating firms receive special reports, briefings, and access to university facilities. Cornell, Michigan, MIT, Wisconsin, Minnesota, and the University of Washington, among others, engage in extensive consortial interactions with industry. The MIT Polymer Processing Program involves a dozen companies, including Xerox, ITT, and General Motors, which pay up to one hundred thousand dollars annually to support about twenty-five projects connected with polymer research. Wisconsin presently has sixteen consortia under way, from plasma processing, robotics design, and cast metals technology to consortia that apply particularly to state industries, such as electrical machine and power technology, to cheese processing. The university has three levels of membership fees, beginning at five thousand dollars to ensure that smaller companies can take part.[8] Industrial associate or affiliate programs are broader in nature than research consortia. Under these programs, several firms pay a fee to have access to research in many areas at the university. This is a particularly useful arrangement for companies interested in gaining an overview of a new field. For a fee, the university provides the company with preferential access to faculty participating in the program, directories of current research, and permission to audit courses and symposia. The number of member companies and the fees involved vary considerably from program to program. MIT has the most extensive associates program, which began in the late 1940s: the 280 firms that participate pay an annual total of nearly $5 million for the privilege.[9]

These and many other examples of the links between universities and industries in general indicate that collaboration is stronger than ever today.[10] Research interactions in the biomedical sciences are very much a part of this trend. The pharmaceutical industry continues to be one of the most research-intensive industries in the United States. Drug-industry research and development expenditures reached multibillion-dollar proportions by the 1980s. For example, the Pharmaceutical Manufacturers Association estimated that companies spent $3.3 billion in 1983—14.4 percent of sales. This industry's comparatively high research intensity is also seen in the number of research and development scientists and engineers per thousand total employees (sixty-two) in the pharmaceutical industry in relation to the proportion of research personnel in another historically research-conscious industry, the chemical industry (forty-one per thousand) and the average for all industries (twenty-seven).[11]

The pharmaceutical industry clearly has the wherewithal to support research in academe, and if it so desires, it also has the research labor to engage in joint projects with university workers. In pharmacy schools alone an announcement of the latest awards and grants to pharmacy faculty indicated that firms funded nearly three dozen grants, worth over $1 million. This is born out even more dramatically by industry's own version of mega-support for research in universities in recent years, through multimillion-dollar, long-term support of one university program by one company. From 1980 to 1983 such major long-term research agreements between universities and companies provided $140 million to thirteen institutions, almost all of which were private universities. Of the seventeen major contracts in effect during this period all but one involved biotechnology.[12] Firms have identified the departments most likely to yield profitable results, and they have paid enormous sums for the privilege of working exclusively with those departments. It is a situation reminiscent of Germany a century ago, when chemical concerns such as Höchst and BASF "invested" in the laboratories of the most promising figures of the time—Hofmann, Wislicenus, Baeyer, and others—for the right to be the first to capitalize on their results and the right to queue up first to hire their students.

Harvard Medical School took part in some of the earliest major research agreements with industry. For example, in 1974 it launched a twelve-year agreement with Monsanto in which the company agreed to support research on cancer up to a total of $24 million. In return, Monsanto would receive limited-term, exclusive licenses on all Harvard patents based on Monsanto-supported research. Similarly, a five-year, $6 million agreement that Harvard signed with Du Pont in 1981 gave the firm exclusive licenses on patents in exchange for funding genetics research. Among other such agreements on biomedical subjects are those between Washington University School of Medicine and Monsanto for the development of specialty products; Georgetown University and Fidia, an Italian drug concern, for the development of a neurosciences institute at the Washington institution; and the University of Kansas and Upjohn for research on drug transport and metabolism.[13] In these and many other cases pharmaceutical companies identify promising research likely to yield profitable results, and they purchase at least a limited-term monopoly on any marketable results that might derive from the academic laboratory. For companies, these arrangements are calculated business risks; while there is no guarantee that the support will produce a commercially successful product, those academic laboratories that are leaders in the field are more likely than most others to produce. Also, because of the exclusive nature of these arrangements, the company stands to benefit more than it would from associates programs, research parks, and other types of interactions between academe and industry. For universities, such agreements certainly provide a steady and bountiful source of research support, but they also entail many risks that can potentially compromise the very nature and functions of the university (see below).

The consultantship continues to be a popular conduit for interactions between the university and company. The pharmaceutical industry still relies heavily on consultants, as it did in the 1920s and 1930s—although there is little evidence to suggest that the Richardsian general consultantship has survived. If anything, we see the reverse situation today, in which certain firms are at least partially shaping research programs in certain academic laboratories. Many companies have one hundred or more consultants on retainer. Traditionally, universities have "permitted" professors up to one day per week for consulting as a means of supplementing salaries that are generally lower than those of their colleagues in industry. However, monitoring consultantships can be difficult.[14] Consultantships can be profitable, a point made clear in an advertisement for a recent seminar on establishing consulting arrangements. The sponsor, the American Association of Professional Consultants, informed prospective participants that they would learn "how to avoid giving away your valuable know-how for free" and "how to profit while serving the small (or impoverished) clients."[15]

Academic scientists have taken the initiative to stimulate contacts between universities and industry in other ways. Unlike the models for university-industry research relationships discussed earlier, these attempts to link academe with industry rely on the latter more as a source for intellectual rather than as a source for financial support (although this is not to say that industry's wealth did not have some influence in generating these interactions). For example, in 1979 the University of Wisconsin School of Pharmacy established the Louis W. Busse Lectures as a tribute to a retiring faculty member who had had close ties with industrial pharmaceutical research throughout his career at Wisconsin. Each year the school invites a distinguished scientist from the drug industry to spend one week lecturing and interacting with graduate students at the pharmacy school. According to the dean who organized the program, the Busse Lectures provide an opportunity for "valuable contact between industrial scientists and our students and faculty."[16] The same institution annually sponsors a National Industrial Pharmaceutical Research Conference, in which academic and industrial scientists present and discuss their latest research. The 1986 conference featured presentations by academic pharmaceutical scientists from Michigan, MIT, Wisconsin, and three other universities and by industrial workers from nine firms, including Genentech, Abbott, and Merck Sharp and Dohme.[17]

In another novel effort by academic and industrial scientists to stimulate collaboration, the Academy of Pharmaceutical Sciences of the American Pharmaceutical Association, in conjunction with the American Association of Colleges of Pharmacy and the Pharmaceutical Manufacturers Association, began a program in 1985 to put industrial scientists in contact with pharmacy schools. This Pharmaceutical Industry Visiting Scientist Program for Colleges of Pharmacy consists of one- or two-day lecture programs by industrial workers in pharmacy schools. The sponsors launched this program to stimulate interest in graduate work among pharmacy students, to give pharmacy schools access to the expertise of industry scientists, to encourage communication between the pharmaceutical industry and pharmacy schools, and to serve as a public-relations vehicle for industry's concerns, such as costs associated with drug discovery.[18]

Ties between academe and industry have brought considerable prosperity to some campuses and communities. This prosperity coupled with the need to find a source to help fill the void created by the Reagan administration's cuts in support for academic research (other than highly specialized projects such as those for the Department of Defense) and higher education and nonprofit organizations in general, has led many federal agencies, national political organizations, and municipal and county governments to attempt to lure industry to academic institutions.[19] These bodies have focused much of their attention on the biotechnology industry in what Nicholas Wade has aptly called the search for the genetic El Dorado on our nation's campuses. Since 1973 the National Science Foundation (NSF) has funded research centers at which a university can collaborate with several firms. The aforementioned MIT Polymer Processing Program began as an NSF-sponsored center, as did the University of Delaware Catalysis Center, among other programs. Typically, the NSF support lasts for five years, after which the center is expected to be self-supporting. The NSF began funding research centers in biotechnology in the early 1980s at Research Triangle Park in North Carolina, Wisconsin, Purdue, Texas, and Minnesota.[20]

Other ways in which the federal government has tried to stimulate interactions between universities and companies include a relaxation on former patent restrictions for universities and tax breaks for industry. By the late 1970s the then Department of Health, Education and Welfare permitted academic institutions to retain patents deriving from federally funded research (HEW had theretofore claimed such patents) if they agreed to exploit their own discoveries. The 1980 Tax Reform Act encouraged companies to invest in university research by permitting them a supplemental tax credit on research and development support paid to academe—that is, in addition to the normal tax deduction for industry on its research expenses.[21] Following an eighteen-month study of the scientific and technical health of American universities, a task force within the

White House Science Council recommended several ways in which industry can contribute to this health. For example, the group suggested that industry and the federal government jointly sponsor graduate fellowships in "specific fields of science, engineering, and mathematics."[22]

A recent declaration by the Democratic National Committee suggests that the encouragement of university-industry research relationships transcends partisan political boundaries. The committee proposed the creation, through a reallocation of extant federal funds, of an indeterminate number of "centers of excellence," which would promote collaboration between industry and universities. At least some of these centers would capitalize on established regional resources to promote economic growth in different parts of the country. For example, the committee suggested that a center in the industrialized Midwest might focus on manufacturing improvements, and a center in the Farm Belt might devote itself to food-related biotechnology.[23]

On the state and local level, many are courting collaboration by providing investigative funding, preliminary construction expenses, and other inducements. For example, in 1984 the state of Virginia appropriated over $30 million to found a Center for Innovative Technology to reinvigorate the state economy by attracting high-technology firms through Virginia colleges and universities. Among other plans, the president of the center has proposed to establish fifteen so-called commonwealth centers to conduct research and cater to the needs of state corporations; to encourage entrepreneurial activities at universities through spin-off business ventures from faculty research; and to form a privately endowed fund to support research in *industry*.[24]

Montgomery County, Maryland, the site of the National Institutes of Health, the Food and Drug Administration, the Howard Hughes Medical Institute, and other key governmental and private biomedical institutions, is organizing an ambitious academic and industrial research complex called the Shady Grove Life Sciences Center, with plans to establish an ancillary Research and Development Village of light manufacturing, business services, housing, and hotels. The Life Sciences Center will be the site of a new Center for Advanced Research in Biotechnology, developed jointly by the University of Maryland and the National Bureau of Standards, and a branch research facility of the Johns Hopkins University that will offer master's degree work in electrical engineering, computer sciences, and technical management. Montgomery County not only has provided three hundred thousand dollars in investigative funding for the research and business complex but will construct the buildings to house the Hopkins facility and the Maryland research center at its own expense. The county expects to recoup the millions it is investing in this complex by selling land to companies, the first of which (Otsuka Pharmaceutical

Company of Japan) opened a biotechnology research laboratory in the area in 1985.[25]

Given the tremendous effort today on the part of individual researchers, their departments and universities, city, county, state, and federal governments, and companies to develop and strengthen ties between the academy and industry, one might be led to believe that the formation of ties between these two estates of science must indeed be the path to a modern-day city of gold. However, all involved parties are vulnerable when estates of an intrinsically different nature enter into such close ties as those discussed in this chapter. For example, if local governments—which presumably operate in the public's interest—promote collaboration, can they genuinely represent the public as a disinterested party, especially if they have invested millions of dollars in the collaborative arrangements? If the situation called for such an action, could they regulate or even prosecute a firm participating in the collaboration in a disinterested way? A feasibility study for the Montgomery County project is a case in point. A consultant hired by Johns Hopkins to project the impact of the proposed Life Sciences Center on traffic congestion in the county concluded that the county could not accommodate the expected surplus traffic. However, the County Planning Board, the Department of Transportation, and the Office of Economic Development lowered the consultant's estimates by one-third so that the projected traffic flow would fall within established limits for development in Montgomery County. Officials felt that the research complex was too important for them to accept the original estimate.[26]

Industry as well could stand to lose from collaboration. For business interests, most modern types of collaboration—with the exception of the major long-term agreements as discussed above—have a major flaw from the outset in that the company usually must share the results of its academic research investment with its competitors. Additionally, even in the case of exclusive arrangements with universities, the threat of intelligence leaks is always present. Hence, many companies, especially in biotechnology, are developing in-house research facilities. Many major firms presently supporting academic research in biotechnology—Lilly, Upjohn, Du Pont, Monsanto, and others—either have their own research facilities in operation or are preparing them. Also, agreements between companies and universities often have some provision for the education of industrial scientists so that industry can take the knowledge as well as the results back with it.[27]

The development of interactions between universities and companies in the 1920s and 1930s revealed how a firm might at first invest in an academic laboratory such as Tatum's department at Wisconsin or Macleod's laboratory at Toronto but then draw back once it established its own research facilities. Companies of course had to maintain contact with universities, but this was easily accomplished through occasional consultantships, fellowships, or even the so-called goodwill grants that Lilly made use of. The relevant question for today is whether universities and their communities are overdeveloping ties to companies that may decide that it is more profitable to focus their support on in-house research. The fate of MIT's Research Laboratory of Applied Chemistry, which was anchored to industry, may be an instructive example for many seeking El Dorado (see fig. 16).[28]

Universities are probably most at risk in the proliferation of research relationships with industry. Concern about the possible ramifications of growing university-industry research relationships prompted a conference of presidents and faculty of five universities (Harvard, Cal Tech, MIT, Stanford, and the University of California system) and representatives of eleven corporations (including Lilly, Du Pont, and Genentech) at Pajaro Dunes, on the California coast, in 1982. Although the conference produced little of substantive interest, the stated premise of Pajaro Dunes is worth reproducing:

Research agreements and other arrangements with industry [must] be so constructed as not to promote secrecy that will harm the progress of science, impair the educational experience of students and postdoctoral fellows, diminish the role of the university as a credible and impartial source, interfere with the choice by faculty members of the scientific questions they pursue, or divert the energies of faculty members and the resources of the university from primary obligations to teaching or research.[29]

A recent survey by a group at the Kennedy School of Government at Harvard suggests that most of the situations that the Pajaro Dunes participants hoped would be avoided in agreements between academe and industry have already begun to manifest themselves in American universities.[30] The group surveyed over twelve hundred faculty members in biotechnology departments at forty of the fifty leading research universities (as measured by federal research support). About one-quarter of these faculty were heading grants from companies, of whom half received a minimum of 50 percent of their total research funding from industry. Clearly, industry has a significant role in the support of biotechnological research at the leading research universities in this country. The survey

---

Figure 16. A newspaper advertisement from Pfizer, 1986, calling attention to its role as a partner in medical research with universities and the federal government (courtesy of Chas. Pfizer and Company).

supported the Pajaro Dunes recommendation four years earlier that collaborative research should not jeopardize the professor's teaching and service functions. Those involved in research connections with industry were as faithful to their teaching and service commitments as those who did not have ties with industry.

Other conclusions from the survey suggested precisely what the Pajaro Dunes conference feared. Regarding the conference's concern about secrecy, one-fourth of the faculty working with industry support said that they were performing research that was the property of the sponsor and that they could not publish this research without the sponsor's permission; only 5 percent of the faculty receiving funds from nonindustrial sponsors claimed that their research was similarly restricted. Furthermore, 30 percent of the industry-supported faculty admitted that their choices of research projects were influenced by the likelihood that they would produce commercial applications, compared with 7 percent of their colleagues.

Finally, the Pajaro Dunes concern that ties with industry not impair the educational experience of graduate students and postdoctoral fellows appears to be a problem at hand as well. An earlier survey of about one hundred biotechnology firms by the same Kennedy School group revealed that one-third of the firms support the training of graduate students or postdoctoral fellows, which probably is not surprising nor in itself a cause for concern. However, one-third of these companies said that students "must work on problems or projects defined by the company, work for the firm during the summer, or work for the company after completing their training."[31] Such an arrangement threatens what otherwise should be a rich, broad, and creative educational experience.

There are equally dangerous risks on the horizon. One risk deals with the ability of industrially supported workers to maintain disinterestedness. Not surprisingly, the more talented researchers tend to attract the most interest from companies looking for a research investment, and they also happen to be those who are likely to serve on peer-review boards to consider grant applications for various funding agencies. One must wonder whether they will be able to avoid having their commercial interests in research inform their decisions on such boards. Also, the fact that many talented and powerful figures are involved in research relationships with industry may dissuade some junior faculty from voicing objections to such relationships. The trend among public and private funding bodies to focus on "productive" research and departments leads one to wonder what will happen to areas of the university that are less mindful of the application of their research. Or as one author on the subject has commented, "The [industrial] grants encourage the hypertrophy of one segment of the university while the other segments are allowed to atrophy."[32]

Responses to the present and future dangers of collaboration between universities and industry as it is practiced today have taken several forms. One group, the Center for Universities and the Public Interest, plans to serve as a watchdog committee to reveal how the growth of military and corporate research in academic institutions has compromised traditional university ideals. A group at Washington University that is working with Monsanto avoids the possibility of graduate students' spending their time on narrow industrial problems by simply not permitting students to work on Monsato-supported research. This may, however, be an unreasonable solution for laboratories with too few postdoctoral fellows to perform the industrial research. The Association of American Universities has begun a systematic study of ways by which academic participants in university-industry research relationships have avoided conflicts of interest.[33]

We cannot necessarily assume that the future of collaborative research is secure simply because it has experienced a renaissance in the past decade. Many social, economic, and scientific factors conducive to joint research between academe and industry must remain in effect if collaborative research is to continue. University scientists, for example, must foster attitudes favorable to, or at least tolerant of, industry. Visions of academic research like that which G. Stanley Hall promoted in the late nineteenth century are inimical to cooperative research with industry. On the other hand, industry must have a favorable or tolerant perception of academic work. Industry, as J. K. Lilly argued, serves as its own endowment, and it certainly has the right to expect a return on its investments in research. But companies must understand that they cannot necessarily expect the same type of return on their investments in academic research as they would expect in industrial research. This of course presupposes that interaction between universities and companies is a good and desirable enterprise. Collaboration is not always a good thing, but it is necessary under present circumstances. Universities, industry, and the public now have to decide how much collaboration is desirable for their needs; how much profit and impartiality they are willing to sacrifice; and which is the best possible course to satisfy the public good.

Abbreviations

>>>-->>>-->>>-->>>-->>>- <<<-<<<-<<<-<<<-<<<-

AL	Abbott Laboratories Archives
AR	Alfred Newton Richards Papers
ASL	Arthur Salomon Loevenhart Papers
ASPET	American Society for Pharmacology and Experimental Therapeutics Archives
AT-SHSW	Arthur Lawrie Tatum Papers, State Historical Society of Wisconsin
AT-UW	Arthur Lawrie Tatum Papers, University of Wisconsin Archives
CL	Chauncey D. Leake Papers
EC	Edwin J. Cohn Papers
ELC	Eli Lilly and Company Archives
ERS	E. R. Squibb and Sons Archives
FB	F. G. Banting Papers
FDA	Food and Drug Administration Papers
HS	Harry Steenbock Papers
HU-PAC	Pernicious Anemia Committee Papers, Harvard University
JA	John Jacob Abel Papers
JM	J. J. R. Macleod Papers
KRF	Kremers Reference Files, University of Wisconsin
LS	Lyndon Frederick Small Papers
MC	Merck and Company Archives
MRC	Medical Research Council Records

NJ	New Jersey State Division of Archives and Records Management
RA	Roger Adams Papers
SW	Selman A. Waksman Papers
TS	Torald Sollmann Papers
UT-IC	Insulin Committee Papers, University of Toronto
UW-P	Dean's Office Files, University of Wisconsin School of Pharmacy
UW-PT	Department of Pharmacology and Toxicology Papers, University of Wisconsin

Notes

➤➤➤-➤➤➤-➤➤➤-➤➤➤-➤➤➤-‹‹‹-‹‹‹-‹‹‹-‹‹‹-‹‹‹

CHAPTER ONE

The Emergence of Biomedical and Industrial Research in America

1. Among the better introductions to these developments are Aaron J. Ihde, *The Development of Modern Chemistry*; Karl E. Rothschuh, *History of Physiology*; B. Holmstedt and G. Liljestrand, eds., *Readings in Pharmacology*; and Hubert A. Lechevalier and Morris Solotorovsky, *Three Centuries of Microbiology*.

2. Robert E. Kohler, *From Medical Chemistry to Biochemistry*, 94.

3. Richard Harrison Shryock, *American Medical Research*, 68–69. On the antivivisectionist movement in Britain see Richard D. French, *Antivivisection and Medical Science in Victorian Society*.

4. Shryock, *American Medical Research*, 70–72; Gerald L. Geison, "Divided We Stand"; Russell C. Maulitz, " 'Physician versus Bacteriologist' "; John Parascandola, "The Search for the Active Oxytocic Principle of Ergot."

5. John Harley Warner, "Physiology," 60–63; Philip J. Pauly, "The Appearance of Academic Biology in Late Nineteenth-Century America"; John F. Fulton, *Physiology*, 102–7.

6. Russell H. Chittenden, *The Development of Physiological Chemistry in the United States*, 27.

7. The definitive study of the development of biochemistry as a discipline is Kohler, *From Medical Chemistry to Biochemistry*. See also Chittenden, *The Development of Physiological Chemistry*; and Stanley L. Becker, "The Emergence of a Trace Nutrient Concept through Animal Feeding Experiments."

8. John Parascandola, "John J. Abel and the Early Development of Pharmacology at the Johns Hopkins University"; John Parascandola and Elizabeth Keeney, *Sources in the History of American Pharmacology*; David L. Cowen, "Materia Medica and Pharmacology."

9. For example, few university chemistry departments adopted biochemistry as a sister of organic, analytical, and other established fields of chemistry. Only a fraction of those departments that did offer biochemistry taught it in a satisfactory way—at least as far as medical schools were concerned. Abel opposed separate Ph.D. programs for

pharmacology; he preferred that the pharmacologist have a solid training in chemistry and physics prior to work leading to the medical degree. An alternative degree-granting source for pharmacology—schools of pharmacy—did not develop on a significant scale until the 1930s (see Robert E. Kohler, "Medical Reform and Biomedical Science," 30; Parascandola, "Abel and the Development of Pharmacology," 523; John Parascandola and John Swann, "Development of Pharmacology in American Schools of Pharmacy").

10. Kohler, "Medical Reform and Biomedical Science."

11. Howard R. Bartlett, "The Development of Industrial Research in the United States," 2:19–25; Kendall Birr, "The Roots of Industrial Research," 27–29; George H. Daniels, *Science in American Society*, 318; Leonard S. Reich, *The Making of American Industrial Research*, 17–18, 20–23, 36.

12. Bartlett, "Industrial Research in the United States," 25–34; Daniels, *Science in American Society*, 318; Raymond F. Bacon, "Industrial Research in America," 226–30; Reich, *American Industrial Research*, 26–27.

13. Bartlett, "Industrial Research in the United States," 25–26, 29–31; Birr, "Roots of Industrial Research," 31–32; Reich, *American Industrial Research*, 27–29.

14. Daniels, *Science in American Society*, 319; see also Reich, *American Industrial Research*, 34–35, 39–40.

15. A. Hunter Dupree, *Science in the Federal Government*, 302–25; Bartlett, "Industrial Research in the United States," 35–37; Birr, "Roots of Industrial Research," 32.

16. Clarence J. West and Ervye Risher, "Industrial Research Laboratories of the United States"; Clarence J. West and Callie Hull, "Industrial Research Laboratories of the United States"; Callie Hull, "Industrial Research Laboratories of the United States," 6th ed.; idem, "Industrial Research Laboratories of the United States," 7th ed.; Birr, "Roots of Industrial Research," 40–41; Franklin S. Cooper, "Location and Extent of Industrial Research Activity in the United States," 2:174 (fig. 44). Note that the tabulation includes consulting laboratories, although the majority of the data pertain to company laboratories. The NRC conducted earlier surveys of industrial research laboratories, but these were not as comprehensive as the 1927 and later surveys.

17. Cooper, "Location and Extent of Industrial Research," 174 (fig. 44). These data should be qualified to the extent that it is difficult to identify, much less quantify, total research staff in a firm. Companies did not necessarily differentiate between the functions of their technical staff and those of their research staff. For example, research could very well have been an occasional function of personnel who also had quite different responsibilities in the plant. This distinction is not clear in the NRC surveys; however, the surveys clearly indicate a trend of increasing research activity in industry between the two world wars.

18. Bartlett, "Industrial Research in the United States," 38.

19. David Charles Mowery, "The Emergence and Growth of Industrial Research in American Manufacturing, 1899–1945," 120.

20. David Charles Mowery, "The Relationship between Intrafirm and Contractual Forms of Industrial Research in American Manufacturing, 1900–1940."

21. Robert Kennedy Duncan, "On Industrial Fellowships," 600–602.

22. Ibid., 602. Although Duncan personally felt that industrialists would not trust

him if he wanted to make some money, many academic scientists and industrialists would take issue with such a belief.

23. Ibid., 602–3; Mowery, "Growth of Research in American Manufacturing," 257–58.

24. John W. Servos, "The Industrial Relations of Science: Chemical Engineering at MIT, 1900–1939."

25. Arnold Thackray, "University-Industry Connections and Chemical Research," 219–22; Merle Curti and Roderick Nash, *Philanthropy in the Shaping of American Higher Education*, 240; Mowery, "Growth of Research in American Manufacturing," 97–102.

26. Thackray, "University-Industry Connections," 220; D. Stanley Tarbell and Ann Tracy Tarbell, *Roger Adams*. See also below, chap. 3.

27. David Charles Mowery, "British and American Industrial Research," 26; Roger L. Geiger, *To Advance Knowledge*, 177; Bartlett, "Industrial Research in the United States," 38; Thackray, "University-Industry Connections," 216.

28. Lance E. Davis and Daniel J. Kevles, "The National Research Fund"; Geiger, *To Advance Knowledge*, 97 ff.; Ronald C. Tobey, *The American Ideology of National Science, 1919–1930*, 200–225.

29. William J. Hale, "Cooperative Research between Industries and Universities," *Annual Survey of American Chemistry*, 1:250–57; idem, ibid. 2:395–97; Albert L. Barrows, "The Relationship of the National Research Council to Industrial Research," 367.

30. Glenn Sonnedecker, "The Rise of Drug Manufacture in America," 75–76; George Urdang, "Retail Pharmacy as the Nucleus of the Pharmaceutical Industry," 334.

31. Georg Meyer-Thurow, "The Industrialization of Invention"; John J. Beer, "Coal Tar Dye Manufacture."

32. Sonnedecker, "Drug Manufacture," 77–79; Jonathan Michael Liebenau, "Medical Science and Medical Industry, 1890–1929," 46–47; David L. Cowen, "The Nineteenth Century German Immigrant and American Pharmacy," 21.

33. Malcolm Keith Weikel, "Research as a Function of Pharmaceutical Industry," 29–36; David L. Cowen, "The Role of the Pharmaceutical Industry," 73; Liebenau, "Medical Science and Medical Industry," 107–9.

34. Liebenau, "Medical Science and Medical Industry," 186–93; the quotation is from p. 186.

35. Weikel, "Research as a Function of Pharmaceutical Industry," 68–79, 97–104; Peter Stechl, "Biological Standardization of Drugs before 1928," 60–82.

36. Jonathan M. Liebenau, "Scientific Ambitions," 4–6.

37. Ibid., 6–10; Weikel, "Research as a Function of Pharmaceutical Industry," 86–89.

38. Weikel, "Research," 67–68, 105–6, 128; Liebenau, "Medical Science and Medical Industry," 19, 109–10, 188–91, 294–95, 334–35, 363; "Contract between H. K. Mulford Co., of Philadelphia, PA., and Dr. Torald Sollmann, Cleveland, Ohio," 1 March 1900, TS.

CHAPTER TWO

The Rise of University-Industry Interactions in Biomedical Research

1. Of course, barriers to cooperative research never dissolved completely. For example, it is not uncommon today to find university researchers who refuse to investigate industry-selected problems.

2. By fundamental (or basic or pure) research I mean learning for its own sake, to supplement the sum understanding in a field without consideration of any other use. When I refer to applied (or practical) research, I mean learning for the sake of utility or public benefit other than pure intellectual elevation.

3. See Walter B. Kolesnik, *Mental Discipline in Modern Education*, 3–29; the quotation is from p. 18.

4. The following relies on Stanley M. Guralnick, "The American Scientist in Higher Education, 1820–1910."

5. Ibid., 111–12, 115–16; Robert Post, "Science, Public Policy, and Popular Precepts." Cf. Nathan Reingold, "Alexander Dallas Bache."

6. Richard Hofstadter and Walter P. Metzger, *The Development of Academic Freedom in the United States*, 370–73 (the quotation is from 373); Joseph Ben-David and Awraham Zloczower, "Universities and Academic Systems in Modern Societies," 50–53.

7. See Guenter B. Risse, "Kant, Schelling, and the Early Search for a Philosophical 'Science' of Medicine in Germany."

8. See, e.g., Ben-David and Zloczower, "Universities and Academic Systems," 53–57.

9. Hofstadter and Metzger, *Development of Academic Freedom*, 372 (quotation), 374; Laurence R. Veysey, *The Emergence of the American University*, 126–27; Ben-David and Zloczower, "Universities and Academic Systems," 49.

10. Beer, "Coal Tar Dye Manufacture," 131 n. 24. See also Meyer-Thurow, "Industrialization of Invention," 365, 368, 376–77; Jeffrey A. Johnson, "Academic Chemistry in Imperial Germany," 506 ff.; and Timothy Lenoir, "The Binding of Scientific Inquiry."

11. Johnson, "Academic Chemistry," 513–14.

12. Veysey, *Emergence of the American University*, 130 (quotation); Merle Curti, *The Growth of American Thought*, 566.

13. Hofstadter and Metzger, *Development of Academic Freedom*, 377–79; Curti, *Growth of American Thought*, 569.

14. Veysey, *Emergence of the American University*, 149.

15. G. Stanley Hall, "Research the Vital Spirit of Teaching," 561–62; 570.

16. However, Lenoir, "Binding of Scientific Inquiry," is a very good start.

17. See Richard Harrison Shryock, "American Indifference to Basic Science during the Nineteenth Century"; and Edmund Janes James, "The Function of the State University." Cf. Nathan Reingold, "American Indifference to Basic Research," which argues persuasively against Shryock's thesis of the sudden emergence of basic research.

18. Hofstadter and Metzger, *Development of Academic Freedom*, 381–82.

19. See, e.g., Robert E. Kohler, *From Medical Chemistry to Biochemistry*; Gerald L. Geison, "Divided We Stand"; and Russell C. Maulitz, " 'Physician versus Bacteriologist.' "

20. Henry Newall Martin, quoted in Geison, "Divided We Stand," 71; Kohler, *From Medical Chemistry to Biochemistry*, 97–101; John J. Abel, "The Methods of Pharmacology," 105.

21. J. J. Abel to W. deB. MacNider, 5 April 1935, JA. I am indebted to John Parascandola for this and all other letters cited from the Abel Papers. For an example of an influential physical scientist's repudiation of commercial work see Owen Hannaway, "The German Model of Chemical Education in America."

22. *Code of Ethics of the American Medical Association*, chap. 2, art. 1, sec. 4, reproduced in Chauncey D. Leake, ed., *Percival's Medical Ethics*, 226.

23. See George E. Folk, *Patents and Industrial Progress*, 152–53, but cf. Richard Harrison Shryock, *American Medical Research*, 140.

24. Hans Zinsser, "Problems of the Bacteriologist," 161.

25. J. J. Abel to S. L. Johnson, 21 September 1935, JA.

26. F. E. Stewart, "Is It Ethical for Medical Men to Patent Medical Inventions?" 586 (Squibb is quoted from his discussion following this paper); F. W. Nitardy, "Long Range Comparative Report (1916–1941)," typescript, 1 July 1941, 43, "Research, 1900–1925," ERS.

27. Williams Haynes, *American Chemical Industry*, 3:481–508, 512–15; Malcolm Keith Weikel, "Research as a Function of Pharmaceutical Industry," 56–57; Jonathan Michael Liebenau, "Medical Science and Medical Industry, 1890–1929," 92–93; *Code of Ethics*, chap. 2, art. 1, sec. 4, in Leake, *Percival's Medical Ethics*, 226.

28. This is precisely what Mulford did (see Liebenau, "Medical Science and Medical Industry," 197).

29. The definitive histories of "patent" medicines and health quackery are James Harvey Young, *The Toadstool Millionaires*; and idem, *The Medical Messiahs*.

30. As late as 1946, K. K. Chen, a well-respected pharmacologist with Lilly, informed a colleague, "As a rule, I do not publish any negative results from various investigations" (K. K. Chen to C. D. Leake, 8 April 1946, box 44, "Lilly Research Laboratories [K. K. Chen], Jan.–June 1946," CL).

31. Hans Molitor, "Merck Institute of Therapeutic Research: Sixth Annual Report (1938)," typescript, 8, box 30, "Merck Institute, 1931–1940," AR.

32. J. J. Abel to [R.] Hatcher, 31 January 1910, JA.

33. Sinclair Lewis, *Arrowsmith*, 132; see also Charles E. Rosenberg, *No Other Gods*, 123–31.

34. R. A. Hatcher to [J.J.] Abel, 28 January 1910, JA. Sollmann himself had worked much more closely with a firm (albeit a respectable pharmaceutical company). Sollmann had concluded an agreement with Mulford in 1900 whereby the firm paid him one hundred dollars monthly and furnished equipment and supplies for his exclusive services to Mulford as a consultant. The agreement lasted for at least six months (see "Contract between H. K. Mulford Co., of Philadelphia, PA., and Dr. Torald Sollmann, Cleveland, Ohio," TS [I thank John Parascandola for this document]).

35. Abel to Hatcher, 31 January 1910, and R. A. Hatcher to [J.J.] Abel, 2 February 1910, JA.

36. W. deB. MacNider to J. J. Abel, 29 May 1931, JA. Abel sometimes counseled his colleagues that cooperative work seemed acceptable to him, as when A. N. Richards sought his advice on a possible consultantship with Merck (see chap. 3).

37. Abel to Hatcher, 31 January 1910. The American firm to which Abel referred

was Parke-Davis, which had hired pharmacologist E. M. Houghton from the University of Michigan in 1895.

38. J. K. Crellin, "Industrial Pharmacy," 107.

39. Stewart, "Is It Ethical to Patent Inventions?" 586; S. J. Meltzer to A. S. Loevenhart, 20 December 1919, box 3, "Personal Correspondence, P–Q," ASL.

40. From art. 3 of the ASPET constitution, reproduced in K. K. Chen, ed., *The American Society for Pharmacology and Experimental Therapeutics*, 184.

41. The development of research in the pharmaceutical industry after World War I has not previously received significant attention from historians. For a brief overview of the subject see John Parascandola, "Industrial Research Comes of Age."

42. Some control chemists and pharmacologists also found time to work on new products, but by and large their primary responsibility was in the control laboratory (see Weikel, "Research as a Function of Pharmaceutical Industry," 52–53).

43. Liebenau, "Medical Science and Medical Industry," 84, 237–79; Ramunas A. Kondratas, "Biologics Control Act of 1902."

44. See, e.g., Liebenau, "Medical Science and Medical Industry," 313–15; and Haynes, *American Chemical Industry*, 3:311–26.

45. Alfred S. Burdick, quoted in Herman Kogan, *The Long White Line*, 119; C. H. Palmer to F. W. Nitardy (plant superintendent at Squibb), 30 March 1922, "M(1): Research and Development, General, 1920s," ERS.

46. J. K. Lilly to E. Lilly and J. K. Lilly, Jr., 27 April 1926, "J. K. Lilly, Jr., Letters to and from Mr. Lilly, 18 Feb. 1926–11 Sept. 1931," XCAc, ELC. See also Josiah K. Lilly, "Comments on Research in Manufacturing Pharmacy," 5–6; and Gene E. McCormick, "Josiah Kirby Lilly, Sr., the Man," 64–65.

47. George W. Merck, "An Essential Partnership," 739 (quotation); Max Tishler, interview by Leon Gortler and John A. Heitmann, 28–29.

48. Kogan, *Long White Line*, 120; Elmer B. Vliet, "The Abbott Story," lecture delivered at the Research-Development-Control Dinner, Abbott Auditorium, [North Chicago, Ill.,] 16 March 1950, typescript, 12, "Abbott—History," AL; Leonard Engel, *Medicine Makers of Kalamazoo*, 91; Merck and Company, *The Merck Corporation: Annual Report, 1931*; "Merck and Co., Inc. and Consolidated Domestic Subsidiaries: Analysis of Research and Development Expenses," typescript, 15 November 1951, box 29, "Budget, 1953," AR; F. W. Nitardy, "Research and Library Work," typescript (unpaginated), 24 March 1931 [6], ERS; E. R. Squibb and Sons, "Annual Report," typescript, 8 April 1931, 49, "Research, 1900–1925," ERS; Eli Lilly and Company, *Lilly Research Laboratories: Dedication*, 118.

49. O. W. Smith to [E. M.] Houghton, 5 February 1924, historical file, Parke-Davis Research Library, Ann Arbor, Michigan (copy in C[38]a, UW-KRF). The members of the committee were E. M. Houghton (chairman), F. O. Taylor, C. H. Briggs, L. T. Clark, O. Kamm, and A. W. Lescohier. The following year, Wilbur Scoville replaced Briggs, and W. E. King joined the committee (see Weikel, "Research as a Function of Pharmaceutical Industry," 124–25).

50. John Francis Marion, *The Fine Old House*, 130; Gabriel P. Becker, "A Study of the History and Development of Abbott Laboratories," 48; Tishler, interview by Gortler and Heitmann, 31–32.

51. Lilly, "Research in Manufacturing Pharmacy," 6; F. W. Nitardy to P. M. Giesy, 11 April 1924, "M(1): Research and Development, General, 1920s," ERS.

52. G. H. A. Clowes to J. K. Lilly and E. Lilly, 25 January 1929, "G. H. A. Clowes, Correspondence, 1925–1956," XRDc, ELC.

53. [G. H. A. Clowes,] "Report of Scientific Research Work for Year Ending November 1st, 1921," typescript, "G. H. A. Clowes—Report of Scientific Research Work, Year Ending 1 Nov. 1921," XRDe, ELC; the quotation is from p. 1.

54. [G. H. A. Clowes,] "Preliminary Report of Research Department for Year Ending October 20th, 1921," typescript, 3–4, "G. H. A. Clowes, Preliminary Report, Research Dept., 1921," XRDe, ELC.

55. J. C. Fisher, "Basic Research in Industry." The drug companies that placed among the top twenty in Fisher's study of the number of basic research publications as a measure of basic research in industry were Merck (ranked 5th, with 90 publications), Lilly (12th, 54), Upjohn (15th, 44), Burroughs Wellcome, U.S. branch (16th, 35), and Abbott and Parke-Davis (19th, 32 each). The author lists American Cyanamid as 4th with 107 publications but does not include Lederle (a subsidiary of Cyanamid), which produced 60 of Cyanamid's publications; I include Lederle among the top 20.

56. Tishler, interview by Gortler and Heitmann, 29.

57. Francis C. Wood, "John F. Anderson"; "Dr. John F. Anderson"; "Testimonial Dinner Tendered by His Friends and Associates in the Scientific Divisions to Dr. Ernest H. Volwiler in Appreciation of His Notable Services to Abbott Laboratories, to Science, and to Mankind since May 1, 1918," [Chicago, Ill.,] 26 March 1959, mimeograph, AL; George H. A. Clowes, Jr., "George Henry Alexander Clowes"; M. E. Krahl, "Obituary: George Henry Alexander Clowes."

58. *American Men of Science*, 8th ed., s.v. "Gudernatsch, Dr. Friedrich"; Tishler, interview by Gortler and Heitmann, 28–29.

59. G. Stanley Hall, quoted in Veysey, *Emergence of the American University*, 125 n. 12; see also Ronald C. Tobey, *The American Ideology of National Science, 1919–1930*, chap. 1.

60. For example, in John Dewey's *Democracy in Education* (1916) we read that "the isolation and exclusiveness of a gang or clique brings its antisocial spirit into relief. But this same spirit is found wherever one group has interests 'of its own' which shut it out from full interaction with other groups, so that its prevailing purpose is the protection of what it has got, instead of reorganization and progress through wider relationships. . . . The essential point is that isolation makes for rigidity and formal institutionalizing of life, for static and selfish ideals within the group" (from John Dewey, *John Dewey*, 223).

61. "Merck Research Laboratory Dedicated"; Eli Lilly Company, *Lilly Research Laboratories: Dedication*. See also *The Field and the Work of the Squibb Institute*; "Squibb Institute for Medical Research Dedicated October 11"; and Abbott Laboratories, *Addresses*.

62. "Merck Research Laboratory Dedicated," 82; G. H. A. Clowes, "Address by Dr. George H. A. Clowes," 53–54.

63. Ernest H. Volwiler, "Introduction"; Lilly, "Research in Manufacturing Pharmacy," 5; "Merck Research Laboratory Dedicated," 82; Carleton Palmer, "Welcome."

64. H. Molitor to [A. N.] Richards, 28 September 1932, box 32, "Hans Molitor, 1932–1933," AR.

65. New Jersey General Assembly, *Acts of the One Hundred and Fourth Legislature of the State of New Jersey*, chap. 157.

66. New Jersey General Assembly, *Acts of the One Hundred and Thirty-ninth Legislature of the State of New Jersey*, chap. 160, sec. 17.

67. Lilly, for example, established the Lilly Laboratory for Clinical Research in the Indianapolis City Hospital in 1926. Originally, the laboratory evaluated clinical reports on Lilly products from outside clinics, but soon it emphasized original investigations (see Kenneth G. Kohlstaedt, ["The Lilly Laboratory for Clinical Research,"] typescript, n.d., "History of the Lilly Laboratory for Clinical Research, 1926–1958," XRDuc, ELC; Leon G. Zerfas, interview by Gene E. McCormick, 6–8, 23, 26–32, 36, 41–42; and E. J. Kahn, Jr., *All in a Century*, 123).

68. Minutes of meetings of the Department of Health of the State of New Jersey, 13 September 1932 and 6 December 1932, NJ (for these and other materials from this collection I am indebted to David Cowen). R. T. Major to A. N. Richards, 29 December 1932, box 30, "Merck Institute, 1931–1940"; A. N. Richards to C. I. Lafferty, 30 December 1932; A. N. Richards to A. H. Lippincott, all in AR.

69. One of the stated purposes of the Merck Institute was reproduced verbatim from the 1915 amendment: "the investigation into the causes, nature and mode of prevention and cure of diseases in men and animals" (from Certificate of Incorporation of the Merck Institute of Therapeutic Research, art. 2, in "Certificate of Incorporation and By-Laws of Merck Institute of Therapeutic Research," mimeograph, 1, n.d., MC).

70. Ibid.; minutes of a meeting of the Department of Health of the State of New Jersey, 10 January 1933, NJ; New Jersey Department of Health, *Fifty-sixth Annual Report*, 19–20; H. Molitor, "Merck Institute of Therapeutic Research: Third Annual Report," typescript, 15 January 1936, 9–11, box 30, "Merck Institute, 1931–1940," AR; Hans Molitor and Michael Kniazuk, "A New Bloodless Method for Continuous Recording of Peripheral Circulatory Changes."

71. C. M. Gruber to H. B. van Dyke, 13 July 1938, Minutes and Records, vol. 5, 1938–39; H. B. van Dyke to C. M. Gruber, 14 July 1938; H. B. van Dyke to G. P. Grabfield, 21 November 1938; G. A. Harrop to G. P. Grabfield, 22 November 1938; C. Gruber to H. B. van Dyke, 21 July 1938; Minutes of the 30th Annual Meeting of the American Society for Pharmacology and Experimental Therapeutics, 26 April 1939, all from ASPET (I thank John Parascandola for documents cited from this collection).

72. The board of trustees (George Merck, George Perkins, and Joseph Rosin) supervised the financial aspects of the institute; the scientific directors (Molitor, Randolph Major, William H. Engels, and Dickinson Richards, a consultant to Merck on medical affairs) determined research problems; and the scientific advisors (A. N. Richards, William B. Castle, and Henry Dakin) offered counsel on the institute's general policies (see Molitor, "Merck Institute: Sixth Annual Report," 18; and *The Merck Institute for Therapeutic Research*, [3]).

73. [H. Molitor,] "Merck Institute of Therapeutic Research: Its Organization at Present and in the Future," typescript, c. January 1935, 4, attached to H. Molitor to [A. N.] Richards, 18 January 1935, box 30, "Merck Institute, 1931–1940," AR.

74. Molitor, "Merck Institute: Organization," 12–14; idem, "Merck Institute of Therapeutic Research: Fifth Annual Report," typescript, c. January 1938, 3–4, box 30, "Merck Institute, 1931–1940," AR; idem, "Merck Institute for Therapeutic Research: Seventh Annual Report," typescript, 19 January 1940, 7–8, ibid.; *Merck Institute for Therapeutic Research*, [28].

75. Molitor, "Merck Institute: Organization," 3, 18; idem, "Merck Institute of Therapeutic Research: Fourth Annual Report," typescript, c. January 1937, 7, box 30, "Merck Institute, 1931–1940," AR; H. Molitor to [A. N.] Richards, 2 December 1938, report, [14], [21], [30], [33], ibid.; Molitor, "Merck Institute: Seventh Annual Report," 10–12; H. Molitor to [A. N.] Richards, 6 March 1936, box 30, "Merck Institute, 1931–1940," AR; Molitor to Richards, 2 December 1938, 8.

76. Molitor to Richards, 2 December 1938, 10–11.

77. Molitor, "Merck Institute: Organization," 1; Molitor to Richards, 2 December 1938, 4.

78. Molitor, "Merck Institute: Fifth Annual Report," 7; Molitor to Richards, 2 December 1938, [15] (listing travel expenses for 1933–38).

79. For a bibliography of institute publications through 1941 see *Merck Institute for Therapeutic Research*, [39–43].

80. Molitor, "Merck Institute: Fifth Annual Report," 7–8.

81. Molitor, "Merck Institute: Sixth Annual Report," 4–5.

82. Molitor, "Merck Institute: Third Annual Report," 19, and idem, "Merck Institute: Sixth Annual Report," 16.

83. Alfred S. Burdick, "Research," 373–74.

84. The Lilly Fellowship for the Study of Chemistry at the Johns Hopkins University, for example, was a philanthropic fellowship. It awarded a thousand-dollar stipend to an Indiana resident for study at the Baltimore university (see Callie Hull and Clarence J. West, "Fellowships and Scholarships for Advanced Work in Science and Technology," 2d ed., 62). One could argue, of course, that such publicized "philanthropic" fellowships improved a firm's image. In terms of a company's research interests, however, such a fellowship was marginally relevant at most.

85. See, e.g., the descriptions of J. K. Lilly fellowships 28 and 29 at the Purdue University College of Pharmacy and the Parke, Davis and Company fellowships in the Department of Chemistry at the Iowa State College of Agriculture and Mechanic Arts in Callie Hull and Clarence J. West, in "Fellowships and Scholarships for Advanced Work in Science and Technology," 3d ed., 67, 120.

86. Several examples can be seen in the arrangements that Wisconsin pharmacologists Arthur Loevenhart and Arthur Tatum made with the many firms with which they collaborated (see chap. 4).

87. See, e.g., F. W. Nitardy (Squibb general superintendent) to P. M. Giesy, 28 August 1923, "M(1): Research and Development, General, 1920s," ERS: "We might contribute to the expenses of people who would . . . in return [keep] us informed on what was going on and what new things were under investigation, so that if anything of particular interest to E. R. Squibb and Sons were under investigation, we would have first hand information on it and could get in touch with the investigator personally if the case should warrant it. This, as you will see, is just for the purpose of linking the House up in some sort of a direct form with all the medical research work that is done in public institutions."

88. Research Information Service, "Fellowships and Scholarships for Advanced Work in Science and Technology"; Hull and West, "Fellowships and Scholarships," 2d and 3d eds.

89. Where information was incomplete, I made some assumptions. For the 1929 survey, I assumed that Upjohn awarded five fellowships at Kalamazoo College, the

number the firm awarded according to the 1923 survey. Also, the 1929 survey did not state the amount of the Squibb fellowships at California, Hopkins, and Wisconsin; thus, the value of these fellowships is not reflected in the last column, although I counted Squibb and its three fellowships. For the 1934 survey, I again assumed that Upjohn offered five fellowships at Kalamazoo College, and I assumed that Parke-Davis offered three fellowships at Iowa State (the number the firm awarded in 1929). Several companies in the 1934 survey did not state the amount of some of their fellowships: Abbott (1), Lilly (2), Parke-Davis (3), and Squibb (1). While I counted the companies and these seven fellowships, the value of the latter is not included in the last column.

90. See, e.g., Tatum's connections with Abbott (chap. 4).

91. E. R. Squibb and Sons, "Annual Report," 8 April 1931, 51. Squibb supported a fellowship at (at least) one private research institution, the Mellon Institute, which is included in the data; however, the bulk of Squibb's fellowships went to academic workers.

92. Engel, *Medicine Makers of Kalamazoo*, 89–90.

93. J. H. Gage to A. N. Richards, 12 December 1938, box 31, "Merck and Co., 1930–1939," AR; [J. K. Lilly,] "Eli Lilly and Company: A History," 75, 91–92, ELC; Minutes of the meeting of the Research Committee, Eli Lilly and Company, 1 July 1942, "Research Committee, 1942," +XRDj, ELC; "Outline of 1943 Research Plan," sec. 6, p. 1, "Research Plans, 1942–1944," ibid.

94. See *Proceedings of the National Conference on Pharmaceutical Research*, which began publication in 1928, and the *Annual Survey of Research in Pharmacy*, which replaced the Conference's *Proceedings* and continued to be published until 1940.

95. Peter Stechl, "Biological Standardization of Drugs before 1928," 223–29. Industry scientists had played a prominent role in a similar committee, the Committee on Physiological Testing of the Scientific Section of the American Pharmaceutical Association, since its inception in 1910 (see M. G. Allmark et al., "A History of the Committee on Physiological Testing").

96. Haynes, *American Chemical Industry*, 4:251–52.

97. W. P. Murphy to A. N. Richards, 6 and 13 September, 9 October 1939; A. N. Richards to W. P. Murphy, 11 September 1939; and A. N. Richards to R. G. Harrison, 11 June 1940, all in box 14, "Murphy's Committee," AR. According to Richards to Harrison, 11 June 1940, the idea for this committee originated with the Du Ponts' personal physician-psychiatrists, who were interested in medical research and "wanted to get some of the duPont money but [they] decided that their claims were scarcely convincing enough to bring home the bacon, and so they conceived the plan of drawing in the medical [researchers]."

98. Murphy to Richards, 9 October 1939.

99. Minutes of Lilly Research Committee meetings, 20 May and 10 July 1942; and report of the Fellowship Committee of the Lilly Research Committee, 1 July 1942, both in "Research Committee, 1942," ELC.

100. "Outline of 1943 Research Plan," sec. 4, pp. 2–3.

101. J. P. Scott to [K. K.] Chen and [H. A.] Shonle, 6 April 1942, "Research Committee, 1942," ELC; minutes of Lilly Research Committee meetings, 20 May, 10 July, 12 November 1942, ibid.; "Outline of 1943 Research Plan," sec. 4, pp. 2–3; minutes of the Executive Committee of the Lilly Research Committee meeting, 8 February 1943, "Re-

search Committee, 1943," +XRDj, ELC; minutes of the Lilly Research Committee meeting, 13 May 1943, ibid.

102. Report of the Committee on Scientific Awards of the Lilly Research Committee, 11 June 1942, "Research Committee, 1942," ELC. On the typical terms of these awards see, e.g., "The Eli Lilly and Company Award in Biological Chemistry."

103. Minutes of the Lilly Research Committee meeting, 10 July 1942; minutes of the Executive Committee of the Lilly Research Committee meeting, 13 August 1942, "Research Committee, 1942," ELC; minutes of the Executive Committee of the Lilly Research Committee meeting, 1 April 1943, "Research Committee, 1943," ELC.

104. Report of the Committee on Contact Visits to Research Centers of the Lilly Research Committee, 6 July 1942, "Research Committee, 1942," ELC; minutes of the Lilly Research Committee meeting, 10 July 1942.

105. Report of the Committee on Delegates to Society Meetings of the Lilly Research Committee, 6 July 1942, "Research Committee, 1942," ELC; minutes of the Lilly Research Committee meeting, 10 July 1942; minutes of the Lilly Research Committee meetings, 20 May and 10 July 1942. Some of these distinguished speakers, however, already had connections with Lilly; for example, Vincent du Vigneaud had held a Lilly grant since 1938.

106. "Outline of 1943 Research Plan," sec. 3, pp. 1–2.

107. John Parascandola, "Academic Pharmacologists and the Pharmaceutical Industry in the United States, 1900–1940"; minutes of the 11th annual meeting of the American Society for Pharmacology and Experimental Therapeutics, Cincinnati, Ohio, 29 December 1919; A. S. Loevenhart to S. J. Meltzer, 19 January 1920; and A. S. Loevenhart et al., circular regarding proposed amendment to the Constitution of the American Society for Pharmacology and Experimental Therapeutics, n.d., all in box 3, "Personal Correspondence, P–Q," ASL.

108. J. J. Abel to W. deB. MacNider, 3 June 1931, JA; see also Abel to MacNider, 5 April 1935.

109. Parascandola, "Academic Pharmacologists and the Pharmaceutical Industry"; Chen, *American Society*, 178–79.

110. Nitardy, "Long Range Comparative Report," 43; R. T. Major, "Report of Research and Development, Merck and Co., Inc., Year of 1937," typescript, 25 March 1938, 17–20, box 31, "Merck and Co., 1930–1939," AR; "Testimonial Dinner to Volwiler," [10]; Nicholas Murray Butler, quoted in H. Steenbock, "The Relations of the Writer to the Wisconsin Research Foundation and the Events Which Led to Its Organization," typescript, January 1926, box 1, "Relation of Writer to Foundation, 1," HS (I am indebted to Jonathan Liebenau for this and other material cited from the Steenbock Papers). See also Shryock, *American Medical Research*, 141.

111. Steenbock, "Relations of the Writer to the Wisconsin Research Foundation"; Shryock, *American Medical Research*, 141; [H. Steenbock,] "The Administration of the Results of Research," typescript, n.d., box 1, "Relation of Writer to Foundation, 1," HS; Michael Bliss, *The Discovery of Insulin*, 131–33; Morris Fishbein, "Medical Patents," 1539–40.

112. Shryock, *American Medical Research*, 88–174; George Rosen, "Patterns of Health Research in the United States, 1900–1906," 211–16; Roger L. Geiger, *To Advance Knowledge*; 176, 191, 246–55.

CHAPTER THREE
The Scientist as General Consultant

1. Unless indicated otherwise, when I refer to a consultant or consultantship, I mean a general consultant or consultantship.

2. Arnold Thackray, "An Academic Genius with Links to Industrial Science." Adams's department produced 544 Ph.D's from 1922 to 1941, and over half of these went into industry (see Roger Adams, "Universities and Industry in Science," 506).

3. D. Stanley Tarbell and Ann Tracy Tarbell, *Roger Adams*, 99, 221–28. Also, eight of Adams's postdoctoral fellows went into the pharmaceutical industry (see ibid., 299–31).

4. Ibid., 103–14, 137–48, 183–95.

5. See L. F. Haber, *The Chemical Industry, 1900*–1930; Williams Haynes, *American Chemical Industry*, vols. 1 and 3; and John Swann, "The Rise of American Synthetic Drug Industry before 1920."

6. Herman Kogan, *The Long White Line*, 85–89; Louis Goodman and Alfred Gilman, *The Pharmacological Basis of Therapeutics*, 847–49. The company introduced, for example, the antiseptic Chlorazene and Halazone, a sterilizing agent for drinking water.

7. Tarbell and Tarbell, *Roger Adams*, 52–57; Roger Adams, "The Manufacture of Organic Chemicals at the University of Illinois"; transactions of the board of trustees of the University of Illinois, 21 July 1916–11 June 1918, 717–18, University of Illinois Archives, Urbana, Ill.

8. Ernest H. Volwiler, interview by John P. Swann, 1. Kogan, *Long White Line*, 93. E. Vliet to W. Southern, 24 March 1984, AL (Abbott hired Vliet as a chemist in 1919). R. Adams to Abbott Alkaloidal Co., 17 September 1917; A. S. Burdick to R. Adams, 25 October 1917; and R. Adams to A. S. Burdick, 3 December 1917, all in box 4, "Procaine, 1917–1918," RA. R. Adams to J. Stieglitz, 22 June 1918, box 4, "1918–1919," ibid. E. Fischer, "C-C-Dialkyl-barbituric Acid and Process of Making Same." Under the Trading with the Enemy Act, Abbott was able to produce this patented drug without seeking the permission of the patentee (who had assigned his patent to a German firm).

9. R. Adams to A. S. Burdick, 6 November 1917, box 4, "Procaine, 1917–1918," RA; Adams to Stieglitz, 22 June 1918; A. S. Burdick to R. Adams, 6 December 1917, box 4, "Procaine, 1917–1918," RA.

10. R. Adams to A. S. Burdick, 6 November and 3 December 1917 and 2 February 1918; and A. S. Burdick to R. Adams, 8 and 20 November 1917, all in box 4, "Procaine, 1917–1918," RA. "Testimonial Dinner Tendered by His Friends and Associates in the Scientific Divisions to Dr. Ernest H. Volwiler in Appreciation of His Notable Services to Abbott Laboratories, to Science, and to Mankind since May 1, 1918," [Chicago, Ill.,] 26 March 1959, mimeograph, 2, AL.

11. A. S. Burdick to R. Adams, 4 October 1917, box 4, "Procaine, 1917–1918," RA; Adams to Burdick, 6 November 1917; Burdick to Adams, 8 November 1917; Adams to Burdick, 3 December 1917; R. Adams to A. S. Burdick, [21] January 1918, box 4, "Procaine, 1917–1918," RA; Alfred Einhorn, "Alkamin Esters of Para-aminobenzoic Acid." Abbott undertook the production of procaine on the same basis as it had the production of barbital (cf. n. 9).

12. Adams to Burdick, 3 December 1917; A. S. Burdick to R. Adams, 10 December 1917, box 4, "Procaine, 1917–1918," RA; Roger Adams and Oliver Kamm, "Beta-bromoethyl Para-nitro-benzoate"; Adams to Burdick, 3 December 1917.

13. Volwiler, interview by Swann, 5; Kogan, *Long White Line,* 104–5; Oliver Kamm, Roger Adams, and Ernest H. Volwiler, "Anesthetic Compound"; Roger Adams and Ernest H. Volwiler, "N-Butyl Esters of Para-amino Benzoic Acid"; Adams to Burdick, 6 November 1917; R. Adams to A. S. Burdick, 26 October 1923, "Roger Adams," AL; Roger Adams, "Cyclopentenyl Compound and Process of Making Same"; Roger Adams and Charles W. Rodewald, "Arsonophenyl Amino Alcohols and the Process of Making the Same."

14. Adams to Stieglitz, 22 June 1918. Adams's reimbursement as a consultant to Abbott, six hundred dollars annually, was a significant addition to his yearly income as an assistant professor at Illinois. Illinois hired Adams in 1916 at a salary of twenty-eight hundred dollars. Toward the end of Adams's consultantship with Abbott, in the late 1960s, the company paid him four thousand dollars annually for his services. He probably also received a salary during his years on the Abbott board (see R. Adams to P. Gerden, 10 March 1967, box 27, "Abbott Laboratories, 1962–1971," RA; and Tarbell and Tarbell, *Roger Adams,* 45).

15. A. S. Burdick to R. Adams, 5 and 20 February 1918, box 4, "Procaine, 1917–1918," RA; Roger Adams, interview by John B. Mellecker.

16. See, e.g., A. S. Burdick to R. Adams, 27 February 1918; and R. Adams to A. S. Burdick, 28 February 1918, both in box 4, "Procaine, 1917–1918," RA.

17. A. S. Burdick to R. Adams, 16 October 1917, RA; A. S. Burdick to Federal Trade Commission, ibid.; Burdick to Adams, 25 October 1917; Burdick to Adams, 20 November 1917; Volwiler, interview by Swann, 1; Kogan, *Long White Line,* 95–96. "Testimonial Dinner to Volwiler" contains a biography of Volwiler and lists his publications, patents, and outside professional activities.

18. E. H. Volwiler to W. A. Southern, January 1984, AL; Volwiler, interview by Swann, 6–7; E. H. Volwiler, "Remarks at a Symposium Honoring Roger Adams," typescript, c. 3 September 1954, 7–8, AL.

19. Tarbell and Tarbell, *Roger Adams,* 112. Adams also consulted with Du Pont, the A. E. Staley Company, Coca-Cola, the M. W. Kellogg Company, and Johnson and Johnson.

20. See, e.g., R. Adams to A. W. Weston, 18 April 1960, box 15, "Abbott Laboratories, Correspondence, 1959–1960," RA; and R. Adams to A. W. Weston, 6 February 1961, L. E. Miller to R. Adams, 15 June 1961, and R. Adams to A. W. Weston, 19 June 1961, all in box 16, "Abbott Laboratories, Correspondence, 1960–1962" RA.

21. Tarbell and Tarbell, *Roger Adams,* 151–67, 199.

22. See, e.g., R. Adams to G. R. Cain, 3 July 1958, box 15, "Abbott Laboratories, Correspondence, 1957–1958," RA; and R. Adams to E. Biekert, 29 June 1959, R. Adams to T. Iwadare, 8 July 1959, and R. Adams, "Report on Japanese Trip," typescript, attached to R. Adams to G. R. Cain, 24 November 1959, all in box 15, "Abbott Laboratories, Correspondence, 1959–1960," RA.

23. E. H. Volwiler to R. Adams, 28 January 1952, "Roger Adams," AL; *Abbott Laboratories Annual Report,* 1952–58.

24. G. R. Cain to R. Adams, 3 August 1959, box 15, "Abbott Laboratories, Correspondence, 1959–1960," RA. See also G. R. Cain to Roger Adams, 10 August 1959,

ibid.; and R. Adams to A. W. Weston, 14 October 1966, and R. Adams to L. T. Cogge-shall, 1 December 1966, both in box 27, "Abbott Laboratories, 1962–1971," RA.

25. Roger Adams, "The Relation of the University Scientist to the Chemical Indus-tries," 367 (quotation); [R. Adams,] "Introductory Remarks," typescript, c. 1950, box 54, "Speeches, 1947–1950," RA. See also Adams, "Universities and Industry in Science," 510; and idem, interview by Mellecker.

26. Adams, "Universities and Industry in Science," 510.

27. See A. N. Richards, "Processes of Urine Formation"; Carl W. Gottschalk, "Dr. A. N. Richards and Kidney Micropuncture"; and Carl F. Schmidt, "Alfred Newton Richards," 287–90, 292–96, 298–300.

28. Schmidt, "Richards," 297; Isaac Starr, Jr., "Other Activities of Dr. Richards' Department."

29. For a summary of CMR-sponsored research during the war see E. C. Andrus et al., eds., *Advances in Military Medicine*, esp. Richards's foreword, pp. xli–liv; see also Chester S. Keefer, "Dr. Richards as Chairman of the Committee on Medical Research."

30. Other notable administrative positions that Richards held included the vice-presidency of the American Philosophical Society, from 1944 to 1947, and member-ship on the Medical Section of the First Hoover Commission on the Organization of the Executive Branch of the United States Government. For a summary of additional biographical information and a list of sources for further material on Richards see John Parascandola and Elizabeth Keeney, *Sources in the History of American Pharmacology*.

31. "Dr. Alfred Newton Richards: Some Observations" (remarks made at a dinner in honor of Alfred Newton Richards in Philadelphia, 25 May 1959, mimeograph), 5, "Alfred Newton Richards," Biographical Files, University of Pennsylvania Archives, Philadelphia, Pennsylvania; A. N. Richards to [J. J.] Abel, 30 August 1930, JA (I am indebted to John Parascandola for this and all other letters that I have used from the Abel Papers). See also Tom Mahoney, *The Merchants of Life*, 195. On the role of one of the Rosengartens—Joseph G.—as a steady benefactor of the University of Pennsyl-vania see Martin Meyerson and Dilys Pegler Winegrad, *Gladly Learn and Gladly Teach*, 185; and Edward Potts Cheyney, *History of the University of Pennsylvania*, 374, 378.

32. Richards to Abel, 30 August 1930.

33. A. N. Richards, quoted in John Francis Marion, *The Fine Old House*, 120.

34. Richards to Abel, 30 August 1930; A. N. Richards to Council of the American Society for Pharmacology and Experimental Therapeutics (ASPET), 4 April 1935, box 10, "American Society for Pharmacology and Experimental Therapeutics," AR; G W. Perkins to A. N. Richards, 3 September 1930, box 31, "Merck and Co., 1930–1939," AR, A. N. Richards to G. W. Perkins, 23 September 1930, box 32, "A. N. R., Merck and Co.," AR. I have not been able to determine the actual amount of Richards's honoraria from Merck.

35. Richards to Abel, 30 August 1930; see also Richards to ASPET Council, 4 April 1935.

36. J. J. Abel to A. N. Richards, 5 September 1930, JA.

37. K. K. Chen, ed., *The American Society for Pharmacology and Experimental Therapeutics*, 158–59; Abel to Richards, 5 September 1930. Abel went on to say, "I also encourage my own men to take positions as pharmacologists with good firms when the conditions are favorable to scientific research, promotion et cetera." Both Chen and Macht worked with Abel.

38. A. N. Richards to E. P. Pick, 18 December 1931; E. P. Pick to A. N. Richards, 20 January 1932; and A. N. Richards to R. T. Major, 3 February 1932, all in box 32, "Hans Molitor, 1932–1933," AR.

39. R. T. Major to A. N. Richards, 12 February 1932, ibid. The quota system of immigration restriction in the United States stemmed from provisional legislation developed in Congress in 1921 that became the Johnson-Reed Act of 1924. The government imposed a ceiling on total annual immigration (150,000) and placed quotas on the number permitted to emigrate from any one country—equal to 2–3 percent of the population born in that country residing in the United States in 1890. Clearly, this act limited particularly those groups who emigrated mostly after 1890, such as eastern and southern Europeans (see Maldwyn Allen Jones, *American Immigration*, 276–79).

40. Jones, *American Immigration*, 251–52; Major to Richards, 12 February 1932.

41. Richards to Abel, 30 August 1930.

42. A. N. Richards to E. P. Pick, 26 February 1932; Hans Molitor to A. N. Richards, 7 March 1932; and G. W. Perkins to H. Molitor, 31 March 1932, all in box 32, "Hans Molitor, 1932–1933," AR.

43. Molitor to Richards, 7 March 1932; Perkins to Molitor, 31 March 1932; A. N. Richards to H. Molitor, 31 March 1932, box 32, "Hans Molitor, 1932–1933," AR.

44. H. Molitor to [A. N. Richards], 15 April 1932; A. N. Richards to R. T. Major, 4 May 1932; A. N. Richards to H. Molitor, 6 May 1932, all in ibid. Additional examples of Richards's involvement in the negotiations with Molitor can be seen in H. Molitor to [A. N. Richards], 26 May and 12 July 1932, ibid.

45. A. N. Richards to J. Wearn, and A. N. Richards to H. Molitor, both 26 September 1932, ibid.

46. See, e.g., A. N. Richards to E. M. K. Geiling, 1 February 1936, ibid.; and Hans Molitor, "Some Undescribed Pharmacological Properties of Bulbocapnine."

47. R. T. M[ajor] to G. W. Merck, 21 January 1933, MC; A. N. Richards to H. Dale, 3 February 1933, box 32, "Merck, Dedication of Research Laboratory, 1933," AR. On Richards's collaboration with Dale see Schmidt, "Richards," 289, 297–98.

48. G. W. Merck to H. H. Dale, 2 February 1933, box 32, "Merck, Dedication of Research Laboratory, 1933," AR; Richards to Dale, 3 February 1933.

49. H. H. Dale to [G. W.] Merck, 20 February 1933, box 32, "Merck, Dedication of Research Laboratory, 1933," AR; Major to Merck, 21 January 1933.

50. See Henry H. Dale, "Academic and Industrial Research in the Field of Therapeutics"; and "Merck Research Laboratory Dedicated." H. H. Dale to [A. N.] Richards, 6 April 1933, box 32, "Merck, Dedication of Research Laboratory, 1933," AR, explains why the British pharmacologist chose not to speak more frankly on U.S. academic and industrial research policies. As a guest in another country, Dale did not feel entitled to take a "critical and superior" attitude in his lecture.

51. A. N. Richards to J. T. Wearn, 7 February 1934, box 31, "Medical Advisor, 1933–1934," AR.

52. See, e.g., G. L. Shibley to A. N. Richards, 16 February and 20 March 1934, and A. N. Richards to H. L. Amoss, 27 April 1934, ibid.; and A. N. Richards to R. T. Major, 9 May 1934, and G. R. Minot to A. N. Richards, 31 May 1934, box 31, "Merck and Co., 1930–1939," AR.

53. See André F. Cournand, "Dickinson Woodruff Richards," 318; and Merck and

Company, "Fifty Years of Merck Research," 65. Dickinson Richards remained a medical adviser to Merck for nearly forty years.

54. For examples of Simonart's prior interest in the research for which he came to Pennsylvania to work under a Merck fellowship see André Simonart, "Étude physiologique de quelques dérivés d'homocholine"; and idem, "Étude physiologique de quelques dérivés d'homocholine: II."

55. Goodman and Gilman, *Pharmacological Basis of Therapeutics*, 349–56.

56. See Randolph T. Major and Joseph K. Cline, "Preparation and Properties of Alpha- and Beta-methylcholine and Gamma-homocholine"; "Preparation and Properties of Alpha- and Beta-methylcholine Derivatives and Salts and Processes for Their Preparation"; and Goodman and Gilman, *Pharmacological Basis of Therapeutics*, 356.

57. G. W. Perkins to A. N. Richards, 11 September 1930, box 31, "Merck and Co., 1930–1939," AR; G. W. Perkins to Trustees of the University of Pennsylvania, 26 September 1930, box 33, "Merck Fellowship Fund, 1930–1934," AR; A. N. Richards to W. Pepper, 18 December 1931 and 6 June 1932, AR; and Isaac Starr, Jr., et al., "Acetyl-beta-methylcholin," 315.

58. André Simonart, "On the Action of Certain Derivatives of Choline," 192–93; Starr et al., "Acetyl-beta-methylcholin," 313–23; W. Osler Abbott, "Acetyl-beta-methylcholin"; Isaac Starr, Jr., "Acetyl-beta-methylcholin."

59. A. N. Richards to R. T. Major, 23 March 1933, and enclosed draft of a letter from G. W. Merck to [W.] Longcope, n.d.; P. C. Ackerman to A. N. Richards, 11 May 1933; A. N. Richards to P. C. Ackerman, 15 May 1933; and Anna M. H. Josephson to A. N. Richards, 12 April 1935, all in box 31, "Merck and Co., Mecholin Correspondence, 1930–1934," AR.

60. Major and Cline, "Beta-methylcholine Derivatives." On Merck's attempts to have the U.S. Patent Office and the American Medical Association Council on Pharmacy and Chemistry approve Mecholyl Chloride see P. N. Leech to R. E. Gruber, 15 August 1934, box 31, "Merck and Co., Mecholin Correspondence, 1930–1934," AR; Council on Pharmacy and Chemistry of the American Medical Association, "Preliminary Report of the Council," 1935; and idem, "New and Nonofficial Remedies," 1935.

61. Chauncey D. Leake and Mei-Yü Chen, "The Anesthetic Properties of Certain Unsaturated Ethers"; Chauncey D. Leake, P. K. Knoefel, and A. E. Guedel, "The Anesthetic Action of Divinyl Oxide in Animals."

62. William L. Ruigh and Randolph T. Major, "The Preparation and Properties of Pure Divinyl Ether"; Randolph T. Major and William L. Ruigh, "Divinyl Ether and Processes for Its Production"; idem, "Means and Composition for the Stabilization of Divinyl Ether"; idem, "Production of Stabilized Divinyl Ether Suitable for General Anesthesia."

63. R. T. Major to A. N. Richards, 9 June 1933, box 33, "Vinethene, 1933–1936," AR.

64. R. T. Majors to A. N. Richards, 9 June 1933; A. N. Richards to R. T. Major, 31 May 1933; and R. T. Major to A. N. Richards, 7 June 1933, all in ibid. S. Goldschmidt to G. W. Perkins, 16 April 1934; A. N. Richards to H. I. MacLean, 23 April 1934, both in box 33, "Merck Fellowship Fund, 1930–1934," AR. R. T. Major to W. Bourne, 2 May 1933; R. T. Major to I. S. Ravdin, 12 April 1934; and P. N. Leech to R. E. Gruber, 26 December 1935, all in box 33, "Vinethene, 1933–1936," AR.

65. Samuel Goldschmidt et al., "Divinyl Ether"; I. S. Ravdin et al., "Divinyl Ether"; Council on Pharmacy and Chemistry of the American Medical Association, "New and Nonofficial Remedies," 1934; idem, "Report of the Council," 1937.

66. Typescript on the University of Pennsylvania's connections with companies on medical research, c. 12 March 1934 (hereafter referred to as the Penn-Merck Agreement), box 33, "Merck Fellowship Fund, 1930–1934," AR; cf. G. W. Perkins to A. N. Richards, 12 March 1934, MC.

67. On the University of Pennsylvania's policy regarding medical patents see A. N. Richards to G. W. Perkins, 9 March 1934, MC; and Fishbein, "Medical Patents," 1540.

68. H. Molitor to [G. W.] Merck, 3 January 1934, MC. I have no evidence that the company executive officers, such as George Merck and George Perkins, shared or rejected Molitor's concerns about the agreement. But Molitor was a respected and distinguished member of Merck's research staff and the director of the Merck Institute for Therapeutic Research; thus, the Merck executives most likely carefully considered his comments and suggestions.

69. Penn-Merck Agreement; H. Molitor to [G. W.] Perkins, 5 March 1934, MC.

70. Molitor to Perkins, 5 March 1934.

71. See A. W. Lescohier to A. L. Tatum and C. S. Hamilton, 10 September 1943; C. S. Hamilton and A. L. Tatum to A. W. Lescohier, 23 September 1943; and A. W. Lescohier to C. S. Hamilton and A. L. Tatum, 11 October and 17 November 1943, all in box 5, folder 5, AT-UW.

72. [H. Molitor,] "Merck Institute of Therapeutic Research: Its Organization at Present and in the Future," typescript, c. January 1935, 11–12, attached to [H. Molitor] to [A. N.] Richards, 18 January 1935; H. Molitor, "Merck Institute of Therapeutic Research: Fourth Annual Report," typescript, [1937], 1, both in box 30, "Merck Institute, 1931–1940," AR. See also A. N. Richards to W. B. Castle, 8 June 1936, box 30, "Business and Research," AR.

73. See Richards to Castle, 8 June 1936; W. B. Castle to A. N. Richards, 13 June 1936; A. N. Richards to W. B. Castle, 16 June 1936; and G. W. Merck to W. B. Castle, 23 June 1936, all in box 30, "Business and Research," AR.

74. Molitor, "Merck Institute: Organization," 12. Richards to Castle, 8 and 16 June 1936. Merck to Castle, 23 June 1936. A. N. Richards to [G. W.] Merck, 27 December 1939; H. Molitor to G. W. Merck et al., 13 December 1937; H. Molitor to A. N. Richards, 7 November 1939; and H. Molitor to [W. B.] Castle et al., 10 May 1940, all in MC.

75. "Richards: Some Observations," 7 (quotation); "The Merck Institute for Therapeutic Research," 1942, mimeograph, 2, 4, MC; H. Molitor to [R. T.] Major, 6 February 1951, box 30, "Consultants, Grants, Fellowships as of Feb., 1951," AR. Richards became a member of the board of trustees of the Merck Institute (as did Castle) in 1950. The three trustees oversaw the financial operations of the Institute (see ibid.; and "Merck Institute for Therapeutic Research," 1942, 4, 63.

76. H. B. Vickery to G. W. Merck, 5 December 1945; G. W. Merck to H. B. Vickery, 25 January 1946; G. W. Merck to A. N. Richards, with attached memorandum; G. W. Merck, memorandum to Committee of Awards, 16 July 1946; and "Merck Fellowships in Natural Sciences Administered by the National Research Council," mimeograph, c. 1947, all in box 13, "Merck Award Committee, 1946–1948," AR.

77. Merck to Richards, 25 January 1936. A. N. Richards to G. Merck, 12 June 1946; G. W. Merck to A. N. Richards, A. B. Hastings, and F. B. Jewett, 16 July 1946; A. N. Richards to D. W. Bronk, 17 October 1946; and A. N. Richards to G. W. Merck, 14 April 1947, all in box 13, "Merck Award Committee, 1946–1948," AR.

78. Henry D. Dakin, a biochemist in a private New York laboratory who did not have an academic appointment, served on the Merck board from 1938 through 1949. Vannevar Bush, the former head of the wartime OSRD, became a board member in 1949 and served throughout Richards's stay; eventually he became chairman of the board. Formerly a professor of electrical engineering at the Massachusetts Institute of Technology, Bush was president of the Carnegie Institution (since 1939) at the time he joined the Merck directors (See Merck and Company, *Annual Report to Stockholders*, 1938–58; Percival Hartley, "Henry Drysdale Dakin"; and *American Men of Science*, 8th ed., s.v. "Bush, Dr. V[annevar]").

79. Merck and Company, *Annual Report to Stockholders*, 1948, 7 (quotation); Minutes of the meeting of the board of directors of Merck and Co., Inc., New York, N.Y., 20 July 1984, box 32, "ANR—Appt.—Bd. of Directors," AR.

80. E. H. O'Brien to J. T. Connor, 2 May 1949; K. Folkers to H. D. Dakin, 9 June 1949; and R. T. Major to A. N. Richards, 23 June 1949, all in box 32, "Publication Policy," AR. "Richards: Some Observations," 18.

81. A. N. Richards to R. T. Major, 4 July 1949, box 32, "Publication Policy," AR.

82. The folders "Scientific Policy Council" and "Policy of Merck, Corporate and Scientific," in box 33, AR, illustrate the council's activities. See, e.g., minutes of the meeting of the Merck Scientific Policy Council, [Rahway, New Jersey,] 14 June 1954, box 33, "Policy of Merck, Corporate and Scientific," AR.

83. G. W. Merck to [G. W.] Perkins et al. (memorandum of meeting with Richards), 25 January 1935, MC; Molitor to Richards, 7 November 1939; Mahoney, *Merchants of Life*, 198–201; Gary L. Nelson, ed., *Pharmaceutical Company Histories*, 83–86.

84. G. W. Merck to [G. W.] Perkins et al. (memorandum of interview with R. R. Williams), 25 January 1935, MC (quotation). G. W. Merck to A. N. Richards, 29 January 1935; J. S. Zinsser to [G. W.] Merck, 28 January 1935; and R. E. Gruber to [G. W.] Merck, 28 January 1935, all in box 31, "Merck and Co., 1930–1939," AR. H. Molitor to [G. W.] Merck et al., and W. L. Sampson to [H.] Molitor, both 28 January 1935, MC.

85. A. N. Richards to H. S. Gasser, 3 October 1939, MC: "I write this note, not with the thought of supporting Major's request [i.e., Randolph Major's request for a sample of tyrothricin], but only to say that as the result of eight years of association I am confident that you can have complete faith in any engagements into which you may see fit to enter with the officers of [Merck]." Hubert A. Lechevalier and Morris Solotorovsky, *Three Centuries of Microbiology*, 478. H. W. Florey et al., *Antibiotics*, 422–42. R. T. Major to A. N. Richards, 14 August 1939; A. N. Richards to [R. T.] Major, 26 August 1939; W. H. Engels to A. N. Richards, 3 October 1939; H. Molitor to [G. W.] Merck, 8 October 1939; and A. N. Richards to R. T. Major, 28 November 1939, all in MC.

86. Merck to Perkins et al. (memorandum of meeting with Richards), 25 January 1935; George W. Merck, "An Essential Partnership."

87. A. N. Richards to H. Molitor, 29 September 1932, box 32, "Hans Molitor,

1932–1933," AR. R. T. Major to A. N. Richards, 29 December 1932; A. N. Richards to C. I. Lafferty, 30 December 1932; and A. N. Richards to A. H. Lippincott, 30 December 1932, all in box 30, "Merck Institute, 1931–1940," AR.

88. Clarence J. West and Ervye Risher, "Industrial Research Laboratories of the United States"; Clarence J. West and Callie Hull, "Industrial Research Laboratories of the United States"; Callie Hull, "Industrial Research Laboratories of the United States," 7th ed.; *The Merck Corporation: Annual Report, 1931*; "Merck and Co., Inc. and Consolidated Domestic Subsidiaries: Analysis of Research and Development Expenses," typescript, 15 November 1951, box 29, "Budget, 1953," AR.

89. Merck to Perkins et al. (memorandum of meeting with Richards), 25 January 1935.

90. "Richards: Some Observations," 7 (quotation); Detlev W. Bronk, "Alfred Newton Richards," 420.

CHAPTER FOUR

The Scientist as Specialist-Consultant

1. J. F. Biehn to A. L. Tatum, 19 October 1929, and A. L. Tatum to J. F. Biehn, 21 October 1929, box 1, "Abbott Laboratories, 1929–1931," AT-UW; O. Kamm to A. L. Tatum, 25 September 1933, box 4, folder 11, AT-UW; O. M. Gruhzit to [O.] Kamm, 15 December 1936, box 4, folder 5, AT-UW; C. D. Leake to H. W. Rhodehamel, 24 January 1940, box 44, "Lilly Research Laboratories, 1933–1940," CL; R. T. Major to C. D. Leake, 20 November 1942, and C. D. Leake to R. T. Major, 24 November 1942, box 47, "Merck and Co. (G. W. Merck, R. T. Major), 1941–1945." CL.

2. Selman A. Waksman, *My Life with the Microbes*, 184; H. Boyd Woodruff, "A Soil Microbiologist's Odyssey," 8; S. A. Waksman to T. Atkeson, 18 November 1950, box 1, SW; R. T. Major, "The Research Program of Merck and Co., Inc.," typescript, 3 December 1938, 7, box 31, "Merck and Co., 1930–1939," AR.

3. Waksman, *My Life with the Microbes*, 200; S. A. Waksman to A. N. Richards, 26 July 1940, box 4, SW. Waksman himself inoculated the flasks with microorganisms, which Merck workers then incubated at the Rahway plant (see Woodruff, "Soil Microbiologist's Odyssey," 7). Hubert A. Lechevalier, "The Search for Antibiotics at Rutgers University," 115, presents a list of the antibiotics that Waksman and his associates isolated.

4. Waksman, *My Life with the Microbes*, 200–201, 251; Harry F. Dowling, *Fighting Infection*, 158–72. While streptomycin was less toxic than actinomycin and the other antibiotics from soil, it was by no means nontoxic (see Dowling).

5. Waksman, *My Life with the Microbes*, 185. Merck released the patents with the provision that it could withhold part of the royalties until its investment in the development of streptomycin was partially reimbursed (Lechevalier, "Antibiotics at Rutgers," 118), although this probably was a pittance compared with what the firm would have made if it had retained the patents.

6. Lechevalier, "Antibiotics at Rutgers," 118–19; Dowling, *Fighting Infection*, 163; Waksman, *My Life with the Microbes*, 185, 252.

7. Lechevalier, "Antibiotics at Rutgers," 119; Woodruff, "Soil Microbiologist's Odyssey," 11; Dowling, *Fighting Infection*, 161–62; and Waksman, *My Life with the Microbes*, 250–54.

8. S. A. Waksman, "Support of Research," comments to be made at a banquet of the American College of Chest Physicians, Atlantic City, N.J., 4 June 1955, 3–4, box 6, "Speech and Article File," SW; see also idem, *My Life with the Microbes*, 184–85, 246.

9. R. T. Major to R. Clothier, 22 April 1949, box 3, SW. "Outside Research Analysis: Research and Development Division," typescript, 10 October 1952, [5,] box 29, "Budget Proposals, 1953," AR (quotation); Scientific Administration Division, Merck, "Grants and Fellowships" (memorandum to Clarke et al.), 29 May 1953, ibid.; C. R. Scholz to S. A. Waksman, 20 June 1946, box 4, SW; S. A. Waksman to C. R. Scholz, 9 July 1946, ibid.

10. William Charles White, "Committee on Drug Addiction of the National Research Council"; Nathan B. Eddy, "Studies of Morphine, Codeine and Their Derivatives," 339; Lyndon F. Small et al., *Studies on Drug Addiction*, iii–vi; William Charles White, "Report of the Committee on Drug Addiction," typescript plus appendixes, October 1934, box 3, "NA, 1934–35," LS.

11. White, "Report of the Committee on Drug Addiction," 5; Eddy, "Studies of Morphine," 340–59; Small et al., *Studies on Drug Addiction*, iv.

12. L. F. Small to J. Rosin, 22 April 1930, box 3, "ME, 1932"; L. F. Small to A. C. Boylston, 27 April 1931, box 2, "MA"; G. W. Merck to E. A. Alderman, 17 April 1931, box 3, "ME, 1932"; Committee on Drug Addiction of the National Research Council, "Preliminary Annual Report, 1933–1934," 4, box 1, "DO–DR"; L. F. Small to J. Rosin, 28 June 1932, box 3, "ME, 1932"; and L. F. Small to J. Rosin, 8 June 1933, box 3, "ME, 1932–1934," all in LS.

13. L. F. Small to J. Rosin, 21 June 1933, ibid.; White, "Report of the Committee on Drug Addiction," 2; L. F. Small to E. Mallinckrodt, 12 February 1935, box 2, "MA–MC," LS; Lyndon F. Small, Kechee C. Yuen, and Louis K. Eilers, "The Catalytic Hydrogenation of the Halogenmorphides."

14. White, "Report of the Committee on Drug Addiction," 3 (quotation); L. F. Small to G. Merck, 4 September 1934, box 3, "ME, 1934–35," LS; Lyndon Frederick Small, "Morphine Derivative and Processes for Its Preparation."

15. "Memorandum Concerning the Appointment of Alkaloid Research Fellows in the Drug Addiction Laboratory at the University of Virginia," n.d., box 1, "DO–DR," LS. J. F. Anderson to J. L. Newcomb, 7 February 1936; L. F. Small to J. F. Anderson, 21 March 1936; and L. F. Small to J. F. Anderson, 6 June 1936, all in box 1, "AM–AR," LS.

16. R. N. Shreve to L. F. Small, 7 April and 4 August 1931, box 2, "MA"; R. N. Shreve to L. F. Small, 23 May 1933, box 4, "SH–SM"; A. C. Boylston to W. C. White, 7 August 1933, box 1, "BL–BR"; and L. F. Small to V. H. Wallingford, 19 December 1934, and L. F. Small to E. Mallinckrodt, 12 February 1935, box 2, "MA–MC," all in LS.

17. White, "Committee on Drug Addiction," 98. L. F. Small to Barrett Co., 28 June 1930; A. G. Stern to L. F. Small, 11 July 1930; F. H. Johnson to L. F. Small, 15 February 1932; and R. C. Quortrup to L. F. Small, 19 September 1932, all in box 1, "BA–BL,"; LS.

18. See, e.g., "Report of the Committee on Drug Addiction," c. November 1936, app. B (budget), box 1, "CO," LS.

19. See H. S. Gasser, "Arthur S. Loevenhart," 317–19; Russell Chittenden, *The Development of Physiological Chemistry in the United States*, 293–97; and A. S. Loevenhart, "Certain Aspects of Biological Oxidation."

20. Daniel Patrick Jones, "The Role of Chemists in Research on War Gases in the

United States during World War I," 113–14, 156–64, 216–22; H. C. Bradley, "Dr. Loevenhart's War Work."

21. Chauncey D. Leake, "Arthur S. Loevenhart," 497; idem, "Cooperative Research," 251–55; M. E. McCaffrey to A. S. Loevenhart, 9 March 1922, box 11, "A. S. Loevenhart," General Files, Dean's Office, Papers of the University of Wisconsin Medical School Administration, University of Wisconsin Archives, Madison, Wisconsin. On the Interdepartmental Social Hygiene Board, established in 1918, see William F. Snow, "Contributions to Medical Science"; and T. A. Storey, "A Summary of the Work of the United States Interdepartmental Social Hygiene Board." On the Public Health Institute of Chicago, established in 1920, see Leake, "Cooperative Research," 253.

22. W. F. Lorenz et al., "The Therapeutic Use of Tryparsamid in Neurosyphilis"; Leake, "Cooperative Research," 255–56; A. S. Loevenhart, "Tryparsamide." Cf. Wade H. Brown, "Tryparsamide."

23. H. L. Schmitz and A. S. Loevenhart, "A Study of Two Series of Procaine Derivatives"; idem, "A Comparative Study of the Local Anesthetic Properties"; Leake, "Arthur S. Loevenhart," 498.

24. A. S. Loevenhart to A. S. Burdick, 4 October 1926, box 1, "Abbott Laboratories, 1926–1927," ASL; A. S. Burdick to A. S. Loevenhart, 13 October 1926, ibid.; Council on Pharmacy and Chemistry of the American Medical Association, *New and Nonofficial Remedies, 1928*, 219–21.

25. Agreement on therapeutic arsenicals between Abbott Laboratories, Frank C. Whitmore, and A. S. Loevenhart (hereafter Abbott-Whitmore-Loevenhart Agreement), c. October 1926, box 1, "Abbott Laboratories, 1926–1927"; and A. S. Loevenhart to A. S. Burdick, 4 November 1926, both in ASL.

26. A. S. Loevenhart to A. Orr, 16 February 1928, box 1, "Commercial Solvents Corp.," ASL; Williams Haynes, *American Chemical Industry*, 4:187–201, 6:85–89, 436.

27. C. L. Gabriel to A. S. Loevenhart, 28 February 1928; A. S. Loevenhart to C. L. Gabriel, 1 March 1928 (quotation); J. C. Woodruff to A. S. Loevenhart, 6 March and 7 April 1928; and A. S. Loevenhart to J. C. Woodruff, 3 April 1928, all in box 1, "Commercial Solvents Corp.," ASL.

28. A. W. Lescohier to A. S. Loevenhart, 12 February 1926, box 1, "Parke, Davis and Co.: Lescohier, A. W., 1926–1929," ASL.

29. Schmitz and Loevenhart, "Study of Two Series of Procaine Derivatives"; idem, "A Comparative Study of the Local Anesthetic Properties"; A. S. Loevenhart to O. Kamm, 30 November and 28 December 1927, and O. Kamm to A. S. Loevenhart, 17 December 1927, all in box 1, "Parke, Davis and Co.: Kamm, O., 1927–1929," ASL.

30. C. W. Muehlberger to A. W. Lescohier, 3 January 1928, box 1, "Parke, Davis and Co.: Lescohier, A. W., 1926–1929," ASL. O. Kamm to [A. W.] Lescohier, 14 May 1928, box 1, "Parke, Davis and Co.: Kamm, O., 1927–1929," ASL. A. W. Lescohier to A. S. Loevenhart, 31 May and 31 December 1928; and A. S. Loevenhart to A. W. Lescohier, 15 February 1929, all in box 1, "Parke, Davis and Co.: Lescohier, A. W., 1926–1929," ASL. William L. Ruigh, "Acid Halides of Carbazole-N-carboxylic Acids and Process for Their Production."

31. Contract on arsenicals for syphilis and trypanosomiasis between Parke, Davis and Company, Frank C. Whitmore, Cliff S. Hamilton, and Arthur S. Loevenhart (here-

after Parke, Davis–Whitmore–Hamilton–Loevenhart Contract), 30 September 1927, box 1, "Parke, Davis and Co.: Lescohier, A. W., 1926–1929," ASL. Trypanosomes (such as the one that causes African sleeping sickness) and the spirochete responsible for syphilis are similar, so much so that the Wisconsin investigators typically examined arsenicals first in trypanosome-infected animals before testing them in syphilitic animals, to obtain a preliminary indication of the value of the compounds under study in syphilis.

32. O. Kamm to A. L. Tatum, 29 December 1930, box 4, folder 10, AT-UW; "Colleges Pay Industry Dividends"; *American Men of Science*, 4th ed., s.v. "Whitmore, Frank C."

33. Parke, Davis–Whitmore–Hamilton–Loevenhart Contract; A. W. Lescohier to A. L. Tatum, 3 July and 26 September 1929, box 5, folder 3, AT-UW.

34. See, e.g., Garrett Arthur Cooper, "The Present Status of Arsenicals in the Treatment of Syphilis"; and Phyllis Magdalene Nelson, "A Comparative Study of Various Agents." Many of the publications are cited in the notes to this chapter.

35. On the Wisconsin group's work on structure-activity relationships with arsenicals see A. G. Young and A. S. Loevenhart, "The Relation of the Chemical Constitution of Certain Organic Arsenical Compounds."

36. "Profile of a Research Scientist"; F. E. Shideman, "A. L. Tatum, Practical Pharmacologist"; John Parascandola and Elizabeth Keeney, *Sources in the History of American Pharmacology*, 52–53.

37. See, e.g., A. L. Tatum, M. H. Seevers, and K. H. Collins, "Morphine Addiction and Its Physiological Interpretation Based on Experimental Evidences."

38. A. L. Tatum, A. J. Atkinson, and K. H. Collins, "Acute Cocaine Poisoning"; A. H. Maloney, R. Fitch, and A. L. Tatum, "Picrotoxin as an Antidote in Acute Poisoning by the Shorter Acting Barbiturates"; Shideman, "A. L. Tatum," 449.

39. F. C. Koch to P. G. Heinemann, 13 June 1925; P. G. Heinemann to F. C. Koch, 16 June 1925; and A. L. Tatum to P. G. Heinemann, 2 and 29 July 1925, 28 July 1926, and 30 June 1927, all in box 1, "Correspondence, 13 Jan. 1922–21 Oct. 1927," AT-SHSW. A. L. Tatum to P. G. Heinemann, 23 May 1928, box 1, "Correspondence, 13 Jan. 1928–5 Oct. 1928," AT-SHSW.

40. C. Browne to Warner-Jenkinson Co., 6 August 1924 (quotation), "General Correspondence, 1919–1937," FDA, quoted in Sheldon Hochheiser, "Synthetic Food Colors in the United States," 88 n. 59; memorandum of interview of L. H. Cone by [C. W.] Crawford, [H. T.] Herrick, and [J. C.] Munch, 15 June 1927, "General Correspondence, 1919–1937," FDA; C. W. Crawford to W. E. Ralph, 9 January 1928, ibid.; Hochheiser, "Synthetic Food Colors," 84–90. On National Aniline see Haynes, *American Chemical Industry*, 6:292–96. I am indebted to Sheldon Hochheiser for the above and for other documents from the Papers of the Food and Drug Administration.

41. Crawford to Ralph, 9 January 1928; and W. M. Ralph to A. L. Tatum, 14 September 1928, both in box 1, "Correspondence, 13 Jan. 1928–5 Oct. 1928," AT-SHSW.

42. W. M. Ralph to A. L. Tatum, 7 November 1928, box 1, "Correspondence, 7 Nov. 1928–28 March 1929," AT-SHSW.

43. See Hochheiser, "Synthetic Food Colors," 71–81.

44. W. M. Ralph to A. L. Tatum, 3 May 1929, box 2, "Correspondence, 2 April 1929–17 September 1929," AT-SHSW; H. T. Herrick to [P. B.] Dunbar, 24 May 1929, "General Correspondence, 1919–1937," FDA; N. G. Barbella and W. T. McClosky to

[P. B.] Dunbar, 24 June 1929, FDA; Haynes, *American Chemical Industry*, 4:231; *Federal Food, Drug and Cosmetic Law Administrative Reports, 1907−1949*, 728.

45. A. L. Tatum to A. S. Burdick, 7 March 1929, box 1, "Abbott Laboratories, 1929−1931," AT-UW (quotation); A. L. Tatum to P. N. Leech, 23 February 1934, box 1, "Abbott Laboratories, 1934," AT-UW; C. Nielsen to A. L. Tatum, 21 February 1929, box 1, "Correspondence, 7 Nov. 1928−28 March 1929," AT-SHSW; A. S. Burdick to A. L. Tatum, 28 February and 26 March 1929, box 1, "Abbott Laboratories, 1929−1931," AT-UW; Abbott Laboratories, *Price List of Pharmaceutical and Biologic Products and Fine Medicinal Chemicals*, 8, 38, copy in KRF; Herman Kogan, *The Long White Line*, 105−6; unlabeled notebook listing Abbott hypnotics sent to Tatum, box 1, General Subject Files, UW-PT.

46. Burdick to Tatum, 26 March 1929; and A. L. Tatum to C. Nielsen, 19 and 27 September 1929, all in box 1, "Abbott Laboratories, 1929−1931," AT-UW.

47. E. H. Volwiler and D. L. Tabern, "5,5-Substituted Barbituric Acids." Carl Nielsen and Henry Spruth, neither of whom was formally trained in pharmacology, conducted the pharmacological investigations at Abbott (see Kogan, *Long White Line*, 127; and Ernest H. Volwiler, interview by John P. Swann, 12).

48. Tatum to Nielsen, 27 September 1929. A. L. Tatum to C. Nielsen, 12 October 1929; and A. L. Tatum to E. H. Volwiler, 30 December 1929, both in box 1, "Abbott Laboratories, 1929−1931," AT-UW. T. W. Pratt, "A Comparison of the Action of Pentobarbital (Nembutal) and Sodium Barbital." Richard H. Fitch and E. E. McCandless, "A Comparison of the Intraperitoneal and Oral Effects of the Barbituric Acid Derivatives." Richard H. Fitch, Ralph M. Waters, and Arthur L. Tatum, "The Intravenous Use of the Barbituric Acid Hypnotics in Surgery." John S. Lundy, "Experience with Sodium Ethyl (1-Methylbutyl) Barbiturate (Nembutal) in More than 2,300 Cases."

49. Volwiler and Tabern, "Barbituric Acids," 1677; H. A. Shonle, Anna K. Keltch, and E. E. Swanson, "Dialkyl Barbituric Acids"; E. H. Volwiler to W. A. Puckner, 2 February 1931, box 1, "Abbott Laboratories, 1929−1931", AT-UW; Council on Pharmacy and Chemistry of the American Medical Association, "Preliminary Report of the Council," 1937.

50. Fitch, Waters, and Tatum, "Barbituric Acid Hypnotics"; Council on Pharmacy and Chemistry, "Preliminary Report," 1937, 505 and n. 1.

51. A. L. Tatum to E. H. Volwiler, 2 December 1929, box 1, "Abbott Laboratories, 1929−1931," AT-UW; cf. E. H. Volwiler to A. L. Tatum, 29 November and 5 December 1929, ibid. Abbott agreed not to publicize the fellowship.

52. See the enclosure in A. L. Tatum to E. H. Volwiler, 4 April 1930, ibid.; and Council on Pharmacy and Chemistry, "Preliminary Report," 1937, 505 n. 1.

53. E. H. Volwiler to A. L. Tatum, 26 March 1931, box 1, "Abbott Laboratories, 1929−1931," AT-UW. E. H . Volwiler to A. L. Tatum, 19 and 22 February 1934; P. N. Leech to E. H. Volwiler, 16 February 1934; and E. H. Volwiler to Council on Pharmacy and Chemistry, 19 February 1934, all in box 1, "Abbott Laboratories, 1934," AT-UW. Tatum to Leech, 23 February 1934. Council on Pharmacy and Chemistry, "Preliminary Report," 1937, 505 (quotation).

54. This information comes from selected correspondence between Abbott personnel and Tatum, most of which is in boxes 2 and 3, AT-SHSW; and box 2, "Abbott Laboratories, Dr. Volwiler, 1941−1953," AT-UW.

55. E. H. Volwiler to A. L. Tatum, 11 October 1933, box 1, "Abbott Laboratories, 1933," AT-UW.

56. T. W. Pratt et al., "Sodium Ethyl(1-Methyl Butyl)Thiobarbiturate," 464–65. H. W. Werner, T. W. Pratt, and A. L. Tatum, "A Comparative Study of Ultrashort-acting Barbiturates." D. L. Tabern to A. L. Tatum, 28 December 1933, box 1, "Abbott Laboratories, 1933," AT-UW. D. L. Tabern to A. L. Tatum, 20 April 1934, (quotation); and E. H. Volwiler to A. L. Tatum, 27 April and 4 June 1934, all in box 1, "Abbott Laboratories, 1934," AT-UW. D. L. Tabern and E. H. Volwiler, "Sulfur-Containing Barbiturate Hypnotics," 1963. A. L. Tatum to E. H. Volwiler, 10 May 1934, box 1, "Abbott Laboratories, 1934," AT-UW (quotation).

57. E. H. Volwiler to A. L. Tatum, 13 July 1938, box 3, "Correspondence, 11 Jan. 1937–27 Dec. 1939," AT-SHSW; E. H. Volwiler to A. L. Tatum, 27 July and 13 October 1938, box 2, "Abbott Laboratories, 1938–1939," AT-UW; E. H. Volwiler to A. L. Tatum, 9 December 1940, box 2, "Abbott Laboratories, 1940–1942," AT-UW.

58. See Roger L. Geiger, *To Advance Knowledge*, 246–55, esp. 249.

59. "Original Contributions by or under the Direction of Arthur L. Tatum," type-script, KRF.

60. The following account of Mapharsen summarizes John Patrick Swann, "Arthur Tatum, Parke-Davis, and the Discovery of Mapharsen as an Antisyphilitic Agent."

61. On earlier experiences with (and rejection of) Mapharsen see Paul Ehrlich and S. Hata, *Die experimentelle Chemotherapie der Spirillosen*, 42, 57, 81, 84, 121–122; P. Ehrlich and A. Bertheim, "Über das salzsaure 3.3'-Diamino-4.4'-dioxyarsenobenzol und seine nächsten Verwandten," 764; and Carl Voegtlin, "The Pharmacology of Arsphenamine (Salvarsan) and Related Arsenicals."

62. A. L. Tatum to O. Kamm and A. W. Lescohier, 2 October 1929, box 4, folder 10, AT-UW; A. L. Tatum to C. S. Hamilton, 18 October 1929, box 1, folder 17, AT-UW; A. L. Tatum to C. S. Hamilton, 24 June 1930, box 2, folder 17, AT-UW; A. L. Tatum, untitled typescript, 23 April 1940, box 6, folder 10, AT-UW.

63. A. L. Tatum to A. W. Lescohier, 25 March 1931, box 5, folder 3, AT-UW; A. L. Tatum and G. A. Cooper, "An Experimental Study of Mapharsen"; O. M. Gruhzit, "Mapharsen ('Arsenoxide') in the Therapy of Experimental Syphilis and Trypanoso-miasis"; A. L. Tatum and G. A. Cooper, "Meta-Amino Para-Hydroxy Phenyl Arsine Oxide as an Antisyphilitic Agent"; O. H. Foerster et al., "Mapharsen in the Treatment of Syphilis"; O. M. Gruhzit and R. S. Dixon, "Mapharsen in Mass Treatment of Syphilis in a Clinic for Venereal Diseases"; L. M. Wieder, O. H. Foerster, and H. R. Foerster, "Mapharsen in the Treatment of Syphilis."

64. Louis Goodman and Alfred Gilman address the advantages of Mapharsen and disadvantages of the arsphenamines in *The Pharmacological Basis of Therapeutics*, 947–50, 956–58. See also Patricia Spain Ward, "The American Reception of Salvarsan," 47–48.

65. A. L. Tatum, "Therapeutic Agent"; Parke, Davis–Whitmore–Hamilton–Loevenhart Contract; A. W. Lescohier to A. L. Tatum, 4 November 1937, box 5, folder 5, AT-UW; O. Kamm to A. L. Tatum, 10 May 1939, box 5, folder 2, AT-UW; A. L. Tatum and C. S. Hamilton to A. W. Lescohier, 23 September 1943, box 5, folder 5, AT-UW.

66. See the statements that accompanied Parke-Davis's checks to Tatum, in box 5, "Professional Financial Matter," AT-SHSW.

67. Kamm to Tatum, 10 May 1939; University of Wisconsin Budgets, University of Wisconsin Archives, Madison, Wisconsin.

68. A. W. Lescohier to A. L. Tatum, 2 December 1947, box 5, folder 5, AT-UW. A. L. Tatum to C. S. Hamilton, 8 January 1948, and C. S. Hamilton to A. L. Tatum, 27 October 1948, both in box 2, folder 22, AT-UW.

69. "Conferences in Detroit, June 19–20, 1936 with Professors Hamilton and Tatum on Arsenicals and Other Cooperative Research Works," 4, box 5, folder 1, AT-UW.

70. Ibid. The major antimalarials at this time, which were useful only for certain phases of the *plasmodia* life cycle in the human, were quinine, pamaquine (prepared by chemists at Bayer and introduced in 1926 at Plasmochin), and quinacrine (introduced as Atabrine in 1930 and also synthesized by Bayer chemists).

71. Macfarlane Burnet, *Natural History of Infectious Disease*, 341; Erwin H. Ackerknecht, *History and Geography of the Most Important Diseases*, 88; A. W. Lescohier to A. L. Tatum, 13 July 1936, box 5, folder 4, AT-UW; "Conferences in Detroit, June 19–20, 1936."

72. A. L. Tatum to A. B. Scott, 4 February 1937, box 6, "Parke, Davis and Co., A. B. Scott, 1931–1937," AT-UW.

73. See folder entitled "Parke, Davis and Co., Grant-in-aid," box 5, UW-PT.

74. Tatum to Scott, 4 February 1937; A. L. Tatum to O. Kamm, 3 March 1937, box 5, "Parke, Davis and Co., O. Kamm, 1937–1941," AT-UW; W. F. Holcomb to [O.] Kamm, 27 March 1937, box 1, "Synthetic Antimalarials," Manuscripts and Publications, UW-PT; L. A. Sweet to A. L. Tatum, box 6, "Parke, Davis and Co., L. A. Sweet and O. Kamm, 1937–1941," AT-UW; W. F. H[olcomb], "Antimalarial Conference, April 11–12–14, 1941, Detroit, Michigan," box 3, "Conferences (Antimalarial)," Professional Organizations, UW-PT; W. F. Holcomb to A. L. Tatum, 18 December 1942, box 4, "Parke, Davis and Co., W. F. Holcomb, 1942, Antimalarials," AT-UW.

75. E. C. Andrus et al., eds., *Advances in Military Medicine*; Frederick Y. Wiselogle, ed., *A Survey of Antimalarial Drugs, 1941–1945*; O. Kamm to Those Cooperating with Parke, Davis and Company on Antimalarial Research, 10 August 1942, box 3, "Corres., 5 Aug. 1942–7 Sept. 1943," AT-SHSW.

76. O. Kamm to A. L. Tatum, 20 June 1940, box 6, "Parke, Davis and Co., L. A. Sweet and O. Kamm, 1937–1941," AT-UW.

77. See, e.g., "Antimalarial Conference, April 11–12–14, 1941," 5; L. A. Sweet to A. L. Tatum, 14 July 1942, and O. Kamm to A. L. Tatum, 23 July 1942, both in box 6, "Parke, Davis and Co., L. A. Sweet and O. Kamm, 1942–1943," AT-UW. Kamm to Those Cooperating; and A. L. Tatum to F. Y. Wiselogle, 20 August 1942, box 3, "Corres., 5 Aug. 1942–7 Sept. 1943," AT-SHSW.

78. "Antimalarial Conference, Chicago, February 1, 1943," box 3, "Conferences (Antimalarial)," Organizations, Meetings and Conferences, UW-PT; Kamm to Tatum, 2 March 1943.

79. Wiselogle, *Survey of Antimalarial Drugs*, 1:398–400, 2:1165; J. H. Burckhalter et al., "Aminoalkylphenols as Antimalarials."

80. W. F. Holcomb to A. L. Tatum, 22 June 1948, box 4, "Parke, Davis and Co., W. F. Holcomb, 1944–1945," AT-UW.

81. A. L. Tatum to H. L. Templeton, 6 October 1931; J. L. Smith to A. L. Tatum, 19 October 1931; and A. L. Tatum to J. L. Smith, 31 December 1931 and 11 March 1932, all in box 3, "Chas. Pfizer and Co., Inc., J. L. Smith, Vice Pres.," AT-UW.

82. A. L. Tatum to J. L. Smith, 29 March 1932; J. L. Smith to A. L. Tatum, 7 April 1932 (quotation); A. L. Tatum to J. L. Smith, 7 May and 6 June 1932; and J. L. Smith to A. L. Tatum, 18 May and 29 June 1932, all in ibid.

83. H. S. Adams to A. L. Tatum, 8 December 1932; and F. W. Heyl to A. L. Tatum, 27 January 1933, both in box 3, "Upjohn Co., Dr. H. S. Adams, 1932–1937," AT-UW.

84. A. L. Tatum to M. L. Kuhs, 21 July 1942, box 1, "Upjohn Company, Grant-in-aid, 1942–1943," UW-PT. N. M. Clausen et al., "A Study of the Similarities of Several Representative Types of Bismuth Preparations," 338 n. 1. A. L. Tatum to G. F. Cartland, 23 November 1933, 3 February and 8 December 1934, and 7 February 1935; and G. F. Cartland to A. L. Tatum, 21 December 1934, all in box 3, "Upjohn Co., Dr. H. S. Adams, 1932–1937," AT-UW.

85. Council on Pharmacy and Chemistry of the American Medical Association, "Report of the Council," 1942. E. G. Upjohn to A. L. Tatum, 27 October 1938, box 3, "Correspondence, 11 Jan. 1937–27 Dec. 1939," AT-SHSW. Tatum to Kuhs, 21 July 1942. M. L. Kuhs to A. L. Tatum, 22 May 1942; and [Agreement between the Upjohn Company and the University of Wisconsin for research on Bismuth in the Chemotherapy of Syphilis], c. July 1942, both in box 1, "Upjohn Company, Grants-in-aid, 1942–1943," UW-PT. N. M. Clausen, B. J. Longley, and A. L. Tatum, "The Quantitative Nature of the Coaction of Bismuth and Arsenical Compounds."

CHAPTER FIVE

The Scientist as Project Researcher

1. Heinrich Biltz, "Uber die Konstitution der Einwirkungsprodukte," 1391–92; Heinrich Biltz and Karl Seydel, "Eine neue Darstellung von Diphenyl-amido-methan (Benzhydryl-amin)"; Arthur W. Dox and Adrian Thomas, "5,5-Diarylbarbituric Acids," 1815; Benjamin V. White, *Stanley Cobb*, 194 (quotation).

2. Tracy J. Putnam and H. Houston Merritt, "Experimental Determination of the Anticonvulsant Properties of Some Phenyl Derivatives"; H. Houston Merritt and Tracy J. Putnam, "A New Series of Anticonvulsant Drugs Tested by Experiments on Animals"; O. M. Gruhzit, "Sodium Diphenyl Hydantoinate."

3. H. Houston Merritt and Tracy J. Putnam, "Sodium Diphenyl Hydantoinate in the Treatment of Convulsive Disorders"; idem, "Sodium Diphenyl Hydantoinate in Treatment of Convulsive Seizures"; idem, "Further Experiences with the Use of Sodium Diphenyl Hydantoinate"; Council of Pharmacy and Chemistry, "Reports of the Council," 1734.

4. T. C. Daniels and Harry Iwamoto, "N^1,N^4-Nicotinyl Derivatives of Sulfanilamide"; Norman Karr et al., "Chemotherapeutic Activity of 4-Nicotinyl-Amino-Benzene-Sulfonamide."

5. Richard Harrison Shryock, *American Medical Research*, 143. C. D. Leake to A. H. Fiske, 10 November 1939; A. H. Fiske to C. D. Leake, 15 November 1939; H. W. Rhodehamel to C. D. Leake, 21 November 1939; and C. D. Leake to [H. W.] Rhodehamel, 25 November 1939, all in box 44, "Lilly Research Laboratories, 1933–1940," CL. Troy C. Daniels, "Therapeutic Agent" (patent assigned to the Research Corporation). It is not clear what Lilly received in return for withdrawing its application—perhaps the promise of a (limited-term) exclusive license if the drug were marketable.

6. E. Lilly to C. D. Leake, 15 January 1940; C. D. Leake to H. W. Rhodehamel, 15

and 29 January, 10 April, and 13 August 1940; and H. W. Rhodehamel to C. D. Leake, 5 February and 2 July 1940, all in box 44, "Lilly Research Laboratories, 1933–1940," CL.

7. The following summary of endocrinology up to the turn of the century is based on Merriley Borrel, "Organotherapy, British Physiology, and Discovery of the Internal Secretions"; idem, "Brown-Séquard's Organotherapy and Its Appearance in America at the End of the Nineteenth Century"; and F. G. Young, "The Evolution of Ideas about Animal Hormones."

8. See, e.g., Gerald Carson, *The Roguish World of Doctor Brinkley*, which relates how one quack made millions from studies on rejuvenation.

9. On attempts to isolate the internal secretion of the pancreas prior to the research at Toronto see Michael Bliss, *The Discovery of Insulin*, 20–44.

10. The synopsis below of the work at Toronto through the spring of 1922 relies on ibid., 45–153. Bliss's study not only is the definitive history of insulin but also stands as a model for future drug histories.

11. Banting and Best, with Macleod present, announced their results through early November 1921 at the meeting of the American Physiological Society at Yale University on 30 December 1921. The first publication of their work, by Banting and Best, appeared in February 1922: "The Internal Secretion of the Pancreas."

12. J. J. R. Macleod, "Insulin and the Steps Taken to Secure an Effective Preparation," 899.

13. Eli Lilly and Company, *A Complete Priced List of the Products of the Lilly Laboratories*, 181–84, copy in KRF; see also Gene E. McCormick, "Insulin," 33.

14. [Contract between the board of governors of the University of Toronto and Eli Lilly and Company for the production of Insulin,] 30 May 1922, "Insulin—Section 5," ELC (this document and some of the others from this archive cited in this chapter appear to be photocopies of documents from the Insulin Committee Papers in the University of Toronto Archives); F. G. Banting, "The History of Insulin," 10; G. H. A. Clowes to J. K. Lilly, 7 July 1945, "J. K. Lilly, 1861–1948—Letters to and from Dr. G. H. A. Clowes, 1920–1945," XBLk, ELC; and Charles H. Best, interview by Gene E. McCormick, 6.

15. G. H. A. Clowes, "The Banting Memorial Address," 53; Bliss, *Insulin*, 98 (see also 104–6); McCormick, "Insulin," 33; F. G. Banting, "The Early Story of Insulin," 19.

16. J. J. R. Macleod, "History of the Researches Leading to the Discovery of Insulin," 306. G. H. A. Clowes to J. J. R. Macleod, 30 March 1922; and J. J. R. Macleod to G. H. A. Clowes, 3 April 1922, both in "Insulin—Section 5," ELC.

17. See, e.g., James Harvey Young, *The Toadstool Millionaires*; and idem, *The Medical Messiahs*.

18. Bliss, *Insulin*, 175; cf. Macleod, "Insulin Preparation," 899.

19. F. G. Banting, C. H. Best, J. B. Collip, J. J. R. Macleod, and J. G. Fitzgerald to R. Falconer, 12 April 1922, quoted in Bliss, *Insulin*, 133.

20. G. H. A. Clowes to J. J. R. Macleod, 30 March, 24 April, and 11 May 1922, "Insulin—Section 5," ELC; Bliss, *Insulin*, 137.

21. A. E. Gooderham (chairman), Robert Falconer, T. A. Russell, and Joseph Flavelle represented the University of Toronto board of governors. J. G. Fitzgerald and R. D. Defries were the delegates from the Connaught Laboratories, and the Toronto faculty on the committee were Macleod, Banting, Best, and Duncan Graham.

22. "From Sea to Sea and Beyond: Insulin and the University of Toronto,

1921–1948," n.d., typescript, 8–12, "Insulin—Section 5," ELC; Best, interview by McCormick, 23; McCormick, "Insulin," 33; Insulin Committee of the University of Toronto, "Insulin," 484.

23. [Contract between Toronto and Lilly,] 30 May 1922; Best, interview by McCormick, 6; Clowes, "Banting Address," 51; E. J. Kahn, Jr., *All in a Century*, 97.

24. J. J. R. Macleod to W. D. Sansum, 21 June 1922, "Potter," UT-IC; J. J. R. Macleod to R. T. Woodyatt, 21 June 1922, "Woodyatt," UT-IC; Bliss, *Insulin*, 270 n. 37.

25. G. H. A. Clowes to J. J. R. Macleod, 5 September 1922, "Lilly and Co.," UT-IC.

26. [Contract between Toronto and Lilly,] 30 May 1922, 2–3.

27. See, e.g., J. J. R. Macleod to G. H. A. Clowes, 12 December 1922, "Insulin—Section 7," ELC.

28. [Contract between Toronto and Lilly,] 30 May 1922, 4.

29. Even Banting, who went to great lengths to ensure that he received credit for the discovery of insulin, wanted no part in the patent application. Only after considerable persuasion did Banting allow his name to appear on the application (see Bliss, *Insulin*, 132–33, 177–78).

30. [Contract between Toronto and Lilly,] 30 May 1922, 5.

31. Kahn, *All in a Century*, 96–97; McCormick, "Insulin," 34; J. K. Lilly to G. H. A. Clowes, 4 August 1922, "J. K. Lilly, 1861–1948—Letters to and from Dr. G. H. A. Clowes, 1920–1945," KBLk, ELC.

32. [Contract between Toronto and Lilly,] 30 May 1922, 2; Banting, "History of Insulin," 10.

33. G. H. A. Clowes to J. J. R. Macleod, 12 August 1922, "Insulin—Section 7," ELC; Clowes to Macleod, 5 September 1922; [F. M. Allen?] Preface. The clinical advisory committee comprised representatives from Toronto and Lilly and several of the leading American specialists: Elliott Joslin (Harvard Medical School and the New England Deaconess Hospital, Boston), Frederick Allen (Psychiatric Institute, Morristown, N.J.), Rollin Woodyatt (Otho Sprague Memorial Institute Laboratory for Clinical Research and the Presbyterian Hospital, Chicago), H. Rawle Geyelin (College of Physicians and Surgeons and Presbyterian Hospital, New York), John Williams (Highland Hospital, Rochester, N.Y.), and Russell Wilder (Mayo Clinic, Rochester, Minn.).

34. On Lilly's insulin work in early June and the first visit of the Toronto scientists, see McCormick, "Insulin," 34; E. Lilly to J. J. R. Macleod, 17 June 1922, "Insulin—Section 6," ELC; and Clowes, "Banting Address," 55. On Lilly's initial improvements on Toronto's method of making insulin see E. Lilly to Macleod, 17 June 1922; and G. H. A. Clowes to J. J. R. Macleod, 20 June 1922, both in "Insulin—Section 6," ELC.

35. G. H. A. Clowes to F. G. Banting, 18 July 1922, FB; Best, interview by McCormick, 7, 13; Bliss, *Insulin*, 133–34.

36. Clowes to Macleod, 12 August 1922; Clowes to Macleod, 5 September 1922; R. T. Woodyatt to J. J. R. Macleod, 10 May 1922, and J. J. R. Macleod to R. T. Woodyatt, 15 May 1922, all in "Woodyatt," UT-IC. W. D. Sansum to J. J. R. Macleod, 15 June 1922 and 18 February 1923, "Potter," UT-IC.

37. The insulin unit was an arbitrary measure of the potency of the hormone, derived from physiological assays on rabbits. It was based on the amount of sample required to produce convulsions (i.e., lowering the blood sugar to such a point of convulsions) in a nondiabetic rabbit within a certain time.

38. G. H. A. Clowes, "Report on Iletin," n.d., typescript, "Insulin—Section 6," ELC; McCormick, "Insulin," 34; E. Lilly to Macleod, 17 June 1922; J. J. R. Macleod to [R. D. Defries,] 14 July 1922, JM; Clowes to Banting, 18 July 1922; J. K. Lilly to J. J. R. Macleod, 22 July 1922, "Insulin—Section 6," ELC; J. K. Lilly to G. H. A. Clowes, 8 August 1922, "J. K. Lilly, 1861–1948—Letters to and from Dr. G. H. A. Clowes, 1920–1945," XBLk, ELC; Clowes to Macleod, 12 August and 5 September 1922.

39. Clowes to Macleod, 5 and 17 September 1922.

40. Clowes, "Report on Iletin"; McCormick, "Insulin," 34; G. H. A. Clowes to J. J. R. Macleod, 17 (quotation) and 23 September 1922, "Insulin—Section 7," ELC.

41. G. H. A. Clowes to J. J. R. Macleod, 20 October 1922, "Insulin—Section 6," ELC.

42. Roscoe Collins Clark, *Threescore Years and Ten*, 59; M. E. Krahl, "Obituary: George Henry Alexander Clowes," 335.

43. Roger J. Williams, *A Textbook of Biochemistry*, 101 (quotation); Jacques Loeb, *Proteins and the Theory of Colloid Behavior*. See also W. J. V. Osterhaut, "Jacques Loeb," xlv–l.

44. G. H. A. Clowes, "Report of Scientific Research Work for Year Ending November 1st, 1921," typescript, 14, "G. H. A. Clowes—Report of Scientific Research Work, Year Ending 1 Nov. 1921," XRDe, ELC; Best, interview by McCormick, 15; Eli Lilly and Company, General Letter No. 30 (6 April 1923), "General Letters to Salesmen Regarding Iletin, 1 Nov. 1922–9 Oct. 1923," XRDe, ELC; [G. Walden,] untitled report on the manufacture of insulin by isoelectric precipitation, n.d., typescript, attached to J. J. R. Macleod to H. H. Dale, 17 January 1923, 1092/23, MRC.

45. [Walden,] untitled report (quotation on p. 8); McCormick, "Insulin," 35.

46. Bliss, *Insulin*, 274 n. 54; Edward A. Doisy, "Philip Anderson Shaffer."

47. McCormick, "Insulin," 34–35; Banting, "History of Insulin," 10; *Journal of Metabolic Research* 2 (1922): 547–985 (the clinical reports on insulin).

48. Macleod to Clowes, 12 December 1922; G. H. A. Clowes to J. J. R. Macleod, 14 December 1922, "Insulin—Section 7," ELC; Eli Lilly and Company, General Letter No. 18 (20 February 1923), "General Letters to Salesmen Regarding Iletin, 1 Nov. 1922–9 Oct. 1923," ELC; McCormick, "Insulin," 35; Banting, "Story of Insulin," 19; G. H. A. Clowes to H. H. Dale, 18 March 1923, 1092/23, MRC; G. H. A. Clowes to J. J. R. Macleod, 2 March 1923, "Unitage and AMA on 'Iletin,'" ELC (quotation).

49. Minutes of the meeting of the Special Advisory Committee on Diabetes (hereafter Insulin Committee minutes), 14 February and 5 March 1923, UT-IC; G. H. A. Clowes to J. J. R. Macleod, 23 February 1923, "Insulin—Section 8," ELC.

50. See, e.g., Eli Lilly and Company, General Letters Nos. 141 (1 November 1922) and 24 (29 March 1923), "General Letters to Salesmen Regarding Iletin, 1 Nov. 1922–8 Oct. 1923," ELC.

51. Macleod to Clowes, 12 December 1922; J. J. R. Macleod to G. H. A. Clowes, 10 January 1923, "Unitage and AMA on 'Iletin,'" ELC; Insulin Committee minutes, 14 February and 5 March 1923; Lilly, General Letters Nos. 13 (20 February 1923) and 24 (29 March 1923); J. J. R. Macleod to G. H. A. Clowes, 10 March 1923, "Lilly and Co.," UT-IC. On the formation of group clinics as a means of economizing in the early twentieth century see George Rosen, *The Structure of American Medical Practice, 1875–1941*, 53–55.

52. H. H. Dale and H. W. Dudley, "Report to the Medical Research Council on Our

Visit to Canada and the United States, Chiefly to Examine the 'Insulin' Treatment of Diabetes," 30 October 1922, 1092/23, MRC. The "practical difficulties" were that (1) insulin had to be administered indefinitely, (2) there was no other dosage form yet available besides the hypodermic injection, and (3) impurities in the extract were causing reactions in some patients.

53. Eli Lilly and Company, General Letter No. 88 (9 October 1923), "General Letters to Salesmen Regarding Iletin, 1 Nov. 1922–9 Oct. 1923," ELC.

54. Lilly to Clowes, 4 August 1922; J. K. Lilly to E. Lilly, 23 January 1923, "Insulin—Section 8," ELC.

55. G. H. A. Clowes to J. J. R. Macleod, 27 September 1922, "Insulin—Section 6," ELC; Insulin Committee minutes, 30 September 1922, UT-IC; J. K. Lilly to E. Lilly, 23 January 1923; G. H. A. Clowes to J. J. R. Macleod, 20 December 1922, "Insulin—Section 8," ELC; McCormick, "Insulin," 35; Elliott P. Joslin, "Address by Dr. Elliott P. Joslin," 40.

56. Dale and Dudley, "Report," 7; G. H. A. Clowes to J. J. R. Macleod, 14 March 1923, "Lilly and Co.," UT-IC; Bliss, *Insulin*, 71–72, 174; Macleod to Clowes, 12 December 1922; H. H. Dale to W. Fletcher, 26 September 1922, 1092/23, MRC (quotation).

57. Bliss, *Insulin*, 146; J. K. Lilly to Macleod, 22 July 1922; Dale to Fletcher, 26 September 1922; Dale and Dudley, "Report," 7. On Dale see W. Feldberg, "Henry Hallett Dale."

58. Insulin Committee minutes, 30 September 1922 (quotation); J. K. Lilly to G. H. A. Clowes, 3 January 1923, "Unsorted," UT-IC; G. H. A. Clowes to J. J. R. Macleod, 8 January 1923, "Unitage and AMA on 'Iletin,' " ELC; Macleod to Clowes, 10 January 1923; Lilly, General Letter No. 13 (20 February 1923); Clowes to Macleod, 14 March 1923; Bliss, *Insulin*, 178–79.

59. Clowes to Macleod, 5 September 1922.

60. J. K. Lilly to Clowes, 3 January 1923.

61. G. H. A. Clowes to J. J. R. Macleod, 7 March 1923; and G. H. A. Clowes to R. D. Defries, 13 March 1923, both in "Lilly and Co.," UT-IC. Clowes to Macleod, 14 March 1923.

62. Clowes to Macleod, 14 March 1923.

63. G. H. A. Clowes to J. J. R. Macleod, 14 April 1923, "Unitage and AMA on 'Iletin,' " ELC.

64. See, e.g., Macleod, "Insulin Preparation," 899–900.

65. Insulin Committee minutes, 16 March 1923, UT-IC; J. J. R. Macleod to G. H. A. Clowes, 16 March 1923, "Lilly and Co.," UT-IC.

66. Insulin Committee minutes, 14 February 1923; Clowes to Macleod, 7 March 1923; F. G. Banting, Charles Herbert Best, and James Bertram Collip, "Extract Obtainable from the Mammalian Pancreas"; George B. Walden, "Purified Antidiabetic Product and Process of Making It."

67. Insulin Committee minutes, 14 February and 2 April 1923, UT-IC; Clowes to Macleod, 5, 23 (quotation), 27 September 1922; G. H. A. Clowes to C. H. Best, 12 September 1922, "Lilly and Co.," UT-IC; Insulin Committee minutes, 30 September 1922; Dale and Dudley, "Report," 7.

68. Insulin Committee minutes, 2 April 1923; Bliss, *Insulin*, 180.

69. On the Council on Pharmacy and Chemistry see, e.g., Morris Fishbein, *A History of the American Medical Association*, 865–86; and James G. Burrow, *AMA*, 74–75, 109–14, 117–18, 126–28.

70. Council on Pharmacy and Chemistry of the American Medical Association, *New and Nonofficial Remedies, 1924*, 16–17.

71. Clowes to Macleod, 14 April 1923.

72. G. H. A. Clowes to J. J. R. Macleod, 8 April 1923, "Lilly and Co.," UT-IC; Bliss, *Insulin*, 276 n. 82. The council reported their approval of Lilly's brand name for insulin in June 1923 (*Journal of the American Medical Association* 80 [1923]: 1851). The Lilly Company officially assigned its isoelectric patent to the Insulin Committee a few days after the patent was granted (see J. K. Lilly to F. L. Hutchinson, 29 December 1924, "Insulin—Section 6," ELC).

73. [Contract between the governors of the University of Toronto and Eli Lilly and Company on insulin,] 30 June 1923, "Insulin Contracts and Patents, 1923–1945"; and "Contract December 1st, 1923," both in XCAl, ELC.

74. [Contract between Toronto and Lilly,] 30 June 1923, 6–9, 14–15, "Contract December 1st, 1923," 2–3.

75. The problems of standardization are documented in the folder "Unitage and AMA on 'Iletin,'" ELC. The reports from the international conferences are in League of Nations, Health Organisation, *The Biological Standardisation of Insulin*.

76. G. B. Walden to G. H. A. Clowes, 26 April 1955, "G. H. A. Clowes, Correspondence to and from, 1940–1947 [*sic*]," XRDc, ELC.

77. Banting, "History of Insulin," 10; Insulin Committee, "Insulin," 486.

78. G. H. A. Clowes, "Address by Dr. George H. A. Clowes," 52–53.

79. Bliss, *Insulin*, 173.

80. Ibid., 240–41.

81. C. H. Best to E. Lilly, 4 June 1954, "Grants (Insulin): Best, Collip, Fisher," XRDng, ELC. E. N. Beesley to F. B. Peck and R. M. Rice, 15 November 1954 (quotation); F. B. Peck to E. N. Beesley, 13 December 1954; E. N. Beesley to C. H. Best, 8 February 1955; E. N. Beesley to J. B. Collip, 8 February 1955; and E. N. Beesley to A. M. Fisher, 8 February 1955, all in "G. B. Walden—Insulin Corres., 1949–1960," XRDq, ELC. W. R. Kirtley to E. N. Beesley, 30 November 1966 and 28 November 1967, and W. R. Kirtley to B. E. Beck, 16 November 1971, all in "Grants (Insulin): Best, Collip, Fisher," XRDng, ELC.

82. "Eli Lilly and Company: A History," typescript, n.d., 69, 76, ELC; Kahn, *All in a Century*, 101 (quotation).

83. William B. Castle, "The Conquest of Pernicious Anemia," 284; idem, "George Richards Minot," 347; Logan Clendening, *Source Book of Medical History*, 502–6.

84. On the development and significance of early vitamin research see Aaron J. Ihde and Stanley L. Becker, "Conflict of Concepts in Early Vitamin Studies"; Aaron J. Ihde, *The Development of Modern Chemistry*, 644–56; and Stanley L. Becker, "The Emergence of a Trace Nutrient Concept through Animal Feeding Experiments." Dietary therapy for anemias was by no means new in the early twentieth century, but it did not attain wide appeal until after the results from Rochester and Harvard appeared (see Castle, "Pernicious Anemia," 291–93).

85. George W. Corner, *George Hoyt Whipple and His Friends*, 62–64, 98–102;

idem, "George Hoyt Whipple"; George H. Whipple, F. S. Robscheit-Robbins, and G. B. Walden, "Blood Regeneration Following Simple Anemia. IV."

86. Corner, *Whipple*, 179–82; idem, "George Hoyt Whipple," 137–38; Castle, "Pernicious Anemia," 292; F. S. Robscheit-Robbins and G. H. Whipple, "Blood Regeneration in Severe Anemia. II."

87. Corner, *Whipple*, 100, 185; George H. Whipple, "Autobiographical Sketch," 266; George H. Whipple, interview by Gene E. McCormick, 4; George H. Whipple, "Pigment Metabolism and Regeneration of Hemoglobin in the Body"; Castle, "Pernicious Anemia," 293.

88. Castle, "Minot," 338–39, 349; idem, "Pernicious Anemia," 294; Maurice B. Strauss, "Of Medicine, Men and Molecules," 619.

89. Castle, "Pernicious Anemia," 294; William B. Castle and Richard P. Stetson, interview by Gene E. McCormick, Lawrence Kass, *Pernicious Anemia*, 24; "Medicine's Living History," 40–41.

90. George R. Minot et al., "Observations on Patients with Pernicious Anemia Partaking of a Special Diet," 72 (quotation), 74; Kass, *Pernicious Anemia*, 39–40; Castle, "Pernicious Anemia," 294; idem, "Minot," 350–51. Minot and Murphy first published their results in August 1926, in George R. Minot and William P. Murphy, "Treatment of Pernicious Anemia by a Special Diet."

91. See, e.g., Stanley L. Becker, "Will Milk Make Them Grow?"

92. Castle, "Minot," 351–52; John T. Edsall, "Edwin Joseph Cohn," 56; Corner, *Whipple*, 183. The first publication on liver fractionation by the Harvard group appeared in 1927: Edwin J. Cohn et al., "The Nature of the Material in Liver Effective in Pernicious Anemia, I." The Rochester group's first report on their study of liver fractions appeared in the same year: G. H. Whipple and F. S. Robscheit-Robbins, "Simple Experimental Anemia and Liver Extracts."

93. See, e.g., A. A. James and N. B. Laughton, "The Control of Blood Pressure with Liver Extracts"; W. J. MacDonald, "Extractives of Liver Possessing Blood Pressure Reducing Properties"; and Ralph H. Major, "The Effects of Hepatic Extract on High Blood Pressure."

94. Leon G. Zerfas, interview by Gene E. McCormick, 13; G. H. A. Clowes to J. H. Mullin, 25 May 1925, ELC.

95. Zerfas, interview by McCormick, 4–6, 8, 13, 15. Kahn, *All in a Century*, 60–61. L. G. Zerfas to G. Minot, 28 October 1926; G. Minot to L. G. Zerfas, 2 November 1926; and L. G. Zerfas to H. Jackson, 21 April 1927, all in "Liver Extract No. 343: Pre-Product Introduction, 1925–1927," ELC.

96. Zerfas to Minot, 28 October 1926; Minot to Zerfas, 2 November 1926; Kahn, *All in a Century*, 61; Zerfas, interview by McCormick, 13, 15–16; George B. Walden, interview by Gene E. McCormick, 15–16; G. H. A. Clowes to J. K. Lilly, 11 July 1927, "Liver Extract No. 343: Pre-Product Introduction, 1925–1927," ELC.

97. Castle, "Minot," 353; E. J. Cohn to Dr. Hörlein, 25 January 1928, "H–I–J," box 2, HU-PAC; Committee on Pernicious Anemia, "Report."

98. See, e.g., G. R. Minot to E. Cohn, 22 April 1927, "Correspondence, George R. Minot et al. regarding anemia, 1927," EC. W. H. Blome to G. R. Minot, 25 June 1927; W. B. Castle to W. H. Blome, 30 June 1927; O. W. Smith to Pernicious Anemia Committee, 1 July 1927; E. H. Volwiler to G. R. Minot, 29 July 1927; and W. B. Castle to E. H. Volwiler, 11 August 1927, all in box 1, HU-PAC. R. H. Hutchinson to W. B. Castle,

"Grants, Fellowships and Awards to Harvard University, 31 May–5 June 1950," XCAc, ELC. Minot to Clowes, 10 April 1928; Minutes, Lilly Research Committee, 1 July 1942 (quotation).

129. G. H. Whipple to E. Lilly, 4 January 1955, "Liver Extract No. 55, 1930–," ELC.

130. G. H. Whipple to R. L. Thompson, 21 April 1953, ibid.; Corner, *Whipple*, 287–88.

131. G. R. Minot to [J. K.?] Lilly, 25 June 1929, "Liver Extract No. 343: 1928 ff.," ELC; L. G. Zerfas to E. Lilly and G. H. A. Clowes, 8 November 1934, "Post-Clinical, Liver Extract 343 and 55; Nobel Prize," ELC. On the work at Harvard in the early 1930s dealing with injectable liver extracts for pernicious anemia see Maxwell Finland and William Castle, *The Harvard Medical Unit at Boston City Hospital*, 1:22, 250.

132. This pernicious anemia principle was not liver extract no. 343 but dessicated hog stomach lining, an innovation stemming in part from William Castle's research on the connection between pernicious anemia and defective gastric digestion, which he began around 1927 (see Kass, *Pernicious Anemia*, 43–44; Strauss, "Medicine, Men and Molecules," 620–21; and Castle, "Pernicious Anemia," 303–4).

133. See Walden, interview by McCormick, 21.

134. Zerfas, interview by McCormick, 35–36.

135. W. P. Murphy to H. Berlin, 17 August 1927, box 1, HU-PAC.

EPILOGUE:
The Search for the Genetic El Dorado

1. Callie Hull and Mary Timms, "Research Supported by Industry." The reader should bear in mind some of the caveats associated with these NRC surveys from chapter 2, such as the reluctance of some firms and academic researchers to give details about or even to mention industry-supported projects. It is also worth noting that many companies in the above survey did not specify the number of grants or fellowships, their value, or the individual universities that received them. Thus, these data should be interpreted, not as absolute, but rather as bare minimums.

2. See, e.g., Denis Prager and Gilbert S. Omenn, "Research, Innovation."

3. Bruce L. R. Smith and Joseph J. Karlesky, *The State of Academic Science*, 1:62–64.

4. Theodore Cooper and Susan Bennett, "Differing Approaches to Biomedical Research," 107; Prager and Omenn, "Research, Innovation," 380.

5. See, e.g., "ACS Ninth Biennial Education Conference"; Robert D. Varrin and Diane S. Kukich, "Guidelines for Industry-sponsored Research"; Lois S. Peters and Herbert I. Fusfeld, "Current U.S. University/Industry Research Connections"; and Prager and Omenn, "Research Innovation."

6. "Attracting the Research Dollar"; Michael Schrage and Nell Henderson, "U-Md. Thrives on High Tech."

7. Ibid.; Peters and Fusfeld, "Current U.S. University/Industry Research Connections," 107; Smith and Karlesky, *The State of Academic Science*, 1:73–74.

8. Peters and Fusfeld, "Current U.S. University/Industry Research Connections," 81–82, 139; Smith and Karlesky, *The State of Academic Science*, 1:68–70; Prager and Omenn, "Research, Innovation," 381–82; Jean Lang, "Partners with Industry."

9. Martin Kenney, *Biotechnology*, 40–41; Peters and Fusfeld, "Current U.S. University/Industry Research Connections," 92–93; Prager and Omenn, "Research, Innovation," 381.

10. See the extensive study by Peters and Fusfeld: "Current U.S. University/Industry Research Connections."

11. "Pharmaceutical R and D Expenditures Estimated at $3.3 Billion for 1983"; Lois S. Peters, "Pharmaceuticals," 191.

12. "Grants and Awards"; Kenney, *Biotechnology*, 55–57.

13. Kenney, *Biotechnology*, 55–69; Smith and Karlesky, *The State of Academic Science*, 1:66; Prager and Omenn, "Research, Innovation," 382; Peters and Fusfeld, "Current U.S. University/Industry Research Connections," 20, 137–38; Don Colburn, "Uneasy Partners in Discovery"; "Upjohn Enlists KU's Help."

14. Peters, "Pharmaceuticals," 192; Kenney, *Biotechnology*, 91–93.

15. See the advertisements that appeared in the *Washington Post*, March 1986.

16. George Zografi, circular letter of 5 April 1978, A(2) "Busse," KRF (quotation); George Zografi to Pharmaceutics Group, 11 January 1979, "Busse Lectures, 1980," Files, Dean's Office, University of Wisconsin School of Pharmacy, Madison, Wisconsin; "First Annual Busse Lecture to Be Presented at U.W.," press release, 18 July 1979, Center for Health Sciences of the University of Wisconsin, ibid.

17. "Pharmaceutical Considerations in the Use of Peptides and Proteins," syllabus, typescript, attached to A. L. Hanson and M. H. Weinswig to Colleagues, January 1986, author's personal files.

18. "Visiting Scientist Program Launched."

19. David E. Sanger, "U.S. Research Sponsorship"; Boyce Rensberger, "R&D Surge Foreseen"; "Year of the Money Scramble," 22–23; D'Vera Cohn and Barbara Vobejda, "Arts, Education Groups"; Barbara Vobejda, "Academia Using Strategy"; D'Vera Cohn, "Cultural Institutions Join Money Hunt." For difficulties in dealing with restrictions that the Department of Defense places on research results see Michael Schrage, "Scientists Defy Pentagon."

20. Nicholas Wade, "Gene Goldrush," 879; Kenney, *Biotechnology*, 41.

21. Kenney, *Biotechnology*, 33; Derek C. Bok, "Business and the Academy," 25. The tax reforms of 1986 eliminated most of these tax breaks.

22. Kim McDonald, "Strength of U.S."

23. Scott Jaschik, "Democrats Urge Network."

24. Lee Hockstader, "Technology Center's Chief Makes a Hit."

25. Nell Henderson, "Montgomery Forms High-Tech Council"; Molly Sinclair, "Hopkins U. Project Advances"; Dinah Wisenberg, "Betting on Biotech."

26. Molly Sinclair, "Hopkins Traffic Report Altered"; idem, "Hopkins U. Project Advances."

27. Barbara J. Culliton, "The Academic-Industrial Complex," 962.

28. See John W. Servos, "The Industrial Relations of Science."

29. Quoted in Barbara J. Culliton, "Pajaro Dunes," 156.

30. David Blumenthal et al., "University-Industry Research Relationships."

31. David Blumenthal et al., "Industrial Support of University Research," 245.

32. Blumenthal et al., "University-Industry Research Relationships," 1365; Bok, "Business and the Academy," 29; Kenney, *Biotechnology*, 72.

33. Wil Lepkowski, "University/Industry Research Ties."

Bibliography

->>>->>>->>>->>>->>> -<<<-<<<-<<<-<<<-<<<

Manuscript Sources

Abbott Laboratories. Archives. North Chicago, Illinois.

Abel, John Jacob. Papers. Alan Mason Chesney Archives, Johns Hopkins University, Baltimore, Maryland.

Adams, Roger. Papers. University of Illinois Archives, Urbana, Illinois.

American Society for Pharmacology and Experimental Therapeutics. Archives. Bethesda, Maryland.

Banting, F. G. Papers. Thomas Fisher Rare Book Library, University of Toronto, Toronto, Canada.

Cohn, Edwin J. Papers. Francis A. Countway Library, Harvard Medical School, Boston, Massachusetts.

Dean's Office, University of Wisconsin School of Pharmacy. Files. Madison, Wisconsin.

Department of Pharmacology and Toxicology, University of Wisconsin Medical School. Papers. University of Wisconsin Archives, Madison, Wisconsin.

Eli Lilly and Company. Archives. Indianapolis, Indiana.

E. R. Squibb and Sons. Archives. New Brunswick, New Jersey.

Food and Drug Administration. Papers. Record Group 88, National Archives, General Archives Division, Suitland, Maryland.

Insulin Committee of the University of Toronto. Papers. University of Toronto Archives, Toronto, Canada.

Kremers Reference Files. F. B. Power Pharmaceutical Library, University of Wisconsin, Madison, Wisconsin.

Leake, Chauncey D. Papers. National Library of Medicine, Bethesda, Maryland.

Loevenhart, Arthur Salomon. Papers. University of Wisconsin Archives, Madison, Wisconsin.

Macleod, J. J. R. Papers. Thomas Fisher Rare Book Library, University of Toronto, Toronto, Canada.

Medical Research Council. Records. National Institute for Medical Research, London, England.

Merck and Company. Archives. Rahway, New Jersey.

New Jersey State Division of Archives and Records Management, Trenton, New Jersey

Pernicious Anemia Committee of Harvard University. Papers. Francis A. Countway Library, Harvard Medical School, Boston, Massachusetts.

Richards, Alfred Newton. Papers. University of Pennsylvania Archives, Philadelphia, Pennsylvania.

Small, Lyndon Frederick. Papers. National Library of Medicine, Bethesda, Maryland.

Sollmann, Torald. Papers. Allen Medical Library, Case Western Reserve University, Cleveland, Ohio.

Steenbock, Harry. Papers. University of Wisconsin Archives, Madison, Wisconsin.

Tatum, Arthur Lawrie. Papers. State Historical Society of Wisconsin, Madison, Wisconsin.

————. University of Wisconsin Archives, Madison, Wisconsin.

Waksman, Selman A. Papers. Division of Manuscripts, Library of Congress, Washington, D.C.

Interviews

Adams, Roger. Interview by John B. Mellecker, New York, 20 November 1964, 12 February 1965, and 15 March 1965. Tape recording, University of Illinois Archives, Urbana, Illinois.

Best, Charles H. Interview by Gene E. McCormick, Best Institute, University of Toronto, 24 September 1968. Transcript, Eli Lilly and Company Archives, Indianapolis, Indiana.

Castle, William B., and Stetson, Richard P. Interview by Gene E. McCormick, Veterans Administration Hospital, West Roxbury, Massachusetts, 3 December 1968. Transcript, Eli Lilly and Company Archives, Indianapolis, Indiana.

Tishler, Max. Interview by Leon Gortler and John A. Heitmann, Wesleyan University Library, 14 November 1983. Transcript, Center for the History of Chemistry, University of Pennsylvania, Philadelphia, Pennsylvania.

Volwiler, Ernest H. Interview by John P. Swann, Abbott Laboratories, North Chicago, Illinois, 18 April 1984. Transcript, A(2) "Volwiler, Ernest H.," Kremers Reference Files, F. B. Power Pharmaceutical Library, University of Wisconsin, Madison, Wisconsin.

Walden, George B. Interview by Gene E. McCormick, Eli Lilly and Company, Indianapolis, Indiana, 5 November 1968. Transcript, Eli Lilly and Company Archives, Indianapolis, Indiana.

Whipple, George H. Interview by Gene E. McCormick, University of Rochester, Rochester, New York, 8 October 1970. Transcript, Eli Lilly and Company Archives, Indianapolis, Indiana.

Zerfas, Leon G. Interview by Gene E. McCormick, Cambry, Indiana, 22 and 25 October 1968. Transcript, Eli Lilly and Company Archives, Indianapolis, Indiana.

Printed Sources

Abbott, W. Osler. "Acetyl-beta-methylcholin: II, The Action on the Gastro-Intestinal Tract of Normal Persons, in Abdominal Distension, and in Certain Other Conditions." *American Journal of the Medical Sciences* 186 (1933): 323–30.

Abbott Laboratories. *Addresses: Dedication of Research Building, Abbott Laboratories, North Chicago, Illinois, October 7, 1938*. North Chicago, 1938.

———. *Annual Report*, 1952–58. North Chicago.

———. *Price List of Pharmaceutical and Biologic Products and Fine Medicinal Chemicals*. North Chicago, 1928.

Abel, John J. "The Methods of Pharmacology, with Experimental Illustrations." *Pharmaceutical Era* 7 (1892): 105–7.

Ackernecht, Erwin H. *History and Geography of the Most Important Diseases*. New York: Hafner, 1965.

"ACS Ninth Biennial Education Conference." *Journal of Chemical Education* 53 (1976): 672–74.

Adams, Roger. "Cyclopentenyl Compound and Process of Making Same." United States Patent 1,715,052, patented 28 May 1929.

———. "The Manufacture of Organic Chemicals at the University of Illinois." *Science* 47 (1918): 225–28.

———. "The Relation of the University Scientist to the Chemical Industries." *Industrial and Engineering Chemistry* 13 (1935): 365–67.

———. "Universities and Industry in Science." Perkin Medal Address to the Society of Chemical Industry, New York, 15 January 1954. *Industrial and Engineering Chemistry* 46 (1954): 506–10.

Adams, Roger, and Kamm, Oliver. "Beta-bromoethyl Para-nitro-benzoate." United States Patent 1,260,289, patented 26 March 1918.

Adams, Roger, and Rodewald, Charles W. "Arsonophenyl Amino Alcohols and the Process of Making the Same." United States Patent 1,801,535, patented 21 April 1931.

Adams, Roger, and Volwiler, Ernest H. "N-Butyl Esters of Para-amino Benzoic Acid." United States Patent 1,440,652, patented 2 January 1923.

[Allen, F. M.?] Preface to *Journal of Metabolic Research* 2, nos. 5 and 6 (1922).

Allen, F. M. "Summary of Publications on Insulin to Date." *Journal of Metabolic Research* 2 (1922): 125–40.

Allen F. M., and Sherrill, James W. "Clinical Observations with Insulin." *Journal of Metabolic Research* 2 (1922): 803–985.

Allmark, M. G.; Anderson, R. C.; Haley, T. J.; Holck, H. G. O.; Harrisson, J. W. E.; Nelson, J. W.; Swoap, O. F.; Weaver, L. C.; and Swinyard, E. A. "A History of the Committee on Physiological Testing, Scientific Section, American Pharmaceutical Association." *Drug Standards* 24 (1956): 200–205.

American Men of Science: A Biographical Directory, Edited by J. McKeen Cattell and Jaques Cattell. 4th ed. New York: Science Press, 1927.

American Men of Science: A Biographical Directory, edited by Jaques Cattell. 8th ed. Lancaster, Pa.: Science Press, 1949.

Andrus, E. C.; Bronk, D. W.; Carden, G. A., Jr.; Keefer, C. S.; Lockwood, J. S.; Wearn, J.

T.; and Winternitz, M. C., eds. *Advances in Military Medicine Made by American Investigators Working under the Sponsorship of the Committee on Medical Research.* 2 vols. Science in World War II. Boston: Little Brown, 1948.

Annual Survey of Research in Pharmacy. Baltimore: John D. Lucas, 1933–40.

"Attracting the Research Dollar." *New York Times*, 9 March 1985.

Bacon, Raymond F. "Industrial Research in America." *Scientific Monthly* 2 (1916): 226–33.

Banting, F. G. "The Early Story of Insulin." In *Lilly Research Laboratories: Dedication*, 14–20. See Eli Lilly and Company.

———. "The History of Insulin." *Edinburgh Medical Journal*, n.s. 36 (1929): 1–18.

Banting, F. G., and Best, C. H. "The Internal Secretion of the Pancreas." *Journal of Laboratory and Clinical Medicine* 7 (1922): 256–71.

Banting, F. G.; Best, Charles Herbert; and Collip, James Bertram. "Extract Obtainable from the Mammalian Pancreas or from the Related Glands in Fishes, Useful in the Treatment of Diabetes Mellitus, and a Method of Preparing It." United States Patent 1,469,994, patented 9 October 1923.

Banting, F. G.; Campbell, W. R.; and Fletcher, A. A. "Insulin in the Treatment of Diabetes Mellitus." *Journal of Metabolic Research* 2 (1922): 547–604.

Barrows, Albert L. "The Relationship of the National Research Council to Industrial Research." In *Research—A National Resource*, 2:365–69. See *Research—A National Resource.*

Bartlett, Howard R. "The Development of Industrial Research in the United States." In *Research—A National Resource*, 2:19–77. See *Research—A National Resource.*

Becker, Gabriel P. "A Study of the History and Development of Abbott Laboratories." Master's thesis, University of Louisville, 1956.

Becker, Stanley L. "The Emergence of a Trace Nutrient Concept through Animal Feeding Experiments." Ph.D. diss., University of Wisconsin, 1968.

———. "Will Milk Make Them Grow? An Episode in the Discovery of the Vitamins." In *Chemistry and Modern Society: Historical Essays in Honor of Aaron J. Ihde*, edited by John Parascandola and James C. Whorton, 61–83. ACS Symposium Series 228. Washington, D.C.: American Chemical Society, 1983.

Beer, John J. "Coal Tar Dye Manufacture and the Origins of the Modern Industrial Research Laboratory." *Isis* 49 (1958): 123–31.

Ben-David, Joseph, and Zloczower, Awraham. "Universities and Academic Systems in Modern Societies." *Archives européennes de sociologie* 3 (1962): 45–84.

Biltz, Heinrich. "Über die Konstitution der Einwirkungsprodukte von Substituierten Harnstoffen auf Benzil und über einige neue Methoden zur Darstellung der 5,5-Diphenyl-hydantoine." *Berichte der Deutschen Chemischen Gesselschaft* 41 (1908): 1391–93.

Biltz, Heinrich, and Seydel, Karl. "Eine neue Darstellung von Diphenyl-amido-methan (Benzhydryl-amin)." *Berichte der Deutschen Chemischen Gesselschaft* 44 (1911): 411–13.

Birr, Kendall. "The Roots of Industrial Research." In *Research and American Industrial Development: A Bicentennial Look at the Contributions of Applied R and D*, by Harold Vagtborg, 24–50. New York: Pergamon Press, 1976.

Bliss, Michael. *The Discovery of Insulin.* Chicago: University of Chicago Press; Toronto: McClelland and Stewart, 1982.

Blumenthal, David; Gluck, Michael; Louis, Karen Seashore; Stoto, Michael A.; and Wise, David. "University-Industry Research Relationships in Biotechnology: Implications for the University." *Science* 232 (1986): 1361–66.

Blumenthal, David; Gluck, Michael; Louis, Karen Seashore; and Wise, David. "Industrial Support of University Research in Biotechnology." *Science* 231 (1986): 242–46.

Bok, Derek C. "Business and the Academy." *Harvard Magazine* 83, no. 5 (1981): 23–35.

Borell, Merriley. "Brown-Séquard's Organotherapy and Its Appearance in America at the End of the Nineteenth Century." *Bulletin of the History of Medicine* 50 (1976): 309–20.

———. "Organotherapy, British Physiology, and Discovery of the Internal Secretions." *Journal of the History of Biology* 9 (1976): 235–68.

Bradley, H. C. "Dr. Loevenhart's War Work." In "The Loevenhart Memorial Meeting: University of Wisconsin Medical School, May 3, 1929." *Quarterly of the Phi Beta Pi Medical Fraternity* 26 (1929): 283–87.

Bronk, Detlev W. "Alfred Newton Richards (1876–1966)." *Perspectives in Biology and Medicine* 19 (1976): 413–22.

Brown, Wade H. "Tryparsamide." *Science* 62 (1925): 350–51.

Burckhalter, J. H.; Tendick, F. H.; Jones, Eldon M.; Jones, Patricia A.; Holcomb, W. F.; and Rawlins, A. L. "Aminoalkylphenols as Antimalarials. II. (Heterocyclic-amino)-alpha-amino-orthocresols. The Synthesis of Camoquin." *Journal of the American Chemical Society* 70 (1948): 1363–73.

Burdick, Alfred S. "Research." Address at the Annual Meeting of the American Pharmaceutical Manufacturers' Association, Greensboro, North Carolina, 18 May 1932. *Proceedings of the American Pharmaceutical Manufacturers' Association,* 1931–32; 365–75.

Burnet, Macfarlane. *Natural History of Infectious Disease.* 3d ed. Cambridge: Cambridge University Press, 1962.

Burrow, James G. *AMA: Voice of American Medicine.* Baltimore: Johns Hopkins Press, 1963.

Campbell, Walter R. "Ketosis, Acidosis and Coma Treated by Insulin." *Journal of Metabolic Research* 2 (1922): 606–35.

Carson, Gerald. *The Roguish World of Doctor Brinkley.* New York: Holt, Rinehart and Winston, 1960.

Castle, William B. "The Conquest of Pernicious Anemia." In *Blood, Pure and Eloquent: A Story of Discovery, of People, and of Ideas,* edited by Maxwell W. Wintrobe, 283–317. New York: McGraw Hill, 1980.

———. "George Richards Minot." *Biographical Memoirs of the National Academy of Sciences* 45 (1975): 337–83.

Chen, K. K., ed. *The American Society for Pharmacology and Experimental Therapeutics, Incorporated: The First Sixty Years, 1908–1969.* N.p.: [American Society for Pharmacology and Experimental Therapeutics,] 1969.

Cheyney, Edward Potts. *History of the University of Pennsylvania, 1740–1940.* Philadelphia: University of Pennsylvania Press, 1940.

Chittenden, Russell H. *The Development of Physiological Chemistry in the United States*. American Chemical Society Monograph Series. New York: Chemical Catalog, 1930.

Clark, Roscoe Collins. *Threescore Years and Ten: A Narrative of the First Seventy Years of Eli Lilly and Company, 1876–1946*. [Indianapolis: Eli Lilly,] 1946.

Clausen, N. M.; Longley, B. J.; Green, R. E.; and Tatum, A. L. "A Study of the Similarities of Several Representative Types of Bismuth Preparations Used in the Therapy of Experimental Syphilis." *Journal of Pharmacology and Experimental Therapeutics* 76 (1942): 338–42.

Clausen, N. M.; Longley, B. J.; and Tatum, A. L. "The Quantitative Nature of the Coaction of Bismuth and Arsenical Compounds in the Therapy of Experimental Syphilis." *Journal of Pharmacology and Experimental Therapeutics* 74 (1942): 324–33.

Clendening, Logan. *Source Book of Medical History*. 1942. Reprint. New York: Dover Publications, 1960.

Clowes, G. H. A. "Address by Dr. George H. A. Clowes." In *Lilly Research Laboratories: Dedication*, 52–55. *See* Eli Lilly and Company.

———. "The Banting Memorial Address." *Proceedings of the American Diabetes Association* 7 (1947): 49–60.

Clowes, George H. A., Jr. "George Henry Alexander Clowes, Ph.D., D.Sc., LL.D. (1877–1958): A Man of Science for All Seasons." *Journal of Surgical Oncology* 18 (1981): 197–217.

Cohn, D'Vera. "Cultural Institutions Join Money Hunt." *Washington Post*, 26 November 1985.

Cohn, D'Vera, and Vobejda, Barbara. "Arts, Education Groups Now Making Millions." *Washington Post*, 24 November 1985.

Cohn, Edwin J.; McMeekin, Thomas L.; and Minot, George R. "The Nature of the Material Effective in Pernicious Anemia. III." *American Journal of Physiology* 90 (1929): 316–17.

———. "The Nature of the Material Effective in Pernicious Anemia. IV." *Journal of Biological Chemistry* 87 (1930): xlix–lii.

Cohn, Edwin J.; Minot, George R.; Alles, Gordon A.; and Salter, William T. "The Nature of the Material in Liver Effective in Pernicious Anemia. II." *Journal of Biological Chemistry* 77 (1928): 325–58.

Cohn, Edwin J.; Minot, George R.; Fulton, John F.; Ulrichs, Hermann F.; Sargent, Florence C.; Weare, John H.; and Murphy, William P. "The Nature of the Material in Liver Effective in Pernicious Anemia. I." *Journal of Biological Chemistry* 74 (1927): lxix–lxxii.

Colburn, Don. "Uneasy Partners in Discovery." *Washington Post*, 23 April 1986.

"Colleges Pay Industry Dividends." *Chemical and Engineering News* 33 (1955): 5038.

Committee on Pernicious Anemia. "Report of the Committee on Pernicious Anemia of the Harvard Medical School." *Journal of the American Medical Association* 93 (1929): 1144.

Cooper, Franklin S. "Location and Extent of Industrial Research Activity in the United States." In *Research—A National Resource*, 2:173–87. *See Research—A National Resource*.

Cooper, Garrett Arthur. "The Present Status of Arsenicals in the Treatment of Syphilis." M.D. thesis, University of Wisconsin, 1935.

Cooper, Theodore, and Bennett, Susan. "Differing Approaches to Biomedical Research: The NIH, the Academic Medical Center, and the Pharmaceutical Industry." In *Biomedical Institutions, Biomedical Funding, and Public Policy*, edited by H. Hugh Fudenberg, 93–113. New York: Plenum Press, 1983.

Corner, George W. "George Hoyt Whipple." *American Philosophical Society Year Book*, 1976, 135–40.

———. *George Hoyt Whipple and His Friends: The Life Story of a Nobel Prize Pathologist*. Philadelphia: J. B. Lippincott, 1963.

———. *Two Centuries of Medicine: A History of the School of Medicine, University of Pennsylvania*. Philadelphia: J. B. Lippincott, 1965.

Council on Pharmacy and Chemistry of the American Medical Association. "New and Nonofficial Remedies." *Journal of the American Medical Association* 80 (1923): 1617, 1851 (insulin).

———. "New and Nonofficial Remedies." *Journal of the American Medical Association* 90 (1928): 385 (liver extract no. 343).

———. "New and Nonofficial Remedies." *Journal of the American Medical Association* 90 (1928): 2102–3 (liver extract no. 343).

———. "New and Nonofficial Remedies." *Journal of the American Medical Association* 102 (1934): 44 (vinyl ether).

———. "New and Nonofficial Remedies." *Journal of the American Medical Association* 105 (1935): 860–61 (acetyl-beta-methylcholine).

———. *New and Nonofficial Remedies, 1924*. Chicago: American Medical Association, 1924.

———. *New and Nonofficial Remedies, 1928*. Chicago: American Medical Association, 1928.

———. "Preliminary Report of the Council." *Journal of the American Medical Association* 105 (1935): 281–83 (acetyl-beta-methylcholine).

———. "Preliminary Report of the Council." *Journal of the American Medical Association* 109 (1937): 504–5 (pentobarbital sodium).

———. "Report of the Council." *Journal of the American Medical Association* 109 (1937): 656–58 (vinyl ether).

———. "Report of the Council." *Journal of the American Medical Association* 118 (1942): 896–97 (Bismuth Ethylcamphorate).

———. "Reports of the Council." *Journal of the American Medical Association* 113 (1939): 1734–35 (Dilantin).

Cournand, André F. "Dickinson Woodruff Richards, 1895–1973: A Survey of His Contributions to the Physiology and Physiopathology of Respiration in Man." *American Journal of Medicine* 57 (1974): 312–19.

Cowen, David L. "Materia Medica and Pharmacology." In *The Education of American Physicians: Historical Essays*, edited by Ronald L. Numbers, 95–121. Berkeley: University of California Press, 1980.

———. "The Nineteenth Century German Immigrant and American Pharmacy." In *Perspektiven der Pharmaziegeschichte: Festschrift für Rudolf Schmitz Zum 65. Geburtstag*, edited by Peter Dilg with the collaboration of Guido Jüttner, Wolf-

Dieter Müller-Jahncke, and Paul U. Unschuld, 13–28. Graz: Akademisch Druck- u. Verlagsanstalt, 1983.

———. "The Role of the Pharmaceutical Industry." In *Safeguarding the Public: Historical Aspects of Medicinal Drug Control*, edited by John B. Blake, 72–82. Baltimore: Johns Hopkins Press, 1970.

Crellin, J. K. "Industrial Pharmacy: A Divisive Force between Medicine and Pharmacy in the Early Twentieth Century." In *Farmacia e industrializacion: Libre homenaje al Doctor Guillermo Folch Jou*, edited by F. Javier Puerto Sarmiento, 105–14. Madrid: Sociedad Española de Historia de la Farmacia, 1985.

Culliton, Barbara J. "The Academic-Industrial Complex." *Science* 216 (1982): 960–62.

———. "Pajaro Dunes: The Search for Consensus." *Science* 216 (1982): 155–56, 158.

Curti, Merle. *The Growth of American Thought*. 3d ed. New York: Harper and Row, 1964.

Curti, Merle, and Nash, Roderick. *Philanthropy in the Shaping of American Higher Education*. New Brunswick, N. J.: Rutgers University Press, 1965.

Dale, Henry H. "Academic and Industrial Research in the Field of Therapeutics." *Science* 77 (1933): 521–27.

Daniels, George H. *Science in American Society: A Social History*. New York: Alfred A. Knopf, 1971.

Daniels, Troy C. "Therapeutic Agent." United States Patent 2,192,828, patented 3 April 1939.

Daniels, Troy C., and Iwamoto, Harry. "N^1,N^4-Nicotinyl Derivatives of Sulfanilamide." *Journal of the American Chemical Society* 62 (1940): 741–42.

Davis, Lance E., and Kevles, Daniel J. "The National Research Fund: A Case Study in the Industrial Support of Academic Science." *Minerva* 12 (1974): 207–20.

Dewey, John. *John Dewey: The Essential Writings*. Edited by David Sidorsky. New York: Harper and Row, Harper Torchbooks, 1977.

"Dr. John F. Anderson, 1871–1958." *Squibb Sales Bulletin* [34] (1958): 541–42.

Doisy, Edward A. "Philip Anderson Shaffer." *Biographical Memoirs of the National Academy of Sciences* 40 (1969): 321–36.

Dowling, Harry F. *Fighting Infection: Conquests of the Twentieth Century*. Cambridge, Mass.: Harvard University Press, 1977.

Dox, Arthur W., and Thomas, Adrian. "5,5-Diarylbarbituric Acids." *Journal of the American Chemical Society* 45 (1923): 1811–16.

Duncan, Robert Kennedy. "On Industry Fellowships." *Journal of Industrial and Engineering Chemistry* 1 (1909): 600–603.

Dupree, A. Hunter. *Science in the Federal Government: A History of Policies and Activities to 1940*. Cambridge, Mass.: Harvard University Press, Belknap Press, 1957; New York: Harper and Row, Harper Torchbooks, 1964.

Eddy, Nathan B. "Studies of Morphine, Codeine and Their Derivatives. I. General Methods." *Journal of Pharmacology and Experimental Therapeutics* 45 (1932): 339–59.

Edsall, John T. "Edwin Joseph Cohn." *Biographical Memoirs of the National Academy of Sciences* 35 (1961): 47–84.

Ehrlich, P., and Bertheim, A. "Über das salzsaure 3.3′-Diamino-4.4′-dioxyarsenobenzol and seine nächsten Verwandten." *Berichte der Deutschen Chemischen Gesselschaft* 45 (1912): 756–66.

Ehrlich, P., and Hata, S. *Die experimentelle Chemotherapie der Spirillosen*. Berlin: Julius Springer, 1910.

Einhorn, Alfred. "Alkamin Esters of Para-aminobenzoic Acid." United States Patent 812,554, patented 13 February 1906.

Eli Lilly and Company. *A Complete Priced List of the Products of the Lilly Laboratories*, no. 41. [Indianapolis,] 1922.

———. *Lilly Research Laboratories: Dedication*. Indianapolis, 1934.

"The Eli Lilly and Company Award in Biological Chemistry." *Industrial and Engineering Chemistry* 26 (1934): 425–26.

Engel, Leonard. *Medicine Makers of Kalamazoo*. New York: McGraw-Hill, 1961.

Federal Food, Drug and Cosmetic Law Administrative Reports, 1907–1949. Food Law Institute Series. Chicago: Commerce Clearing House, 1951.

Feldberg, W. "Henry Hallett Dale, 1875–1968." *Biographical Memoirs of the Fellows of the Royal Society* 16 (1970): 77–174.

The Field and the Work of the Squibb Institute for Medical Research 1, no. 1 (1938).

Finland, Maxwell, and Castle, William. *The Harvard Medical Unit at Boston City Hospital*. 2 vols. in 3. Boston: Harvard Medical School, 1982.

Fischer, Emil. "C-C-Dialkyl-barbituric Acid and Process of Making Same." United States Patent 782,739, patented 14 February 1905.

Fishbein, Morris. *A History of the American Medical Association, 1847–1947*. Philadelphia: W. B. Saunders, 1947.

———. "Medical Patents." *Journal of the American Medical Association* 109 (1937): 1539–43.

Fisher, J. C. "Basic Research in Industry." *Science* 129 (1959): 1653–57.

Fitch, Richard H., and McCandless, E. E. "A Comparison of the Intraperitoneal and Oral Effects of the Barbituric Acid Derivatives." Scientific Proceedings of the American Society for Pharmacology and Experimental Therapeutics, 22d Annual Meeting, Montreal, Canada, 8–11 April 1931. *Journal of Pharmacology and Experimental Therapeutics* 42 (1931): 266–67.

Fitch, Richard H.; Waters, Ralph M.; and Tatum, Arthur L. "The Intravenous Use of the Barbituric Acid Hypnotics in Surgery." *American Journal of Surgery*, n.s. 9 (1930): 110–14.

Fitz, Reginald; Murphy, William P.; and Grant, Samuel B. "The Effect of Insulin on the Metabolism of Diabetes." *Journal of Metabolic Research* 2 (1922): 753–66.

Fletcher, A. A., and Campbell, W. R. "The Blood Sugar Following Insulin Administration and the Symptom Complex—Hypoglycemia." *Journal of Metabolic Research* 2 (1922): 637–49.

Florey, H. W.; Chain, E.; Heatley, N. G.; Jennings, M. A.; Sanders, A. G.; Abraham, E. P.; and Florey, M. E. *Antibiotics: A Survey of Penicillin, Streptomycin, and Other Antimicrobial Substances from Fungi, Actinomycetes, Bacteria, and Plants*. 2 vols. London: Oxford University Press, 1949.

Foerster, O. H.; McIntosh, R. L.; Wieder, L. M.; Foerster, H. R.; and Cooper, G. A. "Mapharsen in the Treatment of Syphilis: A Preliminary Report." *Archives of Dermatology and Syphilology* 32 (1935): 868–92.

Folk, George E. *Patents and Industrial Progress: A Summary, Analysis and Evaluation of the Record on Patents of the Temporary National Economic Committee*. New York: Harper and Row, 1942.

French, Richard D. *Activivisection and Medical Science in Victorian Society.* Princeton: Princeton University Press, 1975.

Fulton, John F. *Physiology.* Clio Medica: A Series of Primers on the History of Medicine, edited by E. B. Krumbhaar, vol. 5. New York: Paul B. Hoeber, 1931.

Gasser, H. S. "Arthur S. Loevenhart." *Science* 70 (1929): 317–21.

Geiger, Roger L. *To Advance Knowledge: The Growth of American Research Universities, 1900–1940.* New York: Oxford University Press, 1986.

Geison, Gerald L. "Divided We Stand: Physiologists and Clinicians in the American Context." In *The Therapeutic Revolution: Essays in the Social History of American Medicine,* edited by Morris J. Vogel and Charles E. Rosenberg, 67–90. Philadelphia: University of Pennsylvania Press, 1979.

Geyelin, H. Rawle; Harrop, George; Murray, Marjorie F.; and Corwin, Eugenia. "The Use of Insulin in Juvenile Diabetes." *Journal of Metabolic Research* 2 (1922): 767–91.

Goldschmidt, Samuel; Ravdin, I. S.; Lucke, Baldwin; Muller, G. P.; Johnston, C. G.; and Ruigh, W. L. "Divinyl Ether: Experimental and Clinical Studies." *Journal of the American Medical Association* 102 (1934): 21–27.

Goodman, Louis, and Gilman, Alfred. *The Pharmacological Basis of Therapeutics.* New York: Macmillan, 1941.

Gottschalk, Carl W. "Dr. A. N. Richards and Kidney Micropuncture." In "Alfred Newton Richards: Scientist and Man," edited by Isaac Starr. *Annals of Internal Medicine* 71, no. 5, supp. 8, pt. 2 (1969): 28–37.

"Grants and Awards." *American Journal of Pharmaceutical Education* 49 (1985): 224–27.

Gruhzit, O. M. "Mapharsen ('Arsenoxide') in the Therapy of Experimental Syphilis and Trypanosomiasis." *Archives of Dermatology and Syphilology* 32 (1935): 848–67.

———. "Sodium Diphenyl Hydantoinate: Pharmacologic and Histopathologic Studies." *Archives of Pathology* 28 (1939): 761–62.

Gruhzit, O. M., and Dixon, R. S. "Mapharsen in Mass Treatment of Syphilis in a Clinic for Venereal Diseases." *Archives of Dermatology and Syphilology* 34 (1936): 432–58.

Guralnick, Stanley M. "The American Scientist in Higher Education, 1820–1910." In *The Sciences in the American Context: New Perspectives,* edited by Nathan Reingold, 99–141. Washington, D.C.: Smithsonian Institution Press, 1979.

Haber, L. F. *The Chemical Industry, 1900–1930: International Growth and Technological Change.* Oxford: Oxford University Press, Clarendon Press, 1971.

Hale, William J. "Cooperative Research between Industries and Universities." *Annual Survey of American Chemistry* 1 (1925–26): 250–57.

———. "Cooperative Research between Industries and Universities." *Annual Survey of American Chemistry* 2 (1927): 395–97.

Hall, G. Stanley. "Research the Vital Spirit of Teaching." *Forum* (New York) 17 (1894): 558–70.

Hannaway, Owen. "The German Model of Chemical Education in America: Ira Remsen at Johns Hopkins (1876–1913)." *Ambix* 23 (1976): 145–64.

Hartley, Percival. "Henry Drysdale Dakin." *Obituary Notices of Fellows of the Royal Society of London* 8 (1952): 129–48.

Haynes, Williams. *American Chemical Industry.* 6 vols. New York: D. Van Nostrand, 1945–54.

Henderson, Nell. "Montgomery Forms High-Tech Council." *Washington Post,* 3 February 1986.

Herwick, R. P. "A Study of Barbiturate Excretion." Scientific Proceedings of the American Society for Pharmacology and Experimental Therapeutics, 21st Annual Meeting, Chicago, Illinois, 26–29 March 1930. *Journal of Pharmacology and Experimental Therapeutics* 39 (1930): 267–68.

Hochheiser, Sheldon. "Synthetic Food Colors in the United States: A History under Regulation." Ph.D. diss., University of Wisconsin, 1982.

Hockstader, Lee. "Technology Center's Chief Makes a Hit." *Washington Post,* 31 July 1986.

Hofstadter, Richard, and Metzger, Walter P. *The Development of Academic Freedom in the United States.* New York: Columbia University Press, 1955.

Holmstedt, B., and Liljestrand, G., eds. *Readings in Pharmacology.* Oxford: Pergamon Press, 1963; New York: Raven Press, 1981.

Hull, Callie. "Industrial Research Laboratories of the United States, Including Consulting Research Laboratories." 6th ed. *Bulletin of the National Research Council,* no. 102 (1938).

————. "Industrial Research Laboratories of the United States, Including Consulting Research Laboratories." 7th ed. *Bulletin of the National Research Council,* no. 104 (1940).

Hull, Callie, and Timms, Mary. "Research Supported by Industry through Scholarships, Fellowships, and Grants." *Chemical and Engineering News* 24 (1946): 2346–2358.

Hull, Callie, and West, Clarence J. "Fellowships and Scholarships for Advanced Work in Science and Technology." 2d ed. *Bulletin of the National Research Council,* no. 72 (1929).

————. "Fellowships and Scholarships for Advanced Work in Science and Technology." 3d ed. *Bulletin of the National Research Council,* no. 94 (1934).

Ihde, Aaron J. *The Development of Modern Chemistry.* New York: Harper and Row, 1964.

Ihde, Aaron J., and Becker, Stanley L. "Conflict of Concepts in Early Vitamin Studies." *Journal of the History of Biology* 4 (1971): 1–33.

Insulin Committee of the University of Toronto. "Insulin: Its Action, Its Therapeutic Value in Diabetes, and Its Manufacture." *Canadian Medical Association Journal* 13 (1923): 480–86.

James, A. A., and Laughton, N. B. "The Control of Blood Pressure with Liver Extracts." *Canadian Medical Association Journal* 15 (1925): 701–2.

James, Edmund Janes. "The Function of the State University." Inaugural address as president of the University of Illinois, 18 October 1905. *Science* 22 (1905): 609–28.

Jaschik, Scott. "Democrats Urge Network of University-Industry Research Centers Aided by U.S. Funds." *Chronicle of Higher Education,* 3 September 1986.

Johnson, Jeffrey A. "Academic Chemistry in Imperial Germany." *Isis* 76 (1985): 500–524.

Jones, Daniel Patrick. "The Role of Chemists in Research on War Gases in the United States during World War I." Ph.D. diss., University of Wisconsin, 1969.

232   Bibliography

Jones, Maldwyn Allen. *American Immigration*. The Chicago History of American Civ-
ilization, edited by Daniel J. Boorstin. Chicago: University of Chicago Press, 1960.
Joslin, Elliott P. "Address by Dr. Elliott P. Joslin." In *Lilly Research Laboratories:
Dedication*, 39–41. *See* Eli Lilly and Company.
Joslin, Elliott P.; Gray, Horace; and Root, Howard F. "Insulin in Hospital and Home."
Journal of Metabolic Research 2 (1922): 651–99.
Kahn, E. J., Jr. *All in a Century: The First 100 Years of Eli Lilly and Company*. [India-
napolis: Eli Lilly, c. 1976.]
Kamm, Oliver; Adams, Roger; and Volwiler, Ernest H. "Anesthetic Compound."
United States Patent 1,358,751, patented 16 November 1920.
Karr, Norman; Murayama, Fumiko; Finnegan, Jack; and Leake, Chauncey D. "Che-
motherapeutic Activity of 4-Nicotinyl-Amino-Benzene-Sulfonamide." Scientific
Proceedings of the American Society for Pharmacology and Experimental Thera-
peutics, 31st Annual Meeting, New Orleans, Louisiana, 13–16 March 1940. *Journal
of Pharmacology and Experimental Therapeutics* 69 (1940): 291.
Kass, Lawrence. *Pernicious Anemia*. Major Problems in Internal Medicine, edited by
Lloyd H. Smith, vol. 7. Philadelphia: W. B. Saunders, 1976.
Keefer, Chester S. "Dr. Richards as Chairman of the Committee on Medical Research."
In "Alfred Newton Richards," 61–70. *See* Gottschalk.
Kenney, Martin. *Biotechnology: The University-Industrial Complex*. New Haven:
Yale University Press, 1986.
Kogan, Herman. *The Long White Line*. New York: Random House, 1963.
Kohler, Robert E. *From Medical Chemistry to Biochemistry: The Making of a Biomed-
ical Discipline*. Cambridge: Cambridge University Press, 1982.
————. "Medical Reform and Biomedical Science: Biochemistry—A Case Study." In
The Therapeutic Revolution, 27–66. *See* Geison.
Kolesnik, Walter B. *Mental Discipline in Modern Education*. Madison: University of
Wisconsin Press, 1958.
Kondratas, Ramunas A. "Biologics Control Act of 1902." In *The Early Years of Federal
Food and Drug Control*, 8–27. Madison: American Institute of the History of
Pharmacy, 1982.
Krahl, M. E. "Obituary: George Henry Alexander Clowes, 1877–1958." *Cancer Re-
search* 19 (1959): 334–36.
Lang, Jean. "Partners with Industry: University-Industry Consortia Support 'Generic'
Research Programs." *On Wisconsin*, March 1986.
League of Nations, Health Organisation. *The Biological Standardisation of Insulin,
Including Reports on the Preparation of the International Standard and the Defini-
tion of the Unit*. Publications of the League of Nations, no. 3. Geneva, 1926.
Leake, Chauncey D. "Arthur S. Loevenhart." *Journal of Pharmacology and Experimen-
tal Therapeutics* 36 (1929): 495–505.
————. "Cooperative Research: A Case Report." *Science* 62 (1925): 251–56.
————, ed. *Percival's Medical Ethics*. Baltimore: Williams and Wilkins, 1927.
Leake, Chauncey D., and Chen, Mei-Yü. "The Anesthetic Properties of Certain Unsaturated Ethers." *Proceedings of the Society for Experimental Biology and Medicine*
28 (1930): 151–54.
Leake, Chauncey D.; Knoefel, P. K.; and Guedel, A. E. "The Anesthetic Action of

Divinyl Oxide in Animals." *Journal of Pharmacology and Experimental Therapeutics* 47 (1933): 5–16.

Lechevalier, Hubert A. "The Search for Antibiotics at Rutgers University." In *The History of Antibiotics: A Symposium*, edited by John Parascandola, 113–23. Madison: American Institute of the History of Pharmacy, 1980.

Lechevalier, Hubert A., and Solotorovsky, Morris. *Three Centuries of Microbiology*. 1965. Reprint. New York: Dover, 1974.

Lenoir, Timothy. "The Binding of Scientific Inquiry and the Growth of Knowledge in Kaiserreich Germany." *Minerva* (in press).

Lepkowski, Wil. "University/Industry Research Ties Still Viewed with Concern." *Chemical and Engineering News* 62, no. 26 (1984): 7–11.

Lewis, Sinclair. *Arrowsmith*. New York: Harcourt Brace Jovanovich, 1925. Reprint. New York: New American Library, Signet Classics, n.d.

Lewis, Winford Lee. "Production of Derivatives of Arsanilic Acids." United States Patent 1,664,123, patented 27 March 1928.

Liebenau, Jonathan Michael. "Medical Science and Medical Industry, 1890–1929: A Study of Pharmaceutical Manufacturing in Philadelphia." Ph.D. diss., University of Pennsylvania, 1981.

———. "Scientific Ambitions: The Pharmaceutical Industry, 1900–1920." *Pharmacy in History* 27 (1985): 3–11.

Lilly, Josiah K. "Comments on Research in Manufacturing Pharmacy." In *Lilly Research Laboratories: Dedication*, 3–6. *See* Eli Lilly and Company.

Loeb, Jacques. *Proteins and the Theory of Colloid Behavior*. New York: McGraw-Hill, 1922.

Loevenhart, A. S. "Certain Aspects of Biological Oxidation." Lecture presented to the Harvey Society, New York, 8 November 1914. *Archives of Internal Medicine* 15 (1915): 1059–71.

———. "Tryparsamide." *Science* 62 (1925): 587–88.

Lorenz, W. F.; Loevenhart, A. S.; Bleckwenn, W. J.; and Hodges, F. J. "The Therapeutic Use of Tryparsamid in Neurosyphilis." *Journal of the American Medical Association* 80 (1923): 1497–1502.

Lundy, John S. "Experience with Sodium Ethyl (1-Methylbutyl) Barbiturate (Nembutal) in More than 2,300 Cases." *Surgical Clinics of North America* 11 (1931): 909–15.

McCormick, Gene E. "Insulin: A Hope for Life." *Tile and Till* 57, no. 2 (1971): 33–36.

———. "Josiah Kirby Lilly, Sr., the Man." *Pharmacy in History* 12 (1970): 57–67.

McDonald, Kim. "Strength of U.S. Said to Depend on Universities." *Chronicle of Higher Education*, 29 January 1986.

MacDonald, W. J. "Extractives of Liver Possessing Blood Pressure Reducing Properties: Report of Clinical Tests." *Proceedings of the Society for Experimental Biology and Medicine* 22 (1924–25): 483–85.

Macleod, J. J. R. "History of the Researches Leading to the Discovery of Insulin." *Bulletin of the History of Medicine* 52 (1978): 295–315.

———. "Insulin and the Steps Taken to Secure an Effective Preparation." *Canadian Medical Association Journal* 12 (1922): 899–900.

Mahoney, Tom. *The Merchants of Life: An Account of the American Pharmaceutical Industry*. New York: Harper, 1959.

Major, Ralph H. "The Effects of Hepatic Extract on High Blood Pressure." *Journal of the American Medical Association* 85 (1925): 251–53.

Major, Randolph T., and Cline, Joseph K. "Preparation and Properties of Alpha- and Beta-methylcholine and Gamma-homocholine." *Journal of the American Chemical Society* 54 (1932): 242–49.

———. "Preparation and Properties of Alpha- and Beta-methylcholine Derivatives and Salts and Processes for Their Preparation." United States Patent 2,040,146 patented 12 May 1936.

Major, Randolph T., and Ruigh, William L. "Divinyl Ether and Processes for Its Production." United States Patent 2,021,872, patented 19 November 1935.

———. "Means and Composition for the Stabilization of Divinyl Ether." United States Patent 2,044,800, patented 23 June 1936.

———. "Production of Stabilized Divinyl Ether Suitable for General Anesthesia." United States Patent 2,044,801, patented 23 June 1936.

Maloney, A. H.; Fitch, R.; and Tatum, A. L. "Picrotoxin as an Antidote in Acute Poisoning by the Shorter Acting Barbiturates." *Journal of Pharmacology and Experimental Therapeutics* 41 (1931): 465–82.

Marion, John Francis. *The Fine Old House.* Philadelphia: SmithKline, 1980.

Maulitz, Russell C. " 'Physician versus Bacteriologist': The Ideology of Science in Clinical Medicine." In *The Therapeutic Revolution*, 91–107. *See* Geison.

"Medicine's Living History: Recollections of Liver Therapy." *Medical World News* 13, no. 33 (1972): 37–44.

Merck, George W. "An Essential Partnership: The Chemical Industry and Medicine." *Industrial and Engineering Chemistry* 27 (1935): 739–41.

Merck and Company. *Annual Report to Stockholders*, 1938–58. Rahway, N. J.

———. "Fifty Years of Merck Research." *Merck Sharp and Dohme International Review* 21, no. 2 (1983).

———. *The Merck Corporation: Annual Report, 1931.* Rahway, N. J., 1931.

Merck Institute for Therapeutic Research. *The Merck Institute for Therapeutic Research.* [Rahway, N.J.,] 1942.

"Merck Research Laboratory Dedicated." *Merck's Report and Price List* 42 (1933): 82–85.

Merritt, H. Houston, and Putnam, Tracy J. "Further Experiences with the Use of Sodium Diphenyl Hydantoinate in the Treatment of Convulsive Disorders." *American Journal of Psychiatry* 96 (1940): 1023–27.

———. "A New Series of Anticonvulsant Drugs Tested by Experiments on Animals." *Archives of Neurology and Psychiatry* 39 (1938): 1003–15.

———. "Sodium Diphenyl Hydantoinate in the Treatment of Convulsive Disorders." *Journal of the American Medical Association* 111 (1938): 1068–73.

———. "Sodium Diphenyl Hydantoinate in Treatment of Convulsive Seizures." *Archives of Neurology and Psychiatry* 42 (1939): 1053–58.

Meyerson, Martin, and Winegrad, Dilys Pegler. *Gladly Learn and Gladly Teach: Franklin and His Heirs at the University of Pennsylvania, 1740–1976.* [Philadelphia:] University of Pennsylvania Press, 1978.

Meyer-Thurow, Georg. "The Industrialization of Invention: A Case Study from the German Chemical Industry." *Isis* 73 (1982): 363–81.

Minot, George R., and Murphy, William P. "Treatment of Pernicious Anemia by a Special Diet." *Journal of the American Medical Association* 87 (1926): 470–76.

Minot, George R.; Murphy, William P.; Fitz, Reginald; and Monroe, Robert D. "Observations on Patients with Pernicious Anemia Partaking of a Special Diet." *Transactions of the Association of American Physicians* 41 (1926): 72–75.

Molitor, Hans. "Some Undescribed Pharmacological Properties of Bulbocapnine." *Journal of Pharmacology and Experimental Therapeutics* 57 (1936): 135–36.

Molitor, Hans, and Kniazuk, Michael. "A New Bloodless Method for Continuous Recording of Peripheral Circulatory Changes." *Journal of Pharmacology and Experimental Therapeutics* 57 (1936): 6–18.

Mowery, David Charles. "British and American Industrial Research: A Comparison, 1900–1950." Paper presented at the Anglo-American Conference on the Decline of the British Economy, Boston University, August 1983.

———. "The Emergence and Growth of Industrial Research in American Manufacturing, 1899–1945." Ph.D. diss., Stanford University, 1981.

———. "The Relationship between Intrafirm and Contractual Forms of Industrial Research in American Manufacturing, 1900–1940." *Explorations in Economic History* 20 (1983): 351–74.

Nelson, Gary L. *Pharmaceutical Company Histories.* 1 vol. to date. Mandan, N. Dak.: Woodbine, 1983–.

Nelson, Phyllis Magdalene. "I. A Comparative Study of Various Agents in the Chemotherapy of Rat Trichomoniasis; II. Trichomonas Foetus: Infection, Immunity, and Chemotherapy." Ph.D. diss., University of Wisconsin, 1938.

New Jersey. Department of Health. *Fifty-sixth Annual Report of the Department of Health of the State of New Jersey, 1933.* Trenton, N.J., 1933.

———. General Assembly. *Acts of the One hundred and Fourth Legislature of the State of New Jersey, and Thirty-sixth under the New Constitution.* Trenton, N.J., 1880.

———. *Acts of the One Hundred and Thirty-ninth Legislature of the State of New Jersey, and Seventy-first under the New Constitution.* Trenton, N.J., 1915.

Osterhaut, W. J. V. "Jacques Loeb." *Journal of General Physiology* 8 (1928): ix–xcii.

Palmer, Carleton. "Welcome." *The Field and the Work of the Squibb Institute for Medical Research* 1, no. 1 (1938): 3.

Parascandola, John. "Academic Pharmacologists and the Pharmaceutical Industry in the United States, 1900–1940." Paper presented at the Johns Hopkins Institute of the History of Medicine, Baltimore, Maryland, 1 December 1983.

———. "Industrial Research Comes of Age: The American Pharmaceutical Industry, 1920–1940." *Pharmacy in History* 27 (1985): 12–21.

———. "John J. Abel and the Early Development of Pharmacology at the Johns Hopkins University." *Bulletin of the History of Medicine* 56 (1982): 512–27.

———. "The Search for the Active Oxytocic Principle of Ergot: Laboratory Science and Clinical Medicine in Conflict." In *Neue Beiträge zur Arzneimittelgeschichte: Festschrift für Wolfgang Schneider zum 70. Geburtstag,* edited by Erika Hickel and Gerald Schröder, 205–27. Veröffentlichungen der Internationalen Gesselschaft für Geschichte der Pharmazie, n.s. 51. Stuttgart: Wissenschaftliche Verlagsgesellschaft, 1982.

Parascandola, John, and Keeney, Elizabeth. *Sources in the History of American Pharmacology*. Madison: American Institute of the History of Pharmacy 1983.

Parascandola, John, and Swann, John. "Development of Pharmacology in American Schools of Pharmacy." *Pharmacy in History* 25 (1983): 95–115.

Pauly, Philip J. "The Appearance of Academic Biology in Late Nineteenth-Century America." *Journal of the History of Biology* 17 (1984): 369–97.

Peters, Lois S. "Pharmaceuticals." *Technology in Society* 5 (1983): 191–96.

Peters, Lois S., and Fusfeld, Herbert I. "Current U.S. University/Industry Research Connections." In *University-Industry Research Relationships: Selected Studies*, 1–161. Report of the National Science Board of the National Science Foundation. [Washington, D.C.: Government Printing Office, c. 1982.]

"Pharmaceutical R and D Expenditures Estimated at $3.3 Billion for 1983." *American Pharmacy*, n.s. 25 (1985): 266.

Post, Robert. "Science, Public Policy, and Popular Precepts: Alexander Dallas Bache and Alfred Beach as Symbolic Adversaries." In *The Sciences in the American Context: New Perspectives* 77–98. *See* Guralnick.

Prager, Denis, and Omenn, Gilbert S. "Research, Innovation, and University-Industry Linkages." *Science* 207 (1980): 379–84.

Pratt, T. W. "A Comparison of the Action of Pentobarbital (Nembutal) and Sodium Barbital in Rabbits as Related to the Detoxicating Power of the Liver." Scientific Proceedings of the American Society for Pharmacology and Experimental Therapeutics, 24th Annual Meeting, Cincinnati, Ohio, 9–12 April 1933. *Journal of Pharmacology and Experimental Therapeutics* 48 (1933): 285.

Pratt, T. W.; Tatum, A. L.; Hathaway, H. R.; and Waters, R. M. "Sodium Ethyl(1-Methyl Butyl)Thiobarbiturate: Preliminary Experimental and Clinical Study." *American Journal of Surgery*, n.s. 31 (1936): 464–66.

Proceedings of the National Conference on Pharmaceutical Research. N.p., 1928–32.

"Profile of a Research Scientist." *Bulletin for Medical Research of the National Society for Medical Research* 8, no. 6 (1954): 7–8.

Putnam, Tracy J., and Merritt, H. Houston. "Experimental Determination of the Anticonvulsant Properties of Some Phenyl Derivatives." *Science* 85 (1937): 525–26.

Rackemann, Francis Minot. *The Inquisitive Physician: The Life and Times of George Richards Minot*. Cambridge, Mass.: Harvard University Press, 1956.

Ravdin, I. S.: Eliason, E. L.; Coates, G. M.; Holloway, T. B.; Ferguson, L. K.; Gill, A. B.; and Cook, T. J. "Divinyl Ether: A Report of Its Further Use as a General Anesthetic." *Journal of the American Medical Association* 108 (1937): 1163–67.

Reich, Leonard S. *The Making of American Industrial Research: Science and Business at GE and Bell, 1876–1926*. Studies in Economic History and Policy: The United States in the Twentieth Century, edited by Louis Galambos and Robert Gallman. Cambridge: Cambridge University Press, 1985.

Reingold, Nathan. "Alexander Dallas Bache: Science and Technology in the American Idiom." *Technology and Culture* 11 (1970): 163–77.

———. "American Indifference to Basic Research: A Reappraisal." In *Nineteenth-Century American Science: A Reappraisal*, edited by George H. Daniels, 38–62. Evanston, Ill.: Northwestern University Press, 1972.

Rensberger, Boyce. "R & D Surge Foreseen." *Washington Post*, 5 January 1986.

Research—A National Resource. 2 vols. Vol. 1. Report of the Science Committee to the National Resources Committee; vol. 2, Report of the National Research Council to the National Resources Planning Board. Washington, D.C.: Government Printing Office, 1938–41.

Research Information Service. "Fellowships and Scholarships for Advanced Work in Science and Technology." Bulletin of the National Research Council, no. 38 (1923).

Richards, A. N. "Processes of Urine Formation." Croonian Lecture to the Royal Society of London, 30 June 1938. Proceedings of the Royal Society of London, ser. B (Biological Sciences), 126 (1938): 398–432.

Rickes, Edward L.; Brink, Norman G.; Koniuszy, Frank R.; Wood, Thomas R.; and Folkers, Karl. "Crystalline Vitamin B_{12}." Science 107 (1948): 396–97.

Risse, Guenter B. "Kant, Schelling, and the Early Search for a Philosophical 'Science' of Medicine in Germany." Journal of the History of Medicine and Allied Sciences 27 (1972): 145–58.

Robscheit-Robbins, F. S., and Whipple, G. H. "Blood Regeneration in Severe Anemia. II. Favorable Influence of Liver, Heart and Skeletal Muscle in Diet." American Journal of Physiology 72 (1925): 408–18.

Rosen, George. "Patterns of Health Research in the United States, 1900–1960." Bulletin of the History of Medicine 39 (1965): 201–21.

————. The Structure of American Medical Practice, 1875–1941. Edited by Charles E. Rosenberg. Philadelphia: University of Pennsylvania Press, 1983.

Rosenberg, Charles E. No Other Gods: On Science and American Social Thought. Baltimore: Johns Hopkins University Press, 1976.

Rothschuh, Karl E. History of Physiology. Translated and edited by Guenter B. Risse. Huntington, N.Y.: Robert E. Krieger, 1973.

Ruigh, William L. "Acid Halides of Carbazole-N-carboxylic Acids and Process for Their Production." United States Patent 2,089,985, patented 17 August 1937.

Ruigh, William L., and Major, Randolph T. "The Preparation and Properties of Pure Divinyl Ether." Journal of the American Chemical Society 53 (1931): 2662–71.

Sanger, David E. "U.S. Research Sponsorship Soars at Universities." New York Times, 8 September 1986.

Schmidt, Carl F. "Alfred Newton Richards." Biographical Memoirs of the National Academy of Sciences 42 (1971): 271–318.

Schmitz, H. L., and Loevenhart, A. S. "A Comparative Study of the Local Anesthetic Properties of Para-amino Benzoyl Di-iso-propyl Amino Ethanol Hydrochloride ('Isocaine'), Cocaine, Procaine and Butyn." Journal of Pharmacology and Experimental Therapeutics 24 (1924): 167–77.

————. "A Study of Two Series of Procaine Derivatives with Reference to the Relationship between Their Pharmacological Action and Chemical Constitution." Journal of Pharmacology and Experimental Therapeutics 24 (1924): 159–66.

Schrage, Michael. "Scientists Defy Pentagon on Research Restrictions." Washington Post, 21 September 1985.

Schrage, Michael, and Henderson, Nell. "U-Md. Thrives on High Tech." Washington Post, 10 March 1986.

Servos, John W. "The Industrial Relations of Science: Chemical Engineering at MIT, 1900–1939." Isis 71 (1980): 531–49.

Shideman, F. E. "A. L. Tatum, Practical Pharmacologist," *Science* 123 (1956): 449.

Shonle, H. A.; Keltch, Anna K.; and Swanson, E. E. "Dialkyl Barbituric Acids." *Journal of the American Chemical Society* 52 (1930): 2440–51.

Shryock, Richard Harrison. "American Indifference to Basic Science during the Nineteenth Century." *Archives internationales d'historie des sciences*, no. 5 (1948): 50–65.

————. *American Medical Research: Past and present.* New York: Commonwealth Fund, 1947.

Simonart, André. "Étude physiologique de quelques dérivés d'homocholine: L'Ether methylique de la gamma-phenylhomocholine." *Archives internationales de pharmacodynamie et de thérapie* 34 (1928): 15–32.

————. "Étude physiologique de quelques dérivés d'homocholine: II, L'Ether methylé d'homocholine; III, Rapports avec les cholines." *Archives internationales de pharmacodynamie et de thérapie* 34 (1928)L 375–90.

————. "On the Action of Certain Derivatives of Choline." *Journal of Pharmacology and Experimental Therapeutics* 46 (1932): 157–93.

Sinclair, Molly. "Hopkins Traffic Report Altered, Saving Project." *Washington Post*, 6 August 1986.

————. "Hopkins U. Project Advances." *Washington Post*, 8 August 1986.

Small, Lyndon Frederick. "Morphine Derivative and Processes for Its Preparation." United States Patent 1,980,972, patented 13 November 1934.

Small, Lyndon Frederick; Eddy, Nathan B.; Mosettig, Erich; and Himmelsbach, C. K. *Studies on Drug Addiction, with Special Reference to Chemical Structure of Opium Derivatives and Allied Synthetic Substances and Their Physiological Action.* Supplement 138 to the Public Health Reports of the Public Health Service, United States Treasury Department. Washington, D.C.: Government Printing Office, 1938.

Small, Lyndon Frederick; Yuen, Kechee C.; and Eilers, Louise K. "The Catalytic Hydrogenation of the Halogenmorphides: Dihydrodesoxymorphine-D." *Journal of the American Chemical Society* 55 (1933): 3863–70.

Smith, Bruce L. R., and Karlesky, Joseph J. *The State of Academic Science.* 2 vols. Vol. 1, *The Universities in the Nation's Research Effort*; vol. 2, *Background Papers.* New York: Change Magazine Press, 1977–78.

Snow, William F. "Contributions to Medical Science Developed under the Auspices of the United States Interdepartmental Social Hygiene Board." *American Journal of Tropical Medicine* 1 (1921): 97–108.

Sonnedecker, Glenn. *Kremers and Urdang's History of Pharmacy.* 4th ed. Philadelphia: J. B. Lippincott, 1976.

————. "The Rise of Drug Manufacture in America." *Emory University Quarterly* 21 (1965): 73–87.

Sperry, Warren M.; Elden, C. A.; Robscheit-Robbins, Frieda S.; and Whipple, G. H. "Blood Regeneration in Severe Anemia. XV. Liver Fractions and Potent Factors." *Journal of Biological Chemistry* 81 (1929): 251–65.

"Squibb Institute for Medical Research Dedicated October 11." *Squibb Sales Bulletin* 14 (1938): 513–21.

Starr, Isaac, Jr. "Acetyl-beta-methylcholin: II, Its Action on Paroxysmal Tachycardia and Peripheral Vascular Disease, with a Discussion of Its Action in Other Conditions." *American Journal of the Medical Sciences* 186 (1933): 330–45.

————. "Other Activities of Dr. Richards' Department: 'Clinical Pharmacology.' " In "Alfred Newton Richards," 41–42. See Gottschalk.

Starr, Isaac, Jr.; Elsom, K. A.; Reisinger, J. A.; and Richards, A. N. "Acetyl-beta-methylcholin: I, The Action on Normal Persons, with a Note on the Action of the Ethyl Ether of Beta-methylcholin." *American Journal of the Medical Sciences* 186 (1933): 313–23.

Stechl, Peter. "Biological Standardization of Drugs before 1928." Ph.D. diss., University of Wisconsin, 1969.

Stewart, F. E. "Is It Ethical for Medical Men to Patent Medical Inventions?" *Journal of the American Medical Association* 29 (1897): 583–87.

Storey, T. A. "A Summary of the Work of the United States Interdepartmental Social Hygiene Board." *Social Hygiene* 7 (1921): 59–76.

Strauss, Maurice B. "Of Medicine, Men and Molecules: Wedlock or Divorce?" *Medicine* 43 (1964): 619–24.

Swann, John. "Arthur Tatum, Parke-Davis, and the Discovery of Mapharsen as an Antisyphilitic Agent." *Journal of the History of Medicine and Allied Sciences* 40 (1985): 167–87.

————. "The Rise of American Synthetic Drug Industry before 1920." C(38)a, Kremers Reference Files, F. B. Power Pharmaceutical Library, University of Wisconsin, Madison, Wisconsin.

Tabern, D. L., and Volwiler, E. H. "Sulfur-Containing Barbiturate Hypnotics." *Journal of the American Chemical Society* 57 (1935): 1961–63.

Tarbell, D. Stanley, and Tarbell, Ann Tracy. *Roger Adams: Scientist and Statesman.* Washington, D.C.: American Chemical Society, 1981.

Tatum, A. L. "Therapeutic Agent." United States Patent 2,092,036, patented 7 September 1937.

Tatum, A. L.; Atkinson, A. J.; and Collins, K. H. "Acute Cocaine Poisoning, Its Prophylaxis and Treatment in Laboratory Animals." *Journal of Pharmacology and Experimental Therapeutics* 26 (1925): 325–35.

Tatum, A. L., and Copper, G. A. "An Experimental Study of Mapharsen (Meta-Amino Para-Hydroxy Phenyl Arsine Oxide) as an Antisyphilitic Agent." *Journal of Pharmacology and Experimental Therapeutics* 50 (1934): 198–215.

————. "Meta-Amino Para-Hydroxy Phenyl Arsine Oxide as an Antisyphilitic Agent." *Science* 75 (1932): 541–42.

Tatum, A. L.; Pfeiffer, C. C.; Kuhs, M. L.; Lorenz, W. F.; and Green, J. T., Jr. "A Study of the Sodium Salt of 3-Amino-4-beta-hydroxyethoxyphenylarsonic Acid in Experimental Syphilis and in Clinical Syphilis and Neurosyphilis." *Journal of Pharmacology and Experimental Therapeutics* 59 (1937): 241–48.

Tatum, A. L.; Seevers, M. H.; and Collins, K. H. "Morphine Addiction and Its Physiological Interpretation Based on Experimental Evidences." *Journal of Pharmacology and Experimental Therapeutics* 36 (1929): 447–75.

Thackray, Arnold. "An Academic Genius with Links to Industrial Science." Review of *Roger Adams: Scientist and Statesman,* by D. Stanley Tarbell and Ann Tracy Tarbell. *Chemical and Engineering News* 60, no. 23 (1982): 41–42.

————. "University-Industry Connections and Chemical Research: An Historical Perspective." In *University-Industry Research Relationship,* 193–233. *See* Peters and Fusfeld.

Tobey, Ronald C. *The American Ideology of National Science, 1919–1930.* Pittsburgh: University of Pittsburgh Press, 1971.

University Laboratory of Physical Chemistry Related to Medicine and Public Health, Harvard University. N.p., 1950.

"Upjohn Enlists KU's Help in Drug-Efficiency Research." *Kansas Alumni,* October 1986.

Urdang, George. "Retail Pharmacy as the Nucleus of the Pharmaceutical Industry." In *Essays in the History of Medicine,* edited by Henry E. Sigerist, 325–46. *Bulletin of the History of Medicine,* supp. 3. Baltimore: Johns Hopkins Press, 1944.

Varrin, Robert D., and Kukich, Diane S. "Guidelines for Industry-sponsored Research at Universities." *Science* 227 (1985): 385–88.

Veysey, Laurence R. *The Emergence of the American University.* Chicago: University of Chicago Press, 1965; Phoenix Books, 1970.

"Visiting Scientist Program Launched as Tripartite Project." *Academy Reporter* (Academy of Pharmaceutical Sciences, American Pharmaceutical Association) 21, no. 2 (1985): 1, 10.

Vobejda, Barbara. "Academia Using Strategy from the Corporate World." *Washington Post,* 25 November 1985.

Voegtlin, Carl. "The Pharmacology of Arsphenamine (Salvarsan) and Related Arsenicals." *Physiological Reviews* 5 (1925): 63–94.

Voegtlin, Carl, and Smith, Homer. "Quantitative Studies in Chemotherapy. II. The Trypanocidal Action of Arsenic Compounds." *Journal of Pharmacology and Experimental Therapeutics* 15 (1920): 475–93.

Volwiler, Ernest H. "Introduction." In *Addresses: Dedication of Research Building, Abbott Laboratories, North Chicago, Illinois, October 7, 1938,* 4. North Chicago: Abbott Laboratories, 1938.

Volwiler, Ernest H., and Tabern, D. L. "5,5-Substituted Barbituric Acids." *Journal of the American Chemical Society* 52 (1930): 1676:–79.

Wade, Nicholas. "Gene Goldrush Splits Harvard, Worries Brokers." *Science* 210 (1980): 878–79.

Waksman, Selman A. *My Life with the Microbes.* London: Robert Hale, 1958.

Walden, George B. "Liver Extract for Secondary Anemia and Process of Making It." United States Patent 1,813,788, patented 7 July 1931.

————. "Purified Antidiabetic Product and Process of Making It." United States Patent 1,520,673, patented 23 December 1924.

Ward, Patricia Spain. "The American Reception of Salvarsan." *Journal of the History of Medicine and Allied Sciences* 36 (1981): 44–62.

Warner, John Harley. "Physiology." In *The Education of American Physicians,* 48–71. *See* Cowen, "Materia Medica."

Weikel, Malcolm Keith. "Research as a Function of Pharmaceutical Industry: The American Formative Period." Master's thesis, University of Wisconsin, 1962.

Werner, H. W.; Pratt, T. W.; and Tatum, A. L. "A Comparative Study of Ultrashort-acting Barbiturates, Nembutal, and Tribromomethanol." *Journal of Pharmacology and Experimental Therapeutics* 60 (1937): 189–97.

West, Clarence J., and Hull, Callie. "Industrial Research Laboratories of the United States, Including Consulting Research Laboratories." 5th ed. *Bulletin of the National Research Council,* no. 91 (1933)

West, Clarence J., and Risher, Ervye. "Industrial Research Laboratories of the United States, Including Consulting Research Laboratories." 3d ed. *Bulletin of the National Research Council,* no. 60 (1927).

West, Randolph. "Activity of Vitamin B$_{12}$ in Addisonian Pernicious Anemia." *Science* 107 (1948): 398.

Whipple, George H. "Address by Dr. George H. Whipple." In *Lilly Research Laboratories: Dedication,* 48–49. *See* Eli Lilly and Company.

———. "Autobiographical Sketch." *Perspectives in Biology and Medicine* 2 (1959): 253–89.

———. Experimental Anemias, Diet Factors and Related Pathologic Changes of Human Anemias." *Journal of the American Medical Association* 91 (1928): 863–67.

———. "Pigment Metabolism and Regeneration of Hemoglobin in the Body." *Archives of Internal Medicine* 29 (1922): 711–31.

Whipple, George H.; Robscheit, F. S.; and Hooper, C. W. "Blood Regeneration Following Simple Anemia. IV. Influence of Meat, Liver and Various Extractives, Alone or Combined with Standard Diets." *American Journal of Physiology* 53 (1920): 236–62.

Whipple, George H., and Robscheit-Robbins, F. S. "Simple Experimental Anemia and Liver Extracts." *Proceedings of the Society for Experimental Biology and Medicine* 24 (1926–27): 860–64.

Whipple, George H.; Robscheit-Robbins, F. S.; and Walden, G. B. "Blood Regeneration in Severe Anemia. XXI. A Liver Fraction Potent in Anemia Due to Hemorrhage." *American Journal of the Medical Sciences* 179 (1930): 628–43.

White, Benjamin V. *Stanley Cobb: A Builder of the Modern Neurosciences.* Boston: Francis A. Countway Library of Medicine, 1984; distributed by University Press of Virginia.

White, William Charles. "Committee on Drug Addiction of the National Research Council." *Science* 73 (1931): 97–98.

Wieder, L. M.; Foerster, O. H.; and Foerster, H. R. "Mapharsen in the Treatment of Syphilis: Further Experiences." *Archives of Dermatology and Syphilology* 35 (1937): 402–13.

Wilder, Russell M.; Boothby, Walter M.; Barborka, Clifford J.; Kitchen, Hubert D.; and Adams, Samuel F. "Clinical Observations on Insulin." *Journal of Metabolic Research* 2 (1922): 701–28.

Williams, John R. "A Clinical Study of the Effects of Insulin in Severe Diabetes." *Journal of Metabolic Research* 2 (1922): 729–51.

Williams, Roger J. *A Textbook of Biochemistry.* New York: D. Van Nostrand, 1938.

Wiselogle, Frederick Y., ed. *A Survey of Antimalarial Drugs, 1941–1945.* 2 vols. in 3. Ann Arbor, Mich.: J. W. Edwards, 1946.

Wisenberg, Dinah. "Betting on Biotech." *Montgomery County Sentinel,* 14 August 1986.

Wood, Francis C. "John F. Anderson, 1871–1958." *Transactions of the Association of American Physicians* 72 (1959): 13–14.

Woodruff, H. Boyd. "A Soil Microbiologist's Odyssey." *Annual Review of Microbiology* 35 (1981): 1–28.

Woodyatt, R. T. "The Clinical Use of Insulin." *Journal of Metabolic Research* 2 (1922): 794–801.

"Year of the Money Scramble: New Financial Realities Challenge Academe." *Chronicle of Higher Education*, 3 September 1986.

Young, A. G., and Loevenhart, A. S. "The Relation of the Chemical Constitution of Certain Organic Arsenical Compounds to Their Action on the Optic Tract." *Journal of Pharmacology and Experimental Therapeutics* 23 (1924): 107–26.

Young, F. G. "The Evolution of Ideas about Animal Hormones." In *The Chemistry of Life: Eight Lectures on the History of Biochemistry*, edited by Joseph Needham, 125–55. Cambridge: Cambridge University Press, 1971.

Young, James Harvey. *The Medical Messiahs: A Social History of Health Quackery in Twentieth Century America.* Princeton: Princeton University Press, 1967.

———. *The Toadstool Millionaires: A Social History of Patent Medicines in America before Federal Regulation.* Princeton: Princeton University Press, 1961.

Zinsser, Hans. "Problems of the Bacteriologist in His Relations to Medicine and the Public Health." Presidential address to the Society of American Bacteriologists, Philadelphia, Pennsylvania, 29 December 1926. *Journal of Bacteriology* 13 (1927): 147–62.

Index

>>>->>>->>>->>>->>>- <<<-<<<-<<<-<<<-<<<

Page numbers in *italic type* refer to photographs

Academic Scientists and the Pharmaceutical Industry

Designed by Ann Walston.

Composed by Professional Book Compositors, Inc.,
in Garamond.

Printed by Edwards Brothers, Inc.,
on 50-lb. Glatfelter Offset,
and bound in Holliston Roxite.